# Orofacial Pain

# Orofacial Pain

## AETIOLOGY, DIAGNOSIS AND TREATMENT

**J.M. Mumford**

PhD, MSc, LDS(Liverpool), MS(Michigan), FDS RCS(England)

Professor of Operative Dental Surgery, University of Liverpool; Consultant in charge of the Conservation Clinics, Liverpool Dental Hospital; Visiting Specialist to the Centre for Pain Relief, Department of Medical and Surgical Neurology, Walton Hospital, Liverpool.

THIRD EDITION

CHURCHILL LIVINGSTONE
EDINBURGH LONDON MELBOURNE AND NEW YORK 1982

CHURCHILL LIVINGSTONE
Medical Division of Longman Group Limited

Distributed in the United States of America by Churchill Livingstone Inc., 19 West 44th Street, New York, N.Y. 10036, and by associated companies, branches and representatives throughout the world.



First edition 1973
  Published under title: *Toothache and related pain*
  First Japanese edition 1974
Second edition 1976
  Published under title: *Toothache and orofacial pain*
  Second Japanese edition 1981
Third edition 1982

ISBN 0 443 02631 9

British Library Cataloguing in Publication Data
Mumford, J.M.
  Orofacial pain. — 3rd ed.
  1. Toothache 2. Facial pain
  I. Title II. Mumford, J.M. Toothache and orofacial pain
  617.6'3 RK305

Library of Congress Catalog Card Number 81-69055

Printed in Singapore by Kyodo Shing Loong Printing Industries Pte Ltd

# Preface

Orofacial pain can be as severe as any pain experienced and includes cases of intractable pain as well as acute pain. The personal, family and social cost of this is enormous, not just in terms of financial loss and cost of treatment but also in the risk of drug addiction, multiple operations and even suicide. The most frequent source of orofacial pain is dental disease and it has been estimated that toothache is suffered for up to five million days, and one million nights' sleep lost as a result of it, in one year, in England and Wales alone. More new patients attending dental hospitals do so because of toothache than for any other reason, and pain is all too frequently a feature of treatment.

This book therefore aims to help the reader develop his understanding of pain in general and orofacial pain in particular, with the object of improving his diagnostic ability and hence treatment. The first few chapters deal with fundamental factors and will provide a useful revision for practitioners, as well as being appropriate for undergraduates from the very beginning of the course. Later chapters deal with orofacial pain as it is encountered in practice, presenting it in a manner which allows the reading of chapters individually if so desired. This presentation, together with the subject index, makes the book also suitable for ready reference.

Liverpool, 1982

J.M.M.

# Acknowledgements


I receive a great deal of help with my research and patients, especially from the following people whom I wish to thank: Mr Alan Newton, Senior Lecturer in Prosthetic Dentistry and Consultant in Restorative Dentistry; Dr W. R. Tyldesley, Reader in Dental Surgery and Pathology, and Consultant Dental Surgeon; Dr David Bowsher, Reader in Neurobiology and Consultant Neurologist; Dr Sampson Lipton, Director of the Centre for Pain Relief and Consultant Anaesthetist, and Mr John Miles, Director of Neurosurgical Studies and Consultant Neurosurgeon in the Regional Centre for Medical and Surgical Neurology, Walton Hospital, Liverpool.

I am grateful to the following organisations and people:

Academic Press Inc. (London) Ltd for permission to use Fig. 16.4.

Munksgaard International Publishers Ltd, Copenhagen, for permission to use Figs. 16.1 and 16.2, modified from the original work.

The Oxford University Press for permission to use, in modified forms, Figs. 3.2 and 18.3.

Pergamon Press for permission to use the following figures from my book on *Endodontics* — Figs. 11.2, 11.5, 11.6, 11.10, 11.12, 11.16, 12.3, 12.4, 12.5, 12.7, 12.8, 12.9, 12.10, 12.11, 12.13, 12.18, 12.22 and 13.6; and from *Archives of Oral Biology* — Figs. 1.11, 6.7, 7.9, 7.11 and 7.12.

The Rockefeller University Press for permission to reproduce Figs. 2.5 and 2.6.

The editor of the *British Dental Journal* for permission to use Figs. 11.6, 11.15, 12.11 and 12.13.

The editor of the *Journal of the British Endodontic Society* for permission to reproduce, in modified form, Figs. 11.3 and 11.4.

The editor of *Pain* for permission to use Fig. 7.8.

The editor of *Proceedings of the Finnish Dental Society* for permission to use Figs. 7.6 and 7.7.

I am also grateful to the following individuals for permission to reproduce their material:

Professor D. J. Anderson of Bristol, England, for Fig. 7.5, modified from his original illustrations.

Professor A. Brodal of Oslo, Norway, for Fig. 3.2, modified from his original illustration.

Drs L. Edwall and L. Olgart of Stockholm, Sweden, for Fig. 7.8, modified from their original illustration.

Dr R. Harris of Sydney, Australia, for Fig. 1.11, modified from his original illustration.

Professor Dr Z. Kunc of Stresovice, Czechoslovakia, for Figs. 3.1, 3.2 and 3.3, modified from his original illustrations.

Mr J. Miles of Liverpool, England, for giving Fig. 16.4 with permission to use it.

Professor V. B. Mountcastle of Baltimore, U.S.A., for permission to reproduce Figs. 2.5 and 2.6.

Dr M. Närhi of Kuopio, Finland, for giving Figs. 7.6 and 7.7 with permission to use them.

Dr P. Pohto of Helsinki, Finland, for giving Fig. 1.12 with permission to use it.

Dr P. Rasmussen of Aarhus, Denmark, for Figs. 16.1 and 16.2, modified from his original illustrations.

Professor P. D. Wall of London, England, for Fig. 4.3.

In addition, my colleagues have kindly allowed me to use some of their illustrations and are acknowledged in the appropriate legends.

When investigating pain cases it is essential to have good radiographs and I must thank Mr Peter Bird and his staff in the Radiological Department of the Liverpool Dental Hospital. Many of their radiographs will be seen throughout the book. I have also been helped by Mr Sydney Bailie of our Department of Medical Illustration, and I thank him for the photographs.

A considerable amount of new typing has been necessary for this edition and I am pleased to have had the willing help of Mrs Ethel Little.

J.M.M.

# Contents

# Introduction

*What is pain?*

Pain is essentially an unpleasant sensation arising in a particular part of the body. It is associated with various activities and bodily changes, and may be described as part of a complex made up of the following features:

1. The unpleasant sensation itself.
2. Withdrawal movements, which may be involuntary, such as flexion of a limb.
3. Vascular changes.
4. Involuntary vocalisation, such as a cry or moan.
5. Startle reaction, the person possibly feeling obliged to explain that he wasn't expecting the pain-producing stimulus.
6. Attempts to reduce the sensation by nursing the affected area, such as by holding the face in the hands in cases of toothache.
7. Activity which produces alternative sensory stimuli, such as by rubbing the affected part, or even knocking his head against a wall.
8. Evaluation of the sensation, possibly leading to an emotional response. Thus, pain in a leg might not seem as important as a pain of comparable intensity in the chest.
9. Central control. The person may withstand the pain of a tooth being drilled without jerking his head away because he accepts that this pain is the lesser of evils. It is even possible for the patient to reduce the pain by concentrating on listening to music or by thinking that the pain is only a sensation which, in the skilled hands of the dentist, does not constitute a threat.
10. The physical and psychological state of suffering is also a feature but needs time to develop, and can only be expected in association with long lasting pain rather than pain of brief duration.

*What is the purpose of pain?*

Pain is usually considered to be a warning of damage, but disease does not necessarily cause pain. For example, carcinoma may not cause pain for a considerable time, and when it does so the warning may be too late to allow effective treatment. At this stage pain only adds to the unpleasantness of the disease, making the patient even worse off than he would have been without it. In the mouth, dental caries and chronic gingivitis all too often do not cause pain, which accounts for the often heard remark, "But my teeth haven't caused me any trouble doctor". On the other hand, pain sometimes occurs in teeth which are apparently quite normal, as a result of stimuli which are not obviously harmful, such as when ice cream lingers on lower incisors. In some cases pain can be very severe following minor stimulation, and even a light touch can cause excruciating pain in idiopathic trigeminal neuralgia.

It has also been suggested that pain is not simply a means of indicating tissue damage but of indicating the rate of tissue damage, e.g. pain occurs when tissue is damaged quickly as by a burn, but not when the damage occurs more slowly as by tuberculosis. This suggestion gains support from the common observation that pain usually occurs with acute conditions rather than chronic ones.

It is beyond the scope of this book to indulge in metaphysical speculation about pain. However, it is certainly conceivable that a limited amount of discomfort and even pain may be desirable to help us appreciate our normally healthy state, always provided that the quantity of pain is not such as to be destructive to the individual. It is here that the clinician comes in, and it is hoped that the book will help him.

# 1

# Innervation of the orofacial tissues

## TRIGEMINAL NERVE

The main sensory supply of this region is the trigeminal nerve with its three great divisions, the ophthalmic, the maxillary and the mandibular, each with many important branches (Fig. 1.1). The nerve has two roots, the sensory root which enters the brain stem at the level of the pons, and the smaller motor root which leaves the pons alongside it. The latter may be joined by a variable number of rootlets (Pelletier, Poulos and Lende, 1974).

Within the cranial cavity the sensory root has an enlargement called the trigeminal ganglion which lies in a depression on the petrous portion of the temporal bone where it is situated laterally to the internal carotid artery and the posterior end of the cavernous venous sinus. The nerve cells which form the sensory part of the trigeminal nerve have their cell bodies in this ganglion except for some in the mesencephalic nucleus (Chapter 3). Though these cells are pseudo-unipolar each, in effect, has two branches, one of which passes via the sensory nerve root to the trigeminal nuclei in the brain (Chapter 3), whilst the other branch contributes to forming the trigeminal nerve. The motor root passes beneath the trigeminal ganglion to join the mandibular division via which it travels to supply the muscles of mastication, the anterior belly of the digastric and mylohyoid muscles, as well as the tensor palati and tensor tympani muscles.

### Ophthalmic nerve

The ophthalmic nerve is the smallest of the three divisions. It passes forwards in the lateral wall of the cavernous sinus to the superior orbital fissure, giving off small branches to the dura mater and the third, fourth and sixth cranial nerves. It has three main branches.

The *lacrimal nerve* goes to the antero-lateral part of the orbit to the conjunctiva and the skin of the upper eyelid laterally (Figs. 1.1,

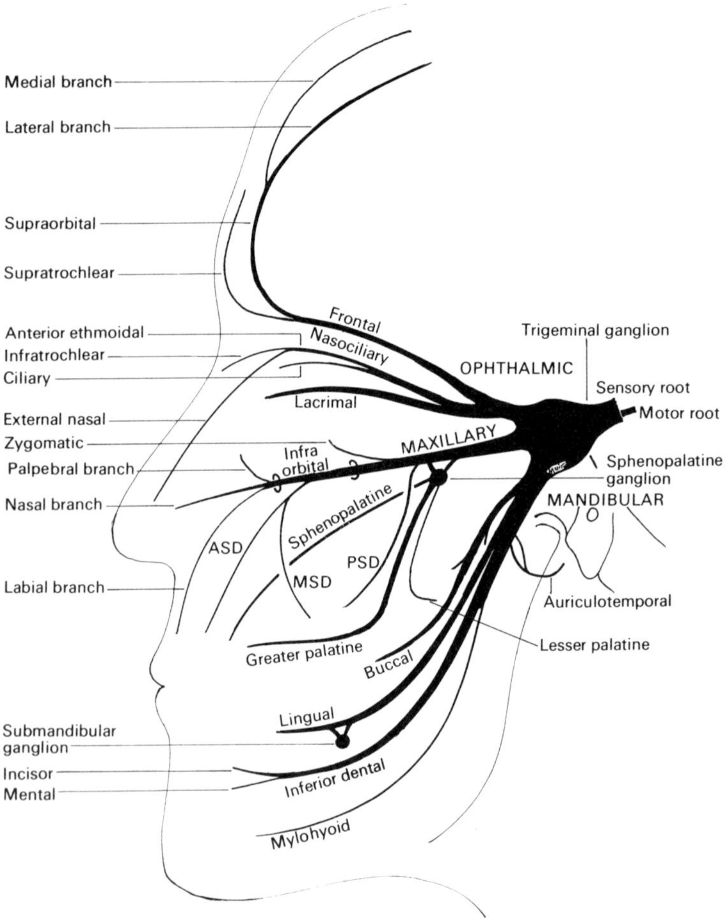


**Fig. 1.1.** Main branches of the trigeminal nerve. ASD, MSD, PSD. Anterior, middle and posterior superior dental nerves.

1.2). It receives secreto-motor fibres from the zygomaticotemporal nerve and delivers them to the lacrimal gland.

The *nasociliary nerve* goes to the antero-medial part of the orbit giving posterior ethmoidal, ciliary and infratrochlear branches. It becomes the anterior ethmoidal nerve which turns medially and terminates by dividing into medial and lateral internal nasal nerves. The latter becomes the external nasal nerve which supplies the skin and mucous membrane of the cartilaginous area of the nose (Fig. 1.2). Sympathetic fibres pass through the nasociliary nerve from the plexus on the internal carotid artery via the ciliary ganglion to

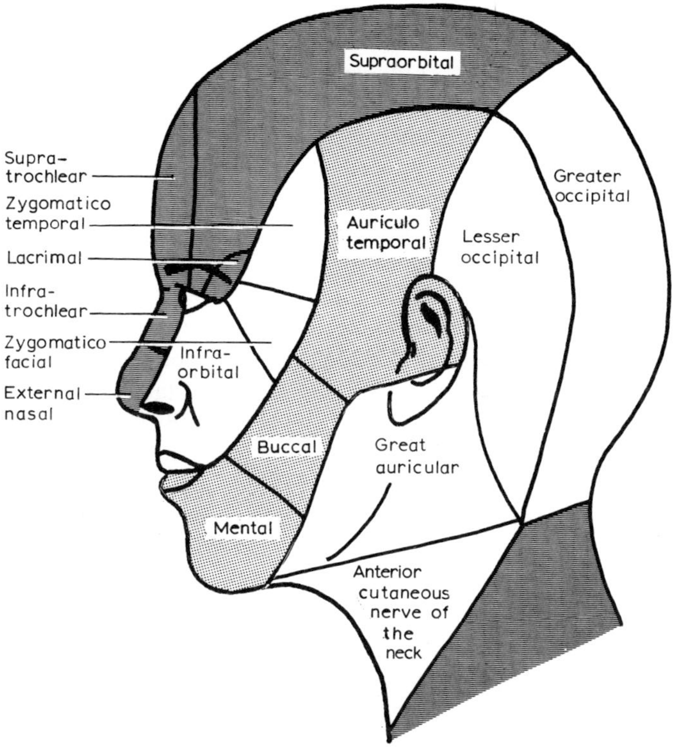


**Fig. 1.2.** Distribution of superficial nerves of the head and neck. (Various authorities show minor variations.)

the dilator muscle of the pupil of the eye. Fibres derived from the oculomotor nerve pass to the sphincter muscle of the pupil.

The *frontal nerve* travels anteriorly and divides into the larger supraorbital branch and smaller supratrochlear branch. The former supplies the skin of the upper eyelid, the forehead and scalp as far back as the vertex of the skull (Fig. 1.2) and also the frontal sinus. The supratrochlear nerve supplies the skin of the forehead in the midline and also the medial part of the upper eyelid.

## Maxillary nerve

The maxillary nerve passes forward in the dura mater (which it supplies) below the cavernous venous sinus, leaves the cranial cavity via the foramen rotundum and reaches the pterygopalatine fossa which it crosses to the inferior orbital fissure where it is named the infraorbital nerve. In the pterygopalatine fossa it sends two short thick roots to the sphenopalatine ganglion (pterygopalatine ganglion) which also receives the nerve of the pterygoid canal, the latter conveying parasympathetic and sympathetic fibres. The following branches are derived from the ganglion.

The *greater palatine nerve* passes through the greater palatine canal to supply the mucoperiosteum of the hard palate as far forward as the incisor teeth where it meets the terminal branches of the long sphenopalatine nerve (Fig. 1.3). It gives branches to the nasal mucous membrane over the inferior concha of the nose, and to the soft palate. The *lesser palatine nerves* also supply the mucous membrane of the soft palate and the tonsil.

The long *sphenopalatine nerve* (nasopalatine nerve) leaves the sphenopalatine ganglion in a medial direction and passes obliquely forwards and downwards along the nasal septum supplying the mucous membrane (Figs. 1.1, 1.3). It reaches the incisive fossa to emerge behind the upper central incisors where its terminals merge with those of its fellow of the opposite side and also with the terminal branches of the greater palatine nerve, supplying the mucous membrane of the hard palate in this area (Fig. 1.3). The *short sphenopalatine nerves* supply the mucous membrane over the superior and middle nasal conchae.

The *zygomatic nerve* leaves the maxillary nerve close to the origin of the posterior superior dental nerve, just before the maxillary becomes the infraorbital nerve. The zygomatic nerve divides into

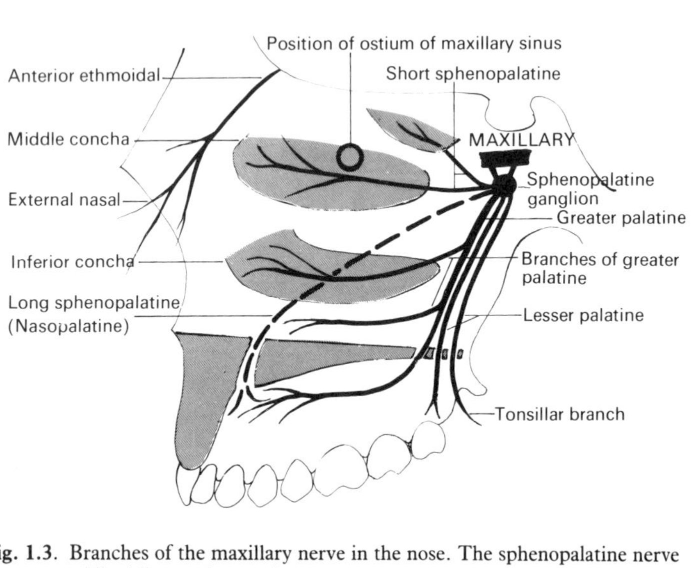


**Fig. 1.3**. Branches of the maxillary nerve in the nose. The sphenopalatine nerve (interrupted line) lies on the nasal septum.

zygomaticotemporal and zygomaticofacial branches which supply the skin areas shown in Fig. 1.2

The *infraorbital nerve* travels in the infraorbital canal where it gives branches to the teeth via the anterior superior dental nerve, and it may also give rise to the middle superior dental nerve (Figs. 1.1, 1.4). These are also known as the anterior and middle superior alveolar nerves.

The *posterior superior dental nerve* (posterior superior alveolar nerve) is given off the maxillary nerve in the pterygopalatine fossa, and is usually represented by two nerves, or sometimes even three (Last, 1973). They descend in the pterygomaxillary fissure to enter the maxilla via the posterior superior dental foramina. They supply the mucous membrane of the maxillary sinus, and the periodontium and pulps of the molar teeth (Fig. 1.4). The pulp of the first molar also receives fibres from the middle superior dental nerve via the mesio-buccal root. Fine terminal branches may overlap with similar branches of the anterior and middle superior dental nerves. (Innervation of the teeth and periodontal tissues is considered more fully later in the chapter.)

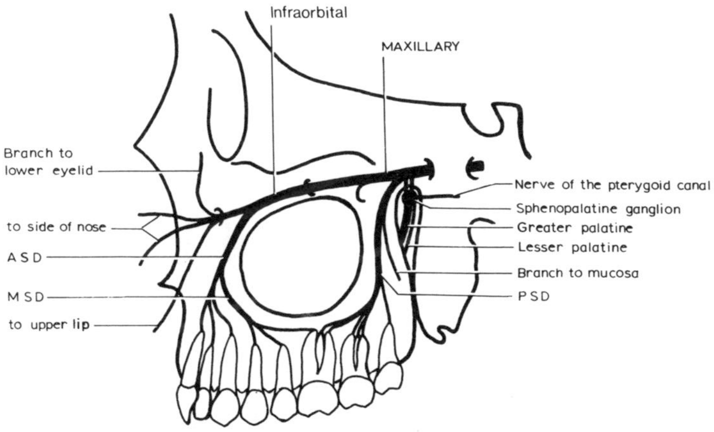


**Fig. 1.4.** The maxillary nerve and its branches.

The *middle superior dental nerve* may be derived directly from the infraorbital nerve or it may be only a branch from the anterior superior dental nerve. It supplies the periodontium and pulps of the premolar teeth and the mesio-buccal root of the first molar, and may join with fine terminal branches of the posterior superior dental nerve.

The *anterior superior dental nerve* is given off in the infraorbital canal. Its branches pass in small bony canals to the periodontium and pulps of the central incisor, lateral incisor and canine teeth. The nerve also supplies the mucous membrane of the adjacent part of the nasal cavity.

On leaving the infraorbital foramen the infraorbital nerve sends branches to the cheek, upper lip, conjunctiva and skin of the lower eyelid, and the skin of the side of the nose (Figs 1.2, 1.4).

## Mandibular nerve

The mandibular nerve is the largest division of the trigeminal nerve. It is composed of sensory fibres from the trigeminal ganglion plus the motor root of the nerve which joins it after leaving the pons and passing beneath the ganglion. The combined nerve leaves the cranial cavity via the foramen ovale and gives off two branches before separating into anterior and posterior parts (Fig. 1.5).

The *nervus spinosus* (meningeal branch) passes through the foramen spinosus in company with the middle meningeal artery. Its anterior branch supplies the dura mater of the middle cranial fossa and part of the anterior cranial fossa and calvarium. Its posterior branch also supplies a twig to the mastoid air cells (Warwick and Williams, 1973). These branches provide part of the neurological basis for referred pain.

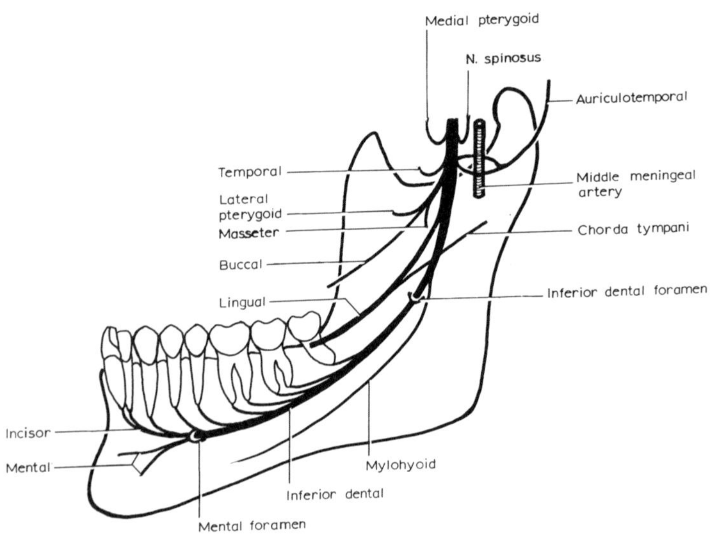


**Fig. 1.5.** The mandibular nerve and its branches.

The *nerve to the medial pterygoid muscle* is a motor nerve which also conveys fibres to the tensor palati and tensor tympani.

The anterior division of the mandibular nerve gives off the following branches.

The *masseteric nerve* is the motor nerve to the masseter and also sends filaments to the temporomandibular joint.

The *deep temporal nerves* are motor nerves to the temporal muscle. There are usually anterior and posterior nerves but there may also be a middle one.

The *two lateral pterygoid nerves* are the motor nerves to the corresponding muscle.

The *buccal nerve* is a sensory nerve supplying the skin and mucous membrane of the cheek down to the buccal sulcus as far as the lower molar teeth (Fig. 1.2). It contains all the fibres for common sensation that are present in the anterior division of the mandibular nerve (Last, 1973).

The posterior trunk gives the following branches.

The *auriculotemporal nerve* supplies the skin over the temple, the temporomandibular joint, the skin of the anterior part of the external auditory meatus plus the tympanic membrane, and the upper part of the auricle (Fig. 1.2). Sympathetic and parasympathetic fibres are conveyed to the parotid gland, the parasympathetic fibres being derived from the glossopharyngeal nerve.

The *lingual nerve* passes laterally to the medial pterygoid muscle close to the posterior end of the mylohyoid line of the mandible where it gives off a gingival branch which supplies the lingual gingiva as far forwards as the midline (Last, 1973). It sweeps forwards and is distributed to the mucous membrane of the anterior two-thirds of the tongue supplying fibres for taste as well as common sensation. It is joined by the chorda tympani branch of the facial nerve carrying parasympathetic and taste fibres (Fig. 1.5). The lingual nerve has branches to and from the submandibular ganglion via which parasympathetic fibres go to the sublingual and submandibular glands. There is a communicating branch to the hypoglossal nerve, and possibly to the inferior dental nerve. The latter could account for incomplete anaesthesia following an inferior dental injection in a small percentage of cases (Rood, 1976).

The *inferior dental nerve* (inferior alveolar nerve) gives a small motor branch to the mylohyoid muscle and the anterior belly of the digastric muscle before it enters the inferior dental canal from which it supplies the pulps and periodontal membranes of the molar and premolar teeth, as well as contributing to the gingival innervation.

The inferior dental nerve may be joined by nerve fibres which enter the bone as components of neurovascular bundles derived from attached muscles such as the masseter and temporalis, those from the latter entering via foramina in the retromolar fossa (Carter and Keen, 1971). Similar connections have been observed from the mylohyoid nerve.

The inferior dental canal contains all of the inferior dental nerve in the majority of cases but its branches sometimes spread so that the canal becomes less distinct. Similarly, although the nerve usually terminates as distinct mental and incisor nerves, the incisor nerve may form a plexus in 34 per cent of cases (Olivier, 1927).

The *incisor nerve* continues within the mandible and supplies the pulps and periodontal membranes of the canine and incisor teeth. It also contributes to the gingival innervation, and may reach the central incisor of the opposite side (Starkie and Stewart, 1931). Some unpublished psychophysical work of the author on human subjects supports this view, and suggests that innervation may cross the midline to the lateral incisor in some cases. This could account for some failures of local anaesthesia. It is even possible that nerve filaments overlap the midline as far as the canine teeth (Anderson and Pearl, 1974) or premolars (Anderson et al, 1977); but these observations derive from experiments on cats. However, Matthews and Lisney (1978), also working on cats, found no evidence for pulpal nerve fibres crossing the midline.

The *mental nerve* leaves the mandible by the mental foramen and supplies the mucous membrane and skin of the lower lip, as well as contributing to the gingival innervation. It also carries a few fibres from the otic ganglion to the glands within the lower lip (Last, 1973).

### Number of nerve fibres

A complete transverse section of a human trigeminal sensory root has been examined by Young (1977). By a combination of counting and calculating he found that there were 124 000 nerve fibres, approximately half being myelinated and half unmyelinated. The unmyelinated were from 0·2–1·3 $\mu$m diameter, and the largest myelinated fibres were up to 11 $\mu$m diameter.

## INNERVATION OF THE TEETH

Nerve fibres enter the tooth via the apical foramen and travel through the pulp as several large bundles in a fairly straight course towards the crown (Figs. 1.6, 1.7).

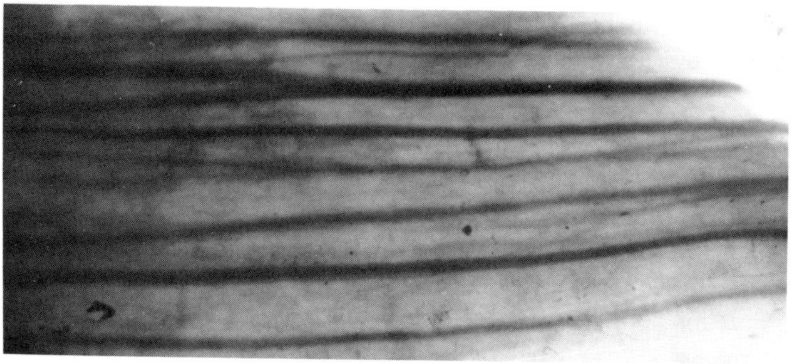

**Fig. 1.6.** Bundles of nerve fibres in the whole pulp of a premolar. The tooth was broken open, the pulp stripped out and the nerves stained with osmium tetroxide. Magnification x 40. (Courtesy of Dr John Appleton.)

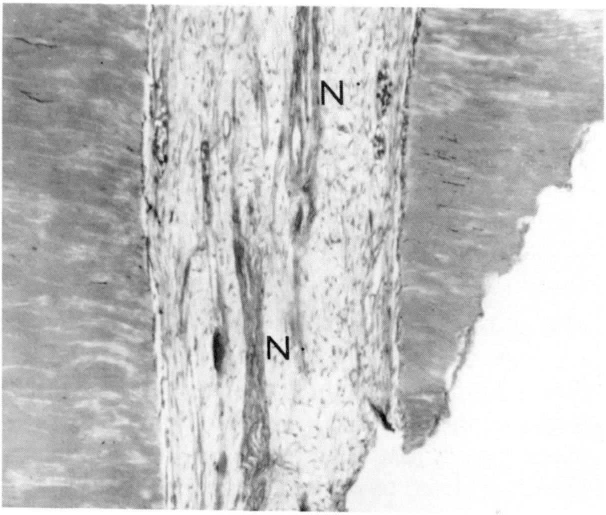


**Fig. 1.7.** Bundles of nerve fibres (N) in a longitudinal section of a pulp. Magnificant x 32.

Few fibres pass to the odontoblastic layer in the root (Arwill, 1958; Fearnhead, 1961; Bernick, 1964) and only occasionally do fibres divide in the pulp canal. On reaching the pulp chamber they spread out towards its roof and walls where they change course abruptly and divide several times in the zone deep to the cell sparse zone (cell free zone of Weil). In incisors and canines nerve fibres go directly to the pulp horns ( Fearnhead, 1961). In teeth with two or more roots a pulp horn is always supplied with nerve fibres entering by the corresponding pulp canal (Engström and Öhman, 1960).

Nerves with branched axons may supply more than one tooth (Lisney and Matthews, 1976).

**Subodontoblastic plexus (plexus of Raschkow)**

This is formed within the coronal part of the pulp by the nerve fibres dividing, spreading out and intertwining. The plexus does not start to form before the level of the cervical part of the pulp. It is present in most permanent teeth when root formation is nearing completion, but is not present in the deciduous teeth at this stage (Fearnhead, 1961).

Within the plexus the nerve fibres are said to lose their myelin sheaths (Fearnhead, 1961; Frank, 1968a, b) but Harris and Griffin (1968) found both myelinated and unmyelinated fibres. In the cat they were mostly unmyelinated, and both types showed changes in diameter, sometimes dramatically (Holland and Nahnybida, 1979).

A marginal nerve plexus on the surface of the predentine has been described by Bradlaw (1936, 1939) and Fearnhead (1961), the fibres being unmyelinated with diameters of 0·1–0·5 $\mu$m. Bernick (1964) described fibres as forming loops in predentine, but Arwill (1958) observed no inter-odontoblastic or supra-odontoblastic plexuses. It seems unnecessary to describe nerve fibres in these zones as part of any plexus.

**Innervation of dentine**

There has been a prolonged controversy about whether or not nerve fibres enter the dentine and it is now accepted that they enter the inner layer of dentine, but the extent of innervation is not fully settled. Older papers have been extensively and painstakingly reviewed by Arwill (1958) to whom the interested reader is referred, but the present position is as follows.

According to Fearnhead (1961) nerve fibres do enter the dentinal tubules, more in the crown than in the root. He considered that between 1 in 200 and 1 in 2000 tubules were innervated, but recent work of Byers (personal communication, 1981) suggests that upto half of the tubules might be innervated.

Various other investigations also show nerves in dentine (Langeland and Yagi, 1972; Roane et al, 1973) but there is still doubt about how far they extend into dentine (Brännström and Garberoglio, 1972).

It is possible that some nerve fibres are coupled with others for it has been shown that sending a nerve impulse into the tooth (antidromically) may result in an impulse away from the tooth (orthodromically) in another nerve fibre (Matthews and Holland, 1975; Matthews, 1977b).

Frank (1966, 1968a) showed electron micrographs of unmyelinated nerve fibres in dentinal tubules. He described the nerve fibres as following, at first, a straight course along the odontoblast process, at which stage the fibre's diameter progressively diminished. Still within the inner dentine its course became more complicated, twisting around the odontoblast process in an irregular spiral. Branches of these nerve fibres could also be seen entering the lateral branches of the dentinal tubules together with branches of the odontoblastic processes (Frank, 1968a, b). At the nerve endings he observed cellular surface specialisations 'which clearly demonstrate a functional relationship between the nerve endings and the odontoblastic process', and 'it can be concluded that we deal here with an intra-dentinal receptor representing a unique type of neurosensitive complex'. Frank's work is excellent, and his conclusion is very interesting but if the odontoblasts have a well defined transduction function and there are neuro-odontoblastic junctions in the dentinal tubules they could presumably occur just as well on the parts of odontoblasts lying within the pulp. Such junctions have not been shown by Avery (1978) or Byers (1979). Moreover, any junction would not necessarily be from odontoblast to nerve, but could function in the reverse direction, allowing the nerve to control the odontoblast. The control of odontogenesis is thought to be an important neural function (Avery and Cox, 1977).

Arwill (1967 found a similar appearance to that described by Frank, but preferred to describe the cells alongside the odontoblasts as associated cells and Arwill *et al.* (1973) suggested that these 'associate cells' are sensory neurones. These cells were rich in mitochondria and contained vesicles from 25–75 nm, the cleft between the cells being 20–25 nm. Both of these sizes happen to be similar to those of synaptic vesicles and synaptic clefts, but the reader should hesitate to think of them in that way (see Chapter 2).

Scott and Tempel (1963) and Scott (1966), using cats, recorded electrical activity from the cut surface of dentine that caused them to postulate the presence of hot and cold receptors in dentine, but their results could be explained by the dentinal tubules acting as microelectrodes and recording events occurring in the pulp. After stimulating the teeth of dogs Matthews (1977) concluded that there were no thermal receptors.

## Role of odontoblasts

It has been suggested that the odontoblasts have a role in mediating pain, and powerful support for this view comes from the physical relationship between them and the nerve fibres as shown by the investigations of Frank described above. The objection has been made that the odontoblasts are derived from mesoderm whereas nerves are derived from ectoderm but, for instance, the outer layers of the pacinian corpuscle are derived from mesoderm. Moreover, it is possible for cells which give rise to odontoblasts in primitive organisms to have emigrated from the neural crest (de Beer, 1947). However, this agreement is not even necessary because the odontoblasts could have a supporting role, and Pringle (1962) takes the view that closely apposed membranes must be considered as a single functional unit. The odontoblasts and/or the dentinal tubules might provide the best environment for the neurones to be excited.

Avery and Rapp (1958, 1959) found specific cholinesterase in the odontoblastic processes with an intense concentration in the odontoblasts themselves. They thought this might indicate a possible pain transmission path through dentine and a 'synapse' in the odontoblastic zone, but they found there was no appreciable amount of acetylcholine in the odontoblasts so that, if the odontoblasts were associated with dentine sensitivity via nerve endings in the pulp, transmission of the impulse would not be mediated by cholinergic activity.

When pain occurs in teeth which are subsequently subjected to microscopic examination, it is frequently found that some odontoblasts have been aspirated into the dentinal tubules, but this is presumably a passive movement caused by pressure changes in the pulpal and dentinal fluids. In fact, it has been shown that when dentine is exposed there can be a fluid flow of 0.6 $\mu l/mm^2/day$ (Johnson, Olgart and Brännström, 1973); this means that a patent tubule could be emptied ten times per day. Such an outward flow could account for aspiration of odontoblasts. Moreover, aspiration of odontoblasts may be found in the absence of pain (Kramer, 1954). Odontoblastic processes are limited to the inner third of coronal dentine (Thomas, 1979), and it may be noted that transmission of stimuli through dentine does not need either nerves or odontoblasts. However, odontoblasts might modulate nerve excitability by changing the composition of extracellular fluid in the area (Byers, 1977). This important aspect of dental pain will be considered in detail in Chapter 7.

### Innervation of enamel

In Arwill's (1958) monograph he quotes a number of investigators as having reported tracing nerve 'elements' into enamel. It is conceivable that if nerve fibres pass well into the dentinal tubules they might reach the dentino-enamel junction, but Frank (1972) states that no nerve fibres are found in the outer dentine, and it is generally accepted that enamel is not innervated.

**Effect of age on innervation of teeth**

The period of tooth development during which nerve fibres enter the tooth is of more than academic interest because it affects the diagnosis of toothache and pulp disease in young people.

By the time dentine starts to form most tooth germs possess one or more fibres, and these increase in number. At the time of root completion the subodontoblastic nerve plexus is present in most permanent teeth, but not in deciduous teeth (Fearnhead, 1961).

Nerve fibres appear to continue to grow after the tooth reaches its final form, even after reaching what might be considered an adequate saturation of the tissue by sensory nerves, and might grow into the dentinal tubules (Fearnhead, 1958). Alternatively, nerve fibres may be enclosed in predentine by advancing years, pathological conditions, or both (Arwill, 1960). As ageing occurs the number of nerve fibres in the pulp is reduced partly because they become involved in calcification (Bernick, 1967).

After extraction of teeth the innervation of the mucosa over the alveolar ridge is said to become diminished in amount and less orderly than in normal gingival tissue. The nerve fibres lie in the deeper parts of the connective tissue but occasional fibres may pass through the epithelium to approach the surface.

**Numbers and types of nerve fibre**

The number of nerve fibres per tooth ranges from 151–1296 (Graf and Björlin, 1951), and each of these might have about 8 terminal branches (Scott, 1966; Harris and Griffin, 1968). In human deciduous canines the mean number of myelinated fibres was 439; of unmyelinated fibres 2521. For permanent canines the corresponding numbers were 361 and 2240 (Johnson and Johns, 1978).

An electronmicroscopic study of one cat canine tooth was made, counting in one complete cross-sectional area of the crown (Beasley and Holland, 1978). There were 3470 nerve fibres, 81 per cent being unmyelinated, and these had a modal diameter of 0·35 μm, the range being 0·1–1·4μm. The myelinated fibres had a modal diameter of 2·5 μm, with a range of 1·0–6·0 μm. The largest myelinated fibres were in the core, and the relative preponderance of unmyelinated fibres increased towards the periphery. This core of myelinated fibres was also found in cats by Johnsen and Karlsson (1974); in deciduous teeth they found 149 unmyelinated fibres and 22 myelinated fibres, whereas in permanent teeth the corresponding figures were 432 and 126 .

The great majority of the myelinated fibres (Fig. 1.8) have diameters which are mainly 2–3 μm (Graf and Bjorlin, 1951; Matthews, Dorman and Bishop, 1959). The larger values they gave, up to 20 μm, are no longer accepted.

In cats the range is 1·3–2·0 μm (Johnsen and Karlsson, 1974) and 1·0–6·0 μm (Beasley and Holland, 1978).

The myelin sheath is formed by Schwann cells (Fig. 1.9) wrapping themselves around the nerve fibres, and sometimes several axons lie in one Schwann cell. Each lamella of myelin is a bimolecular layer of lipids, radially arranged with protein bound on either side (Foster, 1966). In pulpal nerves the width of a single lamella is 0·01 μm, and the total thickness of myelin is from 0·3–1·0 μm (Uchizono and Homma, 1959), or even as thick as 1·5 μm (Matthews, Dorman and Bishop, 1959). Myelination seems to be incomplete prior to closure of the apex, and the number of myelinated axons is greater in older persons (Johnsen and Harshbarger, 1980).

Unmyelinated nerve fibres (Fig. 1.10) have been found by Uchizono and Homma (1959), Miyoshi, Nishijima and Imanishi (1966) and Harris and Griffin (1968). Their diameters range from

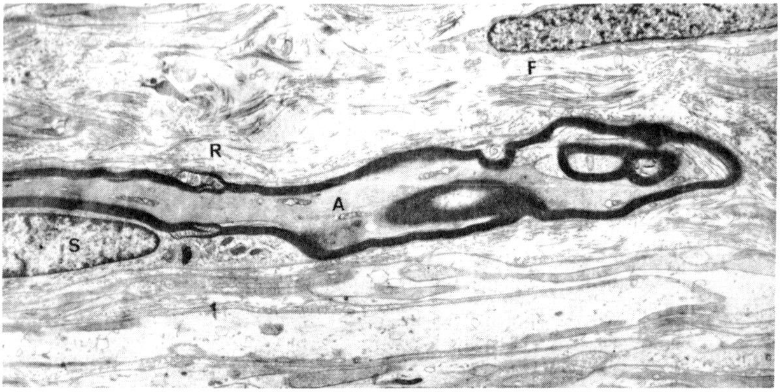


**Fig. 1.8** Myelinated nerve fibre from the pulp of a human tooth. Electron microscope magnification × 7000. In the peripheral nervous system the node of Ranvier is not as open to the external fluid as it is in the central nervous system (Bunge, 1970) or as in conventional diagrams such as Fig. 2.4. A, axon; F, nucleus of fibroblast; R, node of Ranvier; S, nucleus of Schwann cell. (Courtesy of Dr John Appleton).

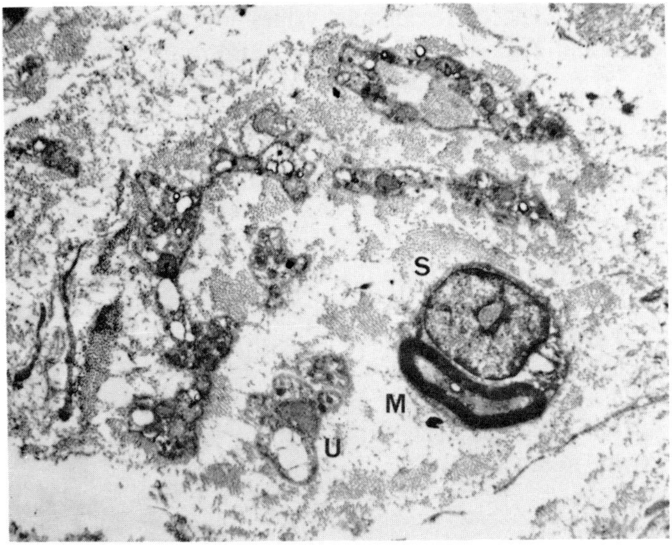


**Fig. 1.9**. Myelinated nerve fibre and Schwann cell from the pulp of a human tooth. Transverse section, electron microscope magnification × 7000. M, myelinated nerve fibre; S, Schwann cell nucleus; U, unmyelinated nerve fibre (Courtesy of Dr John Appleton.)

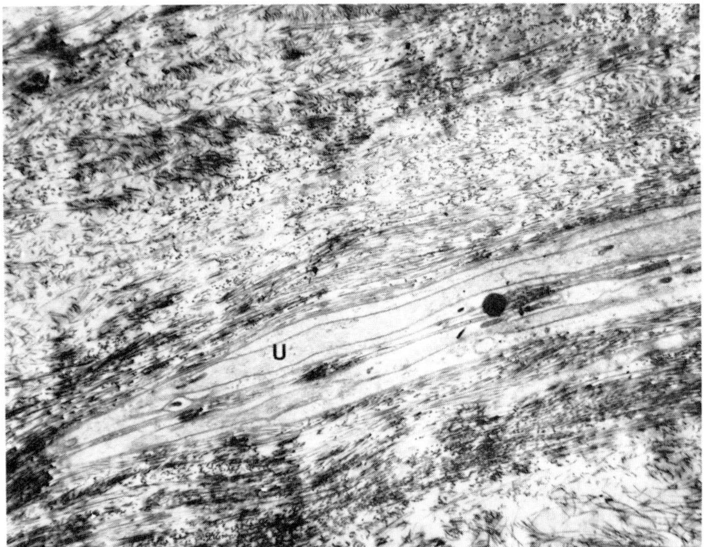


**Fig. 1.10**. Unmyelinated nerve fibre in the pulp of a human tooth. Longitudinal section, electron microscope magnification × 7000. U, unmyelinated fibre (Courtesy of Dr John Appleton.)

0·25–2 μm. The corresponding values in cats were 0·3–4 μm (Johnsen and Karlsson, 1974), and 0·1–1·4 μm (Beasley and Holland, 1978). Johnsen and Karlsson also found that, in cats, permanent teeth had more nerve fibres than did the deciduous teeth. However, if the tooth weight was taken as an indication of the amount of tissue innervated the innervation densities were the same.

In the subodontoblastic plexus Harris and Griffin (1968) found myelinated fibres of 2–5 μm diameter, and unmyelinated fibres of 0·26–1·6 μm diameter with nerve endings which contained vesicles and mitochondria. There were also beaded nerve fibres with axonal expansions, which they thought were apparently concerned with the conduction of pain, and perivascular unmyelinated nerve fibres. They illustrate schematically the nerve endings of a myelinated nerve fibre (Fig. 1.11).

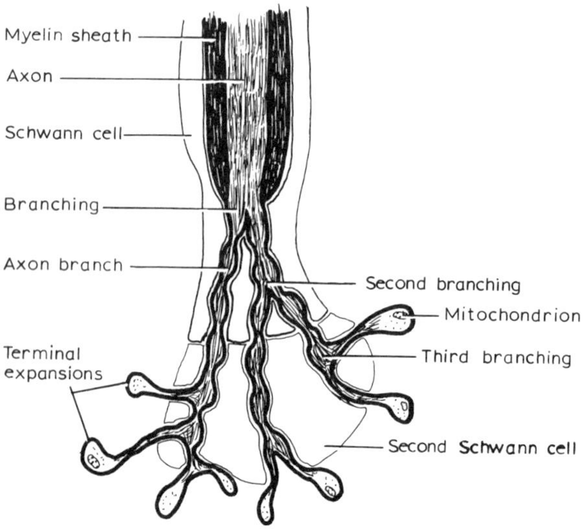


**Fig. 1.11.** Termination of a myelinated nerve. Schematic arrangement as suggested by Harris and Griffin (1968). Modified from their original drawing.

There are autonomic nerve fibres in the pulp (Graf and Björlin, 1950; Matthews, Dorman and Bishop, 1959, Fearnhead, 1961; Harris and Griffin, 1968; Pohto and Antila, 1968a, b, 1972; Pohto, 1972), and they are associated with blood vessels, mainly arterioles (Fig. 1.12). By controlling the arteriole diameter it can be expected that these fibres will play a part in pulpitis. They may

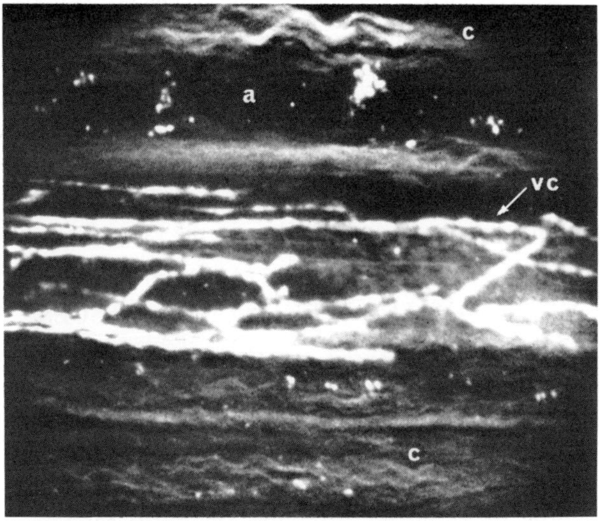


**Fig. 1.12**. Longitudinal section of the pulp of a lower canine (from a cat) showing a sympathetic adrenergic ground plexus on an arteriole. Green-fluorescent nerve terminals with synaptic varicosities (vc). Paraxial arteriole without sympathetic innervation (a). Yellowish auto-fluorescence of collagenous fibres (c). Magnification × 450. (Pohto and Antila, 1968b.)

also modify the excitability of pulpal nerves (Edwall, 1971; Mattews, 1976). It is also possible that some sensory fibres might pass with the autonomic fibres into the sympathetic system (Lewis, 1942) and might mediate pain by this route.

*Conduction velocities of dental nerves*

Since it is difficult to perform these investigations on human subjects, values for animals are given. Electrophysiological studies on human subjects have confirmed the expectation that results would be similar to those found in other mammals (Iggo, 1977). As a basis for comparison it should be noted, as discussed in Chapter 2, that small unmyelinated fibres conduct at 1 metre per sec or less whereas large myelinated fibres conduct at up to 120 metres per second.

Brookhart, Livingston and Haugen (1953) measured the velocity of impulses passing from the canine teeth along the inferior dental nerve of cats, and found values ranging from 30–45 metres per second. There was no suggestion of C-fibre conduction speeds. Matthews and Holland (1975) found conduction velocities of 18–31 metres per second. Anderson and Pearl (1975) found values of 0·1–7·8 metres per second.

Working on dogs, Wagers and Smith (1960) found velocities of 0·8–38 metres per second (mainly 6–20), and Yamada and Sakada (1961) velocities of 40–50 metres per second. Also working with dogs, Funakoshi and Zotterman (1963) found values of 11–17 metres per second; the nerve fibres involved were in the A-delta group, and no activity suggestive of the presence of C fibres was found. Wagers and Smith found only one instance of conduction at 0·8 metres per second which is in the range for C fibres.

## INNERVATION OF THE PERIODONTAL TISSUES

Nerve fibres to the periodontal membrane branch from the bundle entering the pulp or arrive via tiny foramina in the alveolar bone. The latter divide, sending one branch apically and another coronally.

After pulpectomy response to tactile and pressure stimulation is reduced little, if at all (as determined by nerve activity in cats); this was true even after cautery was applied via the pulp canal (Pfaffman, 1939). The distribution of conduction velocities suggests they are type A-alpha somatic afferent fibres (Pfaffman, 1939; Hannam, 1968).

Myelinated fibres, with diameters between 1–6 $\mu$m, lose their myelin sheaths and form several branches of uniform diameter which terminate as axonal swellings 0·5–1·5 $\mu$m in diameter, containing vesicles and mitochondria (Griffin and Harris, 1968). Closely associated with the myelinated fibres are unmyelinated ones with diameters of 0·1–0·6 $\mu$m, and these appear to be type C fibres. The terminal axonal swellings were similar to those seen in the dental pulp by Harris and Griffin (1968).

Loewenstein and Rathkamp (1955) present evidence to suggest that not all pressure receptors are in the periodontal tissues, but some may be located within the dentine, and tactile sensibility may at least partly be mediated via pulpal nerves.

## MASTICATORY CONTROL

Masticatory movements are controlled by sensory feedback from the temporomandibular joints, the muscles of mastication, the oral mucosa and the periodontal membranes. In cases of dental disease noxious stimulation of the dentine and pulp can cause pain and this may influence movement.

Nerve fibres from proprioceptors in the muscles of mastication ascend to the mesencephalic nucleus (Chapter 3) and send collateral branches to the motor nucleus from which motor fibres go to the muscles via the mandibular nerve.There is therefore a two neurone reflex arc; that is, monosynaptic (Kawamura, 1968). He points out that a single motoneurone and its axon innervates a group of from 3–200 muscle fibres, and that in normal mandibular movements motor units of the muscles function successively.

### Facial nerve

This is a mixed nerve, its motor fibres going to the muscles of the face, scalp and neck. Its sensory root (the nervus intermedius) may be considered as a separate nerve, the thirteenth cranial nerve (Last, 1973), which conveys taste fibres reaching it from the anterior two thirds of the tongue via the lingual and chorda tympani nerves, together with fibres mediating general sensation from a small area of the external auditory meatus and the auricle. It also contains efferent parasympathetic fibres which go to the lacrimal gland, salivary glands and the mucous glands of the nose and palate (Fig. 1.13).

### Glossopharyngeal nerve

The glossopharyngeal nerve is a mixed nerve. It conveys motor fibres to the stylopharyngeus muscle and secretory fibres to the posterior third of the tongue and the parotid gland (Fig. 1.13).

It receives fibres from the posterior third of the tongue, some of them mediating common sensation and others the sense of taste. It also receives sensory fibres from the tonsillar region, the pharynx, the soft palate and the posterior palatal arch. The fibres concerned with common sensation probably end in the spinal nucleus of the trigeminal nerve (Brodal, 1969; Warwick and Williams, 1973).

The otic ganglion (see later) is functionally a part of the glossopharyngeal nerve although closely related anatomically to the mandibular nerve.

### Vagus nerve

The vagus nerve contains both sensory and motor fibres, the latter being preganglionic parasympathetic as well as somatic. Its branches are widespread and include those to the pharynx and respiratory system as well as the heart. A branch goes to the floor of the external auditory meatus and the lower part of the tympanic membrane. These sensory fibres eventually end in the trigeminal spinal nucleus, as do the somatic afferent fibres from the glossopharyngeal nerve (Brodal, 1969). This anatomical relationship presumably provides part of the neurological basis for the occurrence of earache when pain from a diseased tooth is referred to the ear.

**Hypoglossal nerve**

This nerve is essentially a motor nerve supplying all the muscles of the tongue including the extrinsic ones. It receives a communicating branch from the lingual nerve, and it seems possible that proprioceptive impulses from the lingual muscles may pass via this to the brain via the hypoglossal nerve (Last, 1973).

**Cervical plexus**

The *lesser occipital nerve* arises from the cervical plexus, its fibres being derived from the second and third cervical nerves, and supplies the skin and fascia of the upper part of the neck and scalp behind the ear (Fig. 1.2).

The *great auricular nerve* is the largest of the cutaneous branches of the cervical plexus, and is composed of fibres of the second and third cervical nerves. Its posterior branch ascends to the skin and fascia behind the ear, where it communicates with both the lesser occipital nerve and the posterior auricular branch of the facial nerve. The middle branch goes to the skin over the lower part of the external ear. The anterior branch passes through the substance of the parotid gland to the skin over it and to the masseter muscle insertion (Romanes, 1964).

The *anterior cutaneous nerve* of the neck also derives its fibres from the second and third cervical nerves, via the cervical plexus, and supplies the skin and fascia in the anterior superior part of the neck (Fig. 1.2).

**Sympathetic nerves**

The nerves of the autonomic system are all efferent, impulses being conveyed along them to the periphery to regulate the body's internal environment; i.e. to maintain homeostasis.

The sympathetic part of this system arises from the thoracic and upper lumbar spinal cord. Its fibres enter the ventral roots of the spinal nerves and leave as the white communicating rami to reach the sympathetic chain. The uppermost part of this, the superior cervical ganglion, sends fibres to the sympathetic nerve plexus about the carotid arteries. From here they are distributed to the skin of the face and other structures. Sympathetic fibres mediate the contraction of smooth muscle fibres in the walls of arteries, and even reach the dental pulp (Fig. 1.12). Here they can produce a pronounced reduction of blood flow (Edwall, 1972). More obviously, the vasoconstriction in skin explains the blanching of a person's face when he is afraid or, sometimes, in pain.

From the internal carotid artery sympathetic fibres pass via the short ciliary nerves to the dilator muscle of the pupil. Others pass via the deep petrosal nerve to the nerve of the pterygoid canal, through the sphenopalatine (pterygopalatine ) ganglion and, via the zygomatic nerve, to the lacrimal gland. Similarly, sympathetic fibres reach the glands of the nasal and palatal mucous membranes (Fig. 1.3).

The sympathetic plexus on the middle meningeal artery sends fibres through the otic ganglion to the parotid gland. Similarly, from the plexus on the facial artery fibres pass through the submandibular ganglion to the sublingual and submandibular glands (Fig. 1.13).

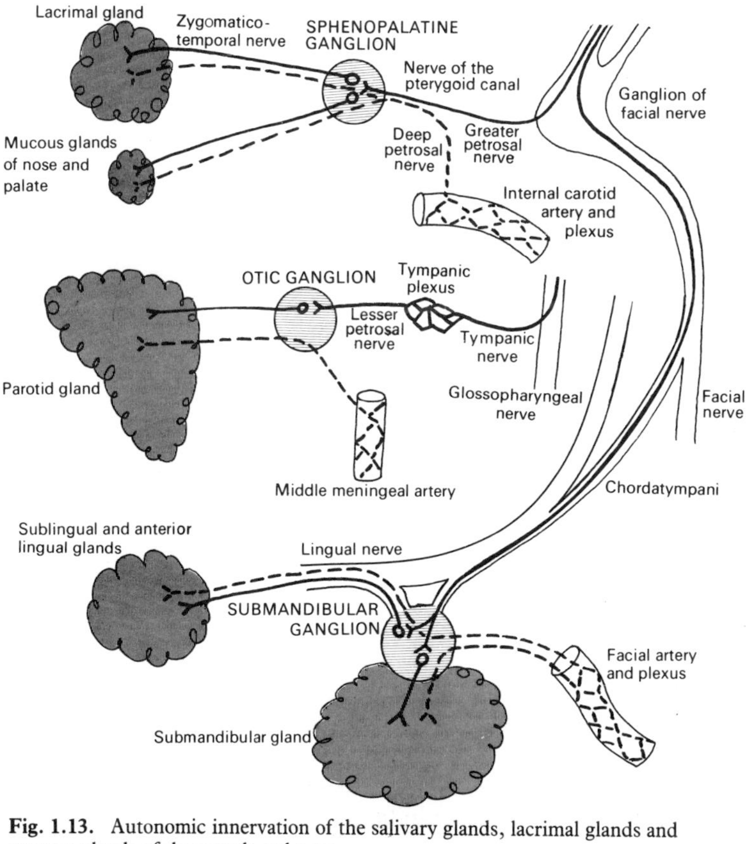


**Fig. 1.13.** Autonomic innervation of the salivary glands, lacrimal glands and mucous glands of the mouth and nose.

A person in a dentist's waiting room (or about to give an after-dinner speech) who suffers from a dry mouth does so because of activity in these fibres. It is part of the 'fight or flight' response, and flight from the dentist's waiting room happens occasionally; the missing patient later excuses himself by rationalising his behaviour, explaining that the toothache had ceased.

The widespread effects of sympathetic activity are partly explained by the fact that its peripheral (postganglionic) fibres originate in the sympathetic ganglion; i.e. much more centrally than the corresponding fibres of the parasympathetic division.

**Autonomic ganglia**

The autonomic ganglia of the head are the ciliary, sphenopalatine, otic and submandibular ganglia. The sympathetic fibres pass through them without synapsing. Sensory fibres also pass straight through these ganglia without synapsing, carrying impulses in the opposite direction towards the brain. Parasympathetic fibres, however, do form synapses in these ganglia which therefore contain the cell bodies of the postganglionic parasympathetic nerves. The proximity of the parasympathetic synapses to the innervated glands explains the localised effects of the parasympathetic fibres.

**Parasympathetic nerves**

The cranial portion of the parasympathetic system is formed by the oculomotor, facial, glossopharyngeal and vagus nerves.

The oculomotor nerve sends fibres to the ciliary ganglion where they form synapses with postganglionic fibres which pass via the short ciliary nerves to the ciliary muscle and the constrictor muscle of the pupil.

Cells in the superior salivatory nucleus in the brain stem give rise to fibres which pass via the sensory root of the facial nerve to the greater petrosal nerve. This joins the deep petrosal nerve which is carrying sympathetic fibres from the internal carotid plexus and the two form the nerve of the pterygoid canal. This passes into the sphenopalatine ganglion. Here, the parasympathetic fibres form synapses and the postsynaptic (postganglionic ) fibres go to the lacrimal gland (Fig. 1.13).

Other cells in the superior salivatory nucleus send fibres via the sensory root of the facial nerve and the chorda tympani to the lingual nerve. From here they pass to the submandibular ganglion where they form synapses. The postsynaptic (postganglionic) fibres are distributed to the submandibular and sublingual glands (Fig. 1.13).

Cells in the inferior salivatory nucleus give rise to fibres which pass via the glossopharyngeal nerve, the tympanic plexus and the lesser petrosal nerve to the otic ganglion. Here they form synapses with neurones which go to the parotid gland via the auriculotemporal nerve.

Sometimes, when a tooth is being drilled, a jet of saliva is seen to spurt from the orifice of the submandibular duct. This depends on neural impulses passing into the central nervous system via the trigeminal system and eventually being relayed to the submandibular glands by the rather tortuous rout briefly described above. However, the neurophysiological mechanisms of this pain-salivary reflex have not yet been fully elucidated (Kawamura and Yamamoto, 1977). (See also Chapter 15.)

Similarly, when a local anaesthetic solution is being injected in the neighbourhood of the upper anterior teeth, neural impulses pass to the brain via the trigeminal system and give rise to parasympathetic neural impulses which activate the lacrimal glands thus bringing tears to the eyes. This does not mean that the patient is being hurt but he may feel embarrassed by the tears so a few words of understanding should be murmured by the operator to keep the patient at ease.

## REFERENCES


Anderson, K. V. and Pearl, G. S. (1974) Transmedian innervation of canine tooth pulp in cats . *Exptl. Neurol.*, **44**, 35–40.

Anderson, K. V. and Pearl, G.S. (1975) C-fiber activity in feline tooth pulp afferents. *Exptl. Neurol.*, **47**, 357–359.

Anderson, K. V., Rosing, H. S. and Pearl, G. S. (1977) Physiological and anatomical studies revealing an extensive transmedian innervation of feline canine teeth. In *Pain in the Trigeminal Region*, ed. Anderson, D.J. and Matthews, B., pp. 149–160. Amsterdam: Elsevier/North Holland.

Arwill, T. (1958) Innervation of the teeth. *Stockholm, Trans. Roy, Schools Dent.*, Stockholm and Umeå.

Arwill T. (1960) The significance of the innervation of the predentine. *Oral Surg.*, **13**, 743–749.

Arwill, T. (1967) Studies on the ultra structure of dental tissues. II: The predentine-pulpal border zone. *Odont. Revy*, **18**, 191–208.

Arwill, T., Edwall, L,. Lilja, J., Olgart, L. and Svensson, S. E. (1973) Ultrastructure of nerves in the dentinal-pulp border zone after sensory and autonomic nerve transection in the cat, *Acta odont. Scand.*, **31**, 273.

Avery , J. K. (1979) Mechanism of reparative dentin formation and pain. In *Mechanism and Control of Pain*, ed. Grossman , L. I., pp. 43–65. New York: Masson.

Avery J. K. and Cox, C. F. (1977) Role of nerves in teeth relative to pain and dentinogenesis. In *Pain in the Trigeminal Region*, ed. Anderson, D. J. and Matthews, B., pp. 37–48. Amsterdam: Elsevier/North Holland.

Avery, J. K. and Rapp, R. (1958) Demonstration of cholinesterase in teeth. *Stain Technol.*, **33**, 31–37.

Avery, J. K. and Rapp, R. (1959) An investigation of the mechanism of neural impulse transmission in human teeth. *Oral Surg.*, **12**, 190–198.

Beasley, W. L. and Holland , G. R. (1978) A quantitative analysis of the innervation of the pulp of the cats canine tooth. *J. comp. Neurol.*, **178**, 487–494.

Beer, G. R. de (1947) The differentiation of neural crest cells into visceral cartilages and odontoblasts in amblyostoma, and a re-examination of the germ layer theory. *Proc. B. Roy. Soc.*, **134**, 377–398.

Bernick, S. (1964) Differences in nerve distribution between erupted and non-erupted human teeth. *J. dent. Res.*, **43**, 406–411.

Bernick, S. (1967) Effect of ageing on the nerve supply to human teeth. *J. dent. Res.*, **46**, 694–699.

Bradlaw, R. (1936) The innervation of teeth *Proc. R. Soc. Med.*, **29**, 507–518.

Bradlaw, R. (1939) The histology and histopathology of the dental innervation. *Proc. R. Soc. Med.*, **32**, 1040–1053.

Brännström, M. and Garberoglio, R. (1972) The dentinal tubules and the odontoblast process. A scanning election microscope study. *Acta odont. Scand.*, **30**, 291–311.

Brodal, A. (1969) *Neurological Anatomy in Relation to Clinical Medicine*, 2nd edition. London: *Oxford Univ. Press.*

Brookhart, J., Livingston, W. K. and Haugen, F. P. (1953) Functional characteristics of afferent fibres from tooth pulp of cat. *J. Neurophysiol.*, **16**, 634–642.

Bunge, P. B. (1970) Structure and function of neuroglia: some recent observations. In *The Neurosciences Second Study Program*, pp. 782–797. New York: Rockfeller Univ. Press.

Byers, M. R. (1979) Large and small trigeminal nerve endings and their associations with odontoblasts in rat molar dentin and pulp. In *Advances in Pain Research and Therapy*, Vol. 3, ed. Bonica, J. J., Liebeskind, J. C. and Albe-Fessard, D. G., pp. 265–270, New York: Raven Press.

Carter, R. B. and Keen, E. N. (1971) The intramandibular course of the inferior dental nerve .*J. Anat.*, **108**, 433–440.

Edwall, L. (1971) *Some Effects of Sympathetic Nerve Activation in Oral Tissues as studied by Tracer Disappearance.* Stockhölm: Kihlström and Söner.

Edwall, L. (1972) Nervous control of blood circulation in the dental pulp and the periodontal tissues. In *Oral Physiology*, ed. Emmelin, N. and Zotterman, Y., pp. 139–149. Oxford: Pergamon.

Engström, H. and Öhman, A. (1960) Studies on the innervation of human teeth. *J. dent. Res.*, **39**, 799–809.

Fearnhead, R. W. (1958) Neurohistology of dentine. *Int. dent. J., Lond.*, **8**, 4–5.

Fearnhead, R. W. (1961) The neurohistology of human dentine. *Proc. R. Soc. Med.*, **54**, 877–884.

Foster, C. L. (1966) *Hewer's Textbook of Histology for Medical Students*, 8th edition. London: Heinemann.

Frank, R. M. (1966) Étude au microscope électronique de l'odontoblaste et du canalicule dentaire humain. *Archs. oral Biol.*, **11**, 179–199.

Frank , R. M. (1968a) Ultrastructural relationship between the odontoblast, its process and the nerve fibre. In *Dentine and Pulp*, ed. Symons, N. B. B., pp. 115–145. London : Livingstone.

Frank, R. M. (1968b) Attachment sites between the odontoblast process and the intradentinal nerve fibre. *Archs. oral Biol.*, **13**, 833–834.

Frank, R. M. Sauvage, C. and Frank, P. (1972) Morphological basis of dental sensitivity. *Int. dent. J. (Lond.)*, **22**, 1–19.

Funakoshi, M. and Zotterman, Y. (1963) A study in the excitation of dental pulp nerve fibres. In *Sensory Mechanisms in Dentine*, ed. Anderson, D. J., pp. 60–72. Oxford: Pergamon.

Graf, W. and Björlin, G. (1950) *Odont. Tidskr.*, **58**, 21. Quoted by Arwill (1958), cited above.

Graf, W. and Björlin, G. (1951) Diameters of nerve fibres in human tooth pulps. *J. Amer. dent. Ass.*, **43**, 186–193.

Griffin, C. J. and Harris, R. (1968) Unmyelinated nerve endings in the periodontal membrane of human teeth. *Archs oral Biol.*, **13**, 1207–1212.

Hannam, A. G. (1968) The conduction velocity of nerve impulses from dental mechanoreceptors in the dog. *Archs. oral Biol.*, **13**, 1377–1383.

Harris, R. and Griffin, C. J. (1968) fine structure of nerve endings in the human dental pulp. *Archs. oral Biol.*, **13**, 773–778.

Holland, C. R. and Nahnybida, L. J. (1979) The ultrastructure of Raschkow's subodontoblastic neural plexus. *J. dent. Res.*, Special issue A, Abstr. 58, p. 215.

Iggo, A. (1977) Cutaneous and subcutaneous sense organs. *Brit. Med. Bull.*, **33**, 97–102.

Johnsen, D. C. and Harshbarger, J. (1980) Quantitation of nerve fibers associated with permanent tooth development. *J. dent. Res.*, Special issue B, Abstr. 414a, p. 990.

Johnsen, D. and Johns, S. (1978) Quantitation of nerve fibres in the primary and permanent canine and incisor teeth in man. *Archs. oral Biol.*, **23**, 825–829.

Johnsen, D. C. and Karlsson, U. L. (1974) Electron microscopic quantitations of feline primary and permanent incisor innervation. *Archs. oral Biol.*, **19**, 671–678.

Johnson, G., Olgart, L. and Brännström, M. (1973) Outward fluid flow under a physiological pressure gradient: Experiments in vitro. *Oral Surg.*, **35**, 238–248.

Kawamura, Y. (1968) Mandibular movement: normal anatomy and physiology and clinical dysfunction. In *Facial Pain and Mandibular Dysfunction*, ed. Schwartz, L. and Chayes, C. M., pp. 37–82. Philadelphia: Saunders.

Kawamura, Y. and Yamamoto, T. (1977) Salivary secretion to noxious stimulation of the trigeminal area. In *Pain in the Trigeminal Region*, ed. Anderson, D. J. and Matthews, B., pp. 395–404. Amsterdam: Elsevier/ North Holland.

Kramer, I. R. H. (1954) The relationship between pain and changes in the dental pulp following the insertion of fillings. *Brit. dent. J.*, **96**, 9–13.

Langeland, K. and Yagi, T. (1972) Investigations on the innervation of teeth. *Int. dent. J. (Lond).*, **22**, 240–269.

Last, R. J. (1966) *Anatomy Regional and Applied*, 4th edition. London: Churchill.

Lewis, T. (1942) Pain. New York: Macmillan.

Lisney, S. J. W. and Matthews, B. (1976) Nerves with branched axons supplying more than one tooth or one tooth and the adjacent mucous membrane. *Proc. Physiol. Soc. July 36P.*

Loewenstein, W. R. and Rathkamp, R. (1955) A study on the pressoreceptive sensibility of the teeth. *J.dent. Res.*, **34**, 287–294.

Matthews, B. (1976) Effects of sympathetic stimulation on the response of intradental nerves to chemical stimulation of dentine. In *Advances in Pain Research and Therapy*, Vol. 1, ed. Bonica, J. J. and Albe-Fessard, D. G., pp. 195–203, New York: Raven Press.

Matthews, B. (1977) Response of intradental nerves to electrical and thermal stimulation of teeth in dogs. *J Physiol. (Lond.)*, **264**, 641–664.

Matthews, B. (1978b) Coupling between nerve terminals in teeth. In *Pain in the Trigeminal Region*, ed. Anderson, D. J. and Matthews, B., pp. 83–93. Amsterdam: Elsevier/North Holland.

Matthews, B. and Holland, G. R. (1975) Coupling between nerves in teeth. *Brain Res.*, **98**, 354–358.

Matthews, B. and Lisney, S. J. W. (1978) Do primary afferents from tooth- pulp cross the midline? *Brain Res.*, **158**, 303–312.

Matthews, J. L., Dorman, H. L. and Bishop, J. G. (1959) Fine structures of dental pulp. *J. dent. Res.*, **38**, 940–946.

Miyoshi, S., Nishijima, S. and Imanishi, I. (1966) Electron microscopy of myelinated and unmyelinated nerve fibres in human dental pulp. *Archs. oral Biol.*, **11**, 845–846.

Olivier, E. (1927) *Annales d'Anatomie pathologique et d'Anatomie normale*, quoted by Starkie and Stewart (see below).
Pelletier, V. A., Poulos, D. A. and Lende, R. A. (1974) Functional localisation in the trigeminal root. *J. Neurosurg.*, **40**, 504–513.
Pfaffman, C. (1939) Afferent impulses from the teeth due to pressure and noxious stimulation. *J. Physiol. (Lond.)*, **97**, 207–219.
Pohto, P. (1972) Sympathetic adrenergic innervation of permanent teeth in the monkey (*Macaca irus*). *Acta odont. Scand.*, **30**, 117–126.
Pohto, P. and Antila, R. (1968a) Demonstration of adrenergic nerve fibres in human dental pulp by histochemical fluorescence method. *Acta odont. Scand.*, **26**, 137–144.
Pohto, P. and Antila, R. (1968b) Acetylcholinesterase and noradrenaline in the nerves of mammalian dental pulps. *Acta odont. Scand.*, **26**, 641–656.
Pohto, P. and Antila, R. (1972) Innervation of blood vessels in the dental pulp. *Int. dent. J. (Lond.)*, **22**, 228–239.
Pringle, J. W. S. (1962) The input element. In *Biological Receptor Mechanisms*, ed. Beament, J. W. L., pp. 1–11. Cambridge: Cambridge Univ. Press.
Roane, J. B., Foreman, D. W., Melfi, R. C. and Marshall, F. J. (1973) An ultrastructural study of dentinal innervation in the adult human tooth. *Oral Surg.*, **35**, 94–104.
Romanes, G. J. (ed) (1964) *Cunningham's Textbook of Anatomy*, 10th edition. New York: Oxford Univ. Press.
Rood, J. P. (1976) The analgesia and innervation of mandibular teeth. *Brit. dent. J.*, **140**, 237–240.
Scott, D. B. (1966) In *Touch, Heat and Pain*, ed. De Reuck, A V. S. and Knight, J., pp. 261–274. London: Churchill.
Scott, D. and Tempel, T. R. (1963) Receptor potentials in response to thermal and other excitation. In *Sensory Mechanisms in Dentine*, ed. Anderson, D. J., pp. 27–46. Oxford: Pergamon.
Starkie, C. and Stewart, D. (1931) The intra-mandibular course of the inferior dental nerve. *J. Anat.*, **65**, 319–323.
Thomas, H. F. (1979) The extent of the odontoblast process in human dentin. *J. dent. Res.*, Special issue D, 2207–2218.
Uchizono, K. and Homma, K. (1959) Electron microscopic studies on nerves of human tooth pulp. *J. dent. Res.*, **38**, 1133–1141.
Wagers, P. W. and Smith, C. M. (1960) Responses in dental nerves of dogs to tooth stimulation and the effects of systemically administered procaine, lidocaine and morphine. *J. Pharmacol. Expt. Therap.*, **103**, 89–105.
Warwick, R. and Williams, P. L. (ed) (1973) *Gray's Anatomy*. Edinburgh: Longman.
Yamada, M. and Sakada, S. (1961) The effects of some chemicals on cervix dentis. *J. dent. Res.*, **40**, 975–987.
Young, R. F. (1977) Fiber spectrum of the trigeminal sensory root of frog, cat and man determined by electron microscopy. In *Pain in the Trigeminal Region*, ed. Anderson, D. J. and Matthews, B., pp. 137–147. Amsterdam: Elsevier/ North Holland.

# 2

# Nerve impulses and their transmission

## Generator potential

When a stimulus is applied to one of the terminal branches of a nerve fibre it sets up an electrical potential change called the generator potential, the magnitude and duration of which depend upon the magnitude and duration of the applied stimulus. The generator potential may be sufficient to cause one or more impulses to start in the nerve fibre or it may be too weak to do so, being of subthreshold intensity. However, two or more subthreshold generator currents can meet where the terminals join and summate both spatially and temporally; if the sum potential change is sufficient an impulse starts in the nerve fibre and passes along it (Sato and Ozeki, 1966).

The nerve impulse is also an electrical potential change, the action potential, but whereas the generator potential is graded an action potential occurs totally or not at all (the all-or-none principle).

## NERVE IMPULSE (ACTION POTENTIAL)

When the nerve fibre (the axon) is at rest its outer surface is positively charged relative to its inner surface, its fluid interior having a relatively low concentration of sodium ions, one-tenth of that outside, whereas there is a high concentration of potassium ions, thirty times that outside (Eccles, 1973). The resulting resting potential is 50–70 mV (Hodgkin, 1967). When the axon is suitably triggered such as by an adequate generator potential its membrane permeability changes and sodium ions pass into it (Fig. 2.1). The interior of the axon at that point becomes positively charged relative to the outside, the total potential swing from the resting to the active state being approximately a tenth of a volt (100 mV). This is the action potential or nerve impulse (Fig. 2.2) and its duration is from 1–50 milliseconds, the duration being least in faster conducting fibres (Walter, 1963). At the crest of the

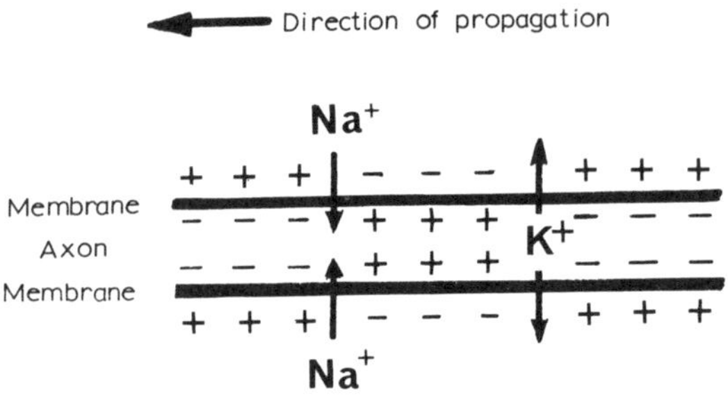


**Fig. 2.1** Diagram of an unmyelinated nerve fibre showing inflow of sodium ions and outflow of potassium ions.

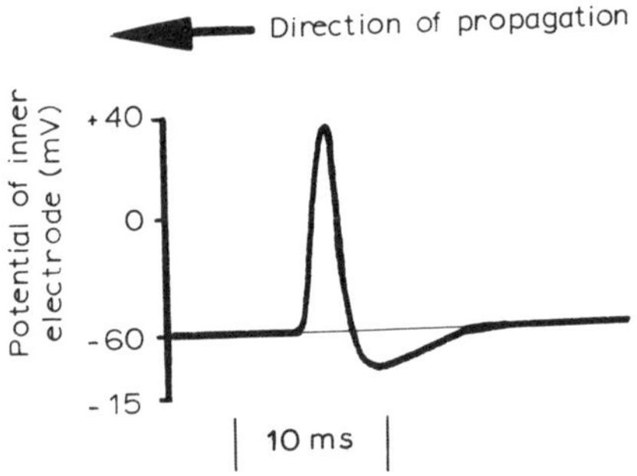


**Fig. 2.2** Action potential.

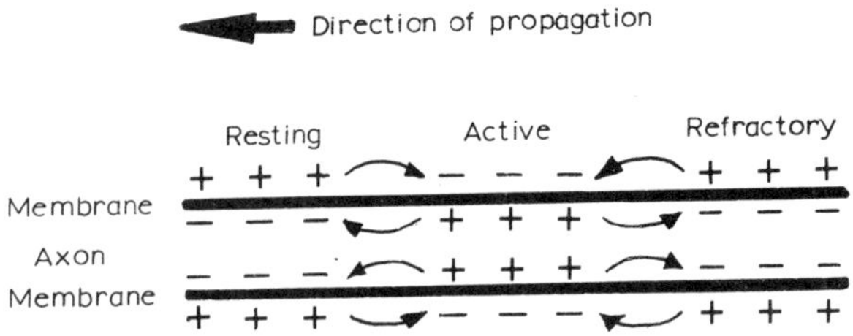


**Fig. 2.3** Diagram of an unmyelinated nerve fibre showing local circuits which cause the wave to be propagated.

action potential the inside of the fibre is 40–50 mV positive to the external solution (Hodgkin, 1967).

The disturbance thus created leads to a change in permeability of adjacent areas of nerve membrane so that the process is repeated, sodium ions enter and the action potential develops here also. This is repeated at adjacent areas all along the membrane (Fig. 2.3). In other words the action potential is propagated along the nerve as a wave of negativity (on the outside) and this can be recorded by an oscilloscope with suitable pick-up electrodes.

When the impulse has passed, the permeability to sodium ions drops and that to potassium ions increases. There is a relatively high concentration of potassium ions within the axon so this increased permeability leads to a rapid outflow of them. Since they are positively charged their outflow restores the interior of the axon to its previous negative state. During this phase a further impulse cannot be set up but this refractory period lasts for only a few milliseconds before the membrane state is restored and a further impulse can be generated.

Each impulse is associated with only minute ionic movements so a nerve fibre can conduct thousands of impulses before it has to restore its sodium and potassium balance. It does this by a process described as the sodium pump, the mechanism of which is not fully understood, but efflux of sodium ions is controlled by metabolic activity which derives its energy from the breakdown of adenosine triphosphate (Katz, 1966).

## Impulse velocity and myelination

The speed of conduction of the nerve impulse is greater in fibres of greater diameter, but increasing the diameter is an inefficient way to increase the velocity because the velocity of conduction increases only with the square root of the diameter (Young, 1966). Fortunately myelination avoids this problem.

Although the axon is nourished and maintained by its cell body and nucleus (for the trigeminal nerve, these are within the trigeminal ganglion), associated with it are Schwann cells which subsidise the axon metabolically although they cannot support it unaided (Katz, 1966). Schwann cells gradually wrap themselves around an axon to form the myelin sheath (Chapter 1) which is an electrical insulator, the cytoplasm of the Schwann cell being gradually squeezed out as myelination progresses. In the central nervous system oligodendroglia provide the myelination (Eccles, 1973).

Each Schwann cell covers the axon over a length of 1–2 mm but the cells do not quite meet each other, thus leaving a gap in the myelin sheath called a node of Ranvier. At a node of Ranvier the axon is bare for a length of about 1 $\mu$m and its electrical resistance is low, so the electrical impulse is able to 'jump' between the nodes (saltatory or jumping conduction) with the result that higher conduction velocities are attained (Fig. 2.4). This is because ionic flow in the tissue fluid and in the axoplasm is much faster than the electrotonic spread along the axon membrane. Moreover, for a given current the small area available will mean a high current density which will therefore be more effective.

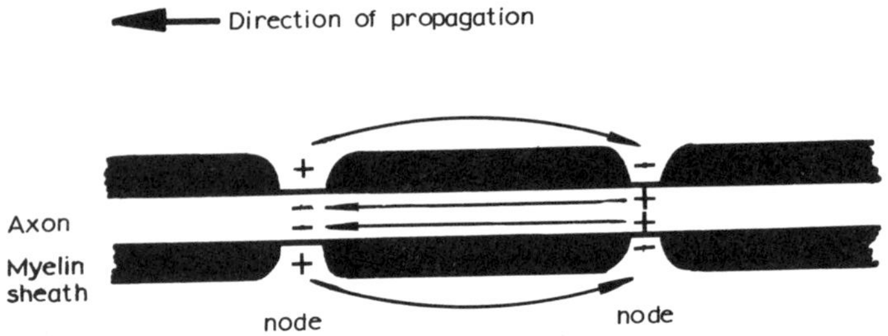


**Fig. 2.4** Diagram of myelinated nerve fibre showing saltatory conduction. Only the nodes of Ranvier are involved in the activity; not the entire length of the nerve membrane.

By myelination and increase in diameter the velocity of the nerve impulse increases from less than 1 metre per second in small unmyelinated nerve fibres to 120 metres per second in large myelinated nerve fibres. This is approximately a direct relationship between velocity and diameter (Bodian, 1967). For a myelinated fibre, its conduction velocity in metres per second is approximately six times its diameter in micrometres.

## Number of impulses and stimulus intensity

The number of impulses passing along a nerve fibre depends upon the intensity of the stimulus applied. If a stimulus of fixed intensity is applied the number of nerve impulses produced is remarkably constant (Fig. 2.5, right). If the stimulus intensity is increased the number of impulses increases (Fig. 2.5, left). Moreover, the number of impulses depends directly on the stimulus intensity (Fig. 2.6).

## Transmission at branches

The nerve impulse has a good safety factor for ensuring its on-

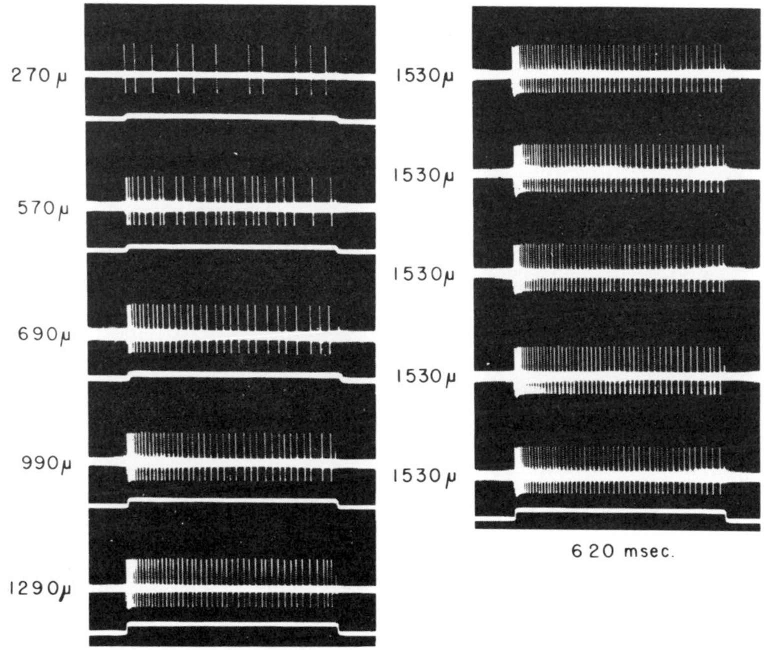


**Fig. 2.5.** Oscillograph records of trains of nerve impulses evoked in a single fibre of the median nerve of a monkey. Records to the left were obtained when the skin was indented to the depths indicated. Those to the right were obtained by repeating a stimulus of one intensity, and show metronome-like repetition of the response. The lower trace of each pair indicates the intensity and duration of the stimulus. (Mountcastle, 1967).

ward transmission and can continue into the branches. It does so at its full value since the process is still all-or-nothing.

**Compound action potential**

A nerve trunk, such as the inferior dental nerve, consists of nerve fibres of different diameters, and impulses are conducted along it in the different fibres at different velocities. If recording electrodes are placed on the nerve trunk at some distance from the point of excitation the fastest impulses arrive and are recorded first, followed by the next fastest impulses until eventually the slowest conducted impulses arrive. The recording of all the impulses is called the compound action potential. The further the impulses have to travel the more separated do they become. It follows that for a single suprathreshold stimulus the action potentials along the different sized nerve fibres will reach the first synapses in a scattered way (in the medulla oblongata for the trigeminal nerve).

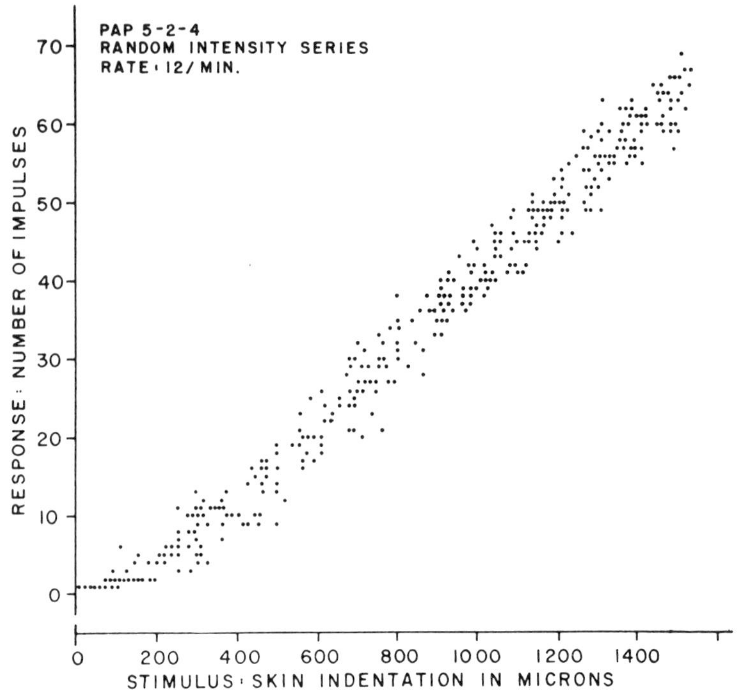


**Fig. 2.6**. Increase in the number of neural impulses as a result of greater stimulus intensity. ( Mountcastle, 1967.)

## SYNAPTIC TRANSMISSION

When the impulse reaches the end of the first nerve fibre it cannot pass directly into the next one for the two are discontinuous, being separated by a narrow zone called the synapse (from Greek, meaning a connection or junction). Although the impulse cannot cross the synapse as an electrical impulse it is transmitted by chemical means. This may seem cumbersome but, as Katz (1967) has pointed out, if the electrical impulse could cross the gap it could also cross sideways to adjacent nerve fibres and this 'crosstalk' between adjacent channels would make the system useless.

On reaching the end of the first neurone the electrical impulse causes the release of a chemical from synaptic vesicles within the axon terminal, and this chemical transmitter diffuses across the synaptic gap to reach the next neurone. The transmitter is acetylcholine at neuromuscular junctions. Noradrenaline and 5-hydroxytryptamine are other substances, and there are now about 30 transmitters known or suspected, with more likely to be recog-

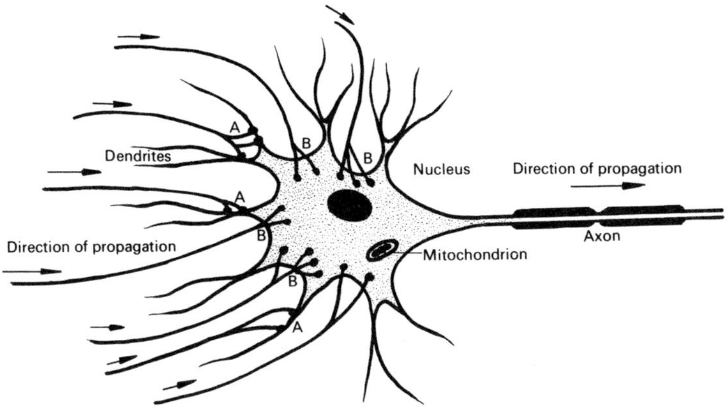


**Fig. 2.7.** Nerve terminals converging on a secondary neurone: A, axo-dendritic synapses; B, axo-somatic synapses.

nised in time (Iversen, 1979). However, an individual neurone acts by the same transmitter at all its synapses (Eccles, 1967). The transmitter crosses the gap between the presynaptic and post-synaptic membranes and causes depolarisation of the latter. If this depolarisation is sufficient it causes a nerve impulse to start in the post-synaptic neurone (Fig. 2.7).

The transmitter depolarising effect lasts a finite time so the effect can build up as further impulses release additional transmitter (temporal summation). Impulses arriving by other neurones can add their share of transmitter so the quantity can also build up in this way, giving spatial summation. In other words, the synapse may be regarded as storing the incoming nerve impulses for a brief period. There is thus an integration of different events at the synapse and thereby an analysis of the incoming information (de Valois, 1966). It is not yet known if the net result of simultaneous synaptic activity is computed by the nerve cell body (perikaryon) or by the major dendrites (Szentàgothai, 1970). Nor is it clear how the integration is affected by the synapse being on, near or away from the cell body (Hubel, 1979).

**Release of transmitter**

The neural impulse reaches the terminal, the sodium and potassium ions being involved as already described. At the terminal, there is a rapid, though transient increase of calcium ions which enables vesicles to fuse with the presynaptic membrane with release of transmitter. The fused vesicle is reclaimed and refilled with transmitter (Stevens, 1979).

Even at rest it appears that small quantities of transmitter are released into the synapse at random intervals, but always in a standard minimum quantity, this being the amount contained in one vesicle (quantal release). The effect of the nerve impulse is to alter the permeability of the axon terminal thus allowing more transmitter to be released. The size of the vesicle is not increased; what is altered is the frequency of the quantal event which increases several hundred thousand times (Katz, 1966).

The function of the transmitter has been emphasised but the process is more complex for other substances having both larger and smaller molecules are released along with the transmitter. The role of these is not yet known but they could, perhaps, produce a more prolonged physiological effect than do the transmitters (Bloom, Iversen and Schmitt, 1970). Such an effect could possibly be involved in fear which is a more prolonged state than the ordinary synaptic events described above (Bloom, Hoffer and Nicoll, 1972). Parkinsonism, depression and Huntington's chorea have also been implicated as transmitter effects.

### Terminal bouton

The terminal bouton (synaptic knob or end bulb) is the swelling at the end of a terminal branch of an axon and it rests on the next neurone to make the synapse (Fig. 2.8). Thousands of these terminal boutons are found on the nerve cell body, on dendrites and

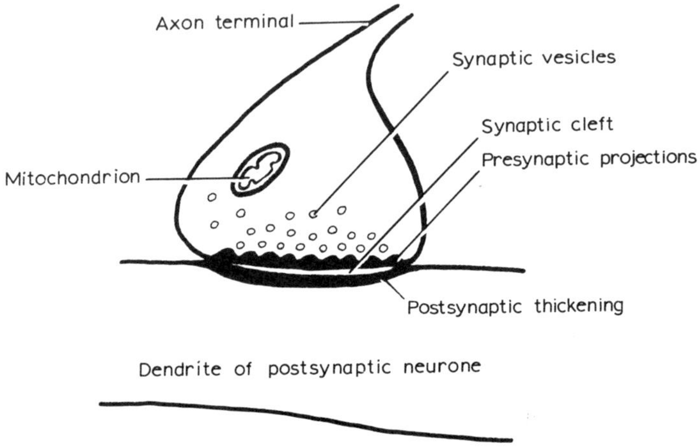


**Fig. 2.8**. Terminal bouton and synapse such as the one represented in **Fig. 2.7** at A. The presynaptic projections might act as guides ushering the nearest vesicle into a release position. (Akert, Gray and Bloom, 1970.)

on axon terminals, thus making axo-somatic, axo-dendritic and axo-axonic synapses. There are so many synapses that they may occupy a considerable area of the cell body, as much as 90 per cent (Bowsher, 1971), leaving the remaining surface for metabolic activity. In its turn, the other neurone gives rise to numerous synapses, from a thousand to ten thousand, according to Stevens (1979). The boutons vary in size from 0·5–30 $\mu$m in diameter. The synaptic vesicles are from 30–60 $\mu$m in diameter (Brodal, 1969; Akert, Gray and Bloom, 1970), and may hold several thousand molecules of transmitter (Stevens, 1979). The synaptic cleft is 200 nanometres across (Stevens, 1979).

**Inhibitory synapses**

The synapses described above are excitatory, but inhibitory synapses occur, and are of two kinds. At postsynaptic inhibitory synapses the transmitter is either glycine or gamma amino butyric acid (GABA) (Eccles, 1973). It diffuses across the synaptic cleft to reach the postsynaptic membrane making it less excitable (i.e. hyperpolarised). It is the commonest inhibitory transmitter in the central nervous system (Iversen, 1979).

The second type of inhibitory synapse is presynaptic, occurs in the central nervous system, and is an important factor in whether or not pain is experienced. Some nerve terminals end on other nerve terminals just as they are about to synapse (axo-axonic synapse). (Fig. 2.9). The effect of impulses in the former is to stabilise the latter so that impulses in them have less effect than usual, with the result that less than the normal amount of transmitter is produced. A recent view of this arrangement is that the presynaptic inhibitory fibre (an interneurone) releases its transmitter, enkephalin, which crosses the synaptic cleft to the primary sensory neurone, inhibiting the release of its transmitter, substance P (Iversen, 1979). However, this effect may turn out to be postsynaptic (Fig. 4.5).

Presynaptic inhibition can occur from fibres carrying their impulses in the same direction from the periphery to the brain — forward inhibition. Impulses descending from the brain also exercise presynaptic control on fibres with ascending impulses — feedback inhibition (Békésy, 1967). It is this control which may allow pain not to be felt in a damaged area when the person is concentrating on something else, such as a football match.

Whereas axons can transmit impulses in both directions, synapses transmit only one way, in which respect they resemble electrical rectifiers.

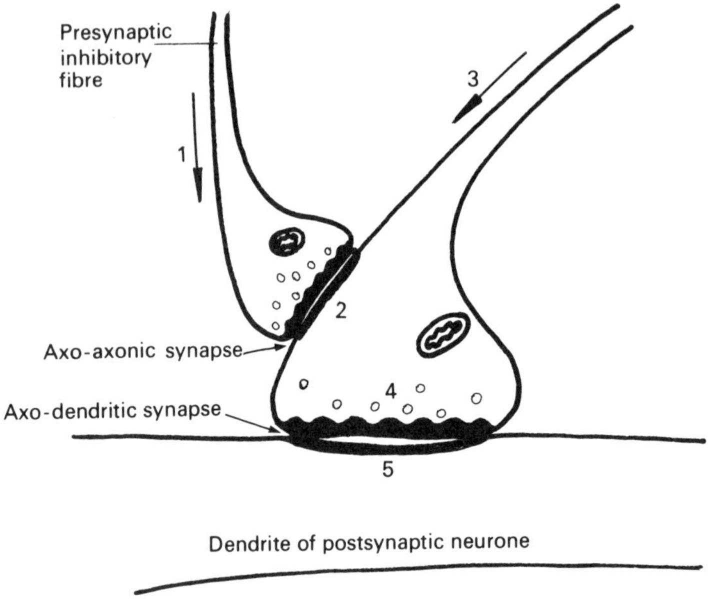


**Fig. 2.9.** Presynaptic inhibition. Impulses passing along the presynaptic inhibitory fibre (1) depolarise the excitatory terminal (2). Because of this the action potential in the latter (3) is diminished in size and less transmitter is produced (4). There is therefore less chance of exciting the postsynaptic neurone (5).

*Facilitation*

Transmission at a synapse may be made easier by the fact that earlier transmission across the synapse has been successfully accomplished within a recent brief period. This may be because the synaptic vesicles have moved in the nerve terminal to a position from which they can more readily be released or that the gating mechanism in the postsynaptic membrane is associated with a conformational change in its protein that is not yet restored. Other possible explanations are that the synaptic area might have enlarged or the number of synapses might have increased. It seems possible that facilitation could be a factor in prolonging pain, including some kinds of toothache.

**Adaptation**

When a constant stimulus is applied the number of nerve impulses produced gradually diminishes until they cease altogether. This is a property of the receptor rather than of the nerve itself, and it has the possible function of protecting the nervous system from being overloaded with incoming impulses which may in any case be redundant in the informational sense. Adaptation is of some importance when human teeth are stimulated (Chapter 5).

**Rapid axonal transport**

Rapid axonal transport is the process in which certain materials move from the nerve cell body along the axon to its terminals (and also in the reverse direction), and the transport rate may be 400 mm a day. Though not fully understood this will presumably have an influence on transmission and it is interesting that Byers et al (1975) have found that axonal transport in the infraorbital nerve (of the rat) can be arrested by immersion in 1–4 per cent lignocaine hydrochloride.

## FURTHER TRANSMISSION

It is theoretically possible for a single nerve impulse to be transmitted from the site of origin along successive nerves via the intermediate synapses right through to the cortex, there to produce excitation of cortical cells. Mountcastle and Powell (1969) considered this likely and pointed out that the threshold for cortical response could therefore be set by the threshold of the sensory receptors in the periphery. This cortical activity is often assumed to lead to perception of the peripheral event, though whether this is so is not known; it would at least require the person to be attentive to the possibility of it occurring. However, it is most unlikely that a single impulse could have bearing on pain perception. If it could then pain would occur from any odd spontaneous discharge, a condition that would be intolerable. Perception of pain probably necessitates a volley of impulses, probably in a number of adjacent fibres.

**Transmission time for impulses mediating pain**

The difficulty in finding this time is that further time is needed for the subject to record that he has perceived the painful sensation, the total of the two times being called the reaction time. After applying painful stimuli to human teeth, Naylor (1963) found the reaction time to be 175 milliseconds. Also investigating human teeth, Newton and Mumford (unpublished) obtained a similar result. For a single visual stimulus the reaction time is 180 milliseconds, provided the subject is prepared for it, but as long as 300 milliseconds if the subject is not warned (Craik, 1959).

The reaction time also depends upon the intensity of stimulation, being shorter with stronger stimuli (Lele, Sinclair and Weddell, 1954).

These two influencing factors of attention and intensity of stimulation explain why a patient reacts faster in some cases, such as when hot gutta percha is applied to a tooth to test its vitality. There may also be increased physical activity so that the patient 'jumps' in the chair.

It might be supposed that half of the reaction time would be the time needed for perception but much of the time is taken up by cerebral processes including synaptic delays. According to Craik conduction of the nerve impulse to the brain accounts for only 10 milliseconds, conduction away from the brain along the motor nerves another 10 milliseconds, which leaves most of the delay accounted for by cerebral processes, including synaptic delays which Craik states to be 0·7 milliseconds each. In an adult human being the distance from the pulpo-dentinal junction of a lower canine tooth to the cerebral cortex is approximately 33 cm (a very crude estimate). This may seem a greater distance than expected but the nerve fibres have to travel the length of the trigeminal nerve and then downwards in the medulla before passing upwards via the thalamus to the cortex. Taking a conduction velocity of 15 metres per second (Funakoshi and Zotterman, 1963) this would need a transmission time of 25 milliseconds. Allowing this time both inwards and outwards leaves about 125 milliseconds involved in cerebral processing and synaptic delays. The figure of 25 milliseconds compares well with the range of transmission times given by Darian-Smith (1966) for tactile sensation in the cat, namely 3·5–18 milliseconds. Also for monkeys, from the tooth pulp, which were 13·6–24·9 milliseconds (Biedenbach et al, 1979).

Following peripheral stimulation it is possible to record electrical changes at the cerebral cortex, the evoked cortical response, and this might be regarded as providing a more reliable indication of the time needed for perception to occur, but this physical effect is not necessarily the same as the subject perceiving the stimulus (Chapter 3). The neural mechanisms of perception are unknown and presumably very complicated.

**Nerve impulse as a signal**

The impulse is conveyed along the nerve fibre without decrement; in other words its amplitude remains the same, as does its shape. What does change is the number of impulses passing in a given time, so this is a frequency modulated signalling system. Since the fibre follows the all-or-none principle the impulse occurs as a discrete entity, and for this reason the signalling has been regarded as digital, but it is now regarded as a time sampled analogue system (Milsum, 1966; Bullock, 1967; Elias, 1967). In other words, the cells higher up receive a flux which is averaged over a period of time and over a certain area of space (Gray, 1966a). The system is, of course, limited at its higher frequencies by the refractory period. The latter is about 0·5 milliseconds, so the maximum theoretical frequency is approximately 1000 per second, although the normal working range is much less than this, being about 5–100 impulses per second (Hodgkin, 1967).

It was assumed for a long time that messages could not differ in the number and frequency of the impulses but patterns in impulse trains may have additional significance, as may various other factors (Bullock, 1967, 1970). Moreover, this is only for one nerve fibre. A nerve trunk contains thousands of fibres, and the transmission of information depends on the distribution of activity throughout the population (Gray, 1966b). This offers further opportunity for coding, including the frequency profile of impulses within the population (Mountcastle, 1967).

The signal is also influenced by convergence which allows temporal and spatial summation. There are also opportunities for modulating the signal as described in Chapter 4.

A human tooth contains 250 fibres or more (Chapter 1) and this, with the pulse durations and refractory periods, sets an upper limit on the channel capacity, but the possibilities for coding information are still considerable.

From the foregoing discussion it will be seen that one way of looking at the problem of toothache is to realise that information about the state of the tooth is sent towards the brain in a frequency modulated, time sampled analogue multichannel information system. It is supposed that the first impulses reaching the brain give information regarding the site and modality of the sensation, and further impulses give information about its intensity, the number of impulses being a function of stimulus intensity. The additional impulses could also continue to give information regarding the site of sensation to make sure that this important information arrives and is recognised.

Since there are so many nerve fibres in the dental pulp, with different thresholds and conduction rates, the amount of information that might be derived from one pulp is enormous (in a cybernetic sense). This means that a patient should be able to describe a pain and its site in great detail. Yet the information available is poor; above threshold levels there is a sensation which is essentially unpleasant, at graded intensity, coming from a site which is only approximately localised, perhaps not even to the correct tooth. In an informational sense this means that most of the nerve fibres in the pulp are being wasted, that they are redundant. Presumably, this is because of a considerable amount of correlated activity due to the overlapping receptor fields of the nerves within the tooth. Another factor will be the branching of nerve fibres to go to more than one tooth, and to a tooth and the adjacent gingiva, as described in Chapter 1.

In these circumstances it seems possible that the central decoding mechanism is only using part of the incoming information and suppressing the rest, as suggested by Darian-Smith and Johnson (1977).

## REFERENCES

Akert, K., Gray, E. G. and Bloom, F. E. (1970) Structure of specialized junctions. *Neurosci. Res. Prog. Bull.*, **8**, 336–360.

Békésy, G. von (1967) *Sensory Inhibition*. Princeton: Princeton Univ. Press.

Biedenbach, M. A., Van Hassel, H. J. and Brown, A. C. (1979) Tooth pulp-driven neurons in somatosensory cortex of primates: role in pain mechanisms including a review of the literature. *Pain*, 7, 31–50.

Bloom, F. E., Hoffer, B. J. and Nicoll, R. A. (1972) Amino acids and poly-peptides in synaptic function: retrospective prospects. *Neurosci. Res. Prog. Bull.*, **10**, 213–218.

Bloom, F. E., Iversen, L. L. and Schmitt, F. O. (1970) Macromolecules in synaptic functions. *Neurosci. Res. Prog. Bull.*, **8**, 325–455.

Bodian, D. (1967) Neurons, circuits, and neuroglia. In *The Neurosciences*, ed. Quarton, G. C., Melnechuck, T. and Schmitt, F. O., pp. 6–24. New York: Rockefeller Univ. Press.

Bowsher, D. (1971) Personal communication. 26 May 1971.

Brodal, A. (1969) *Neurological Anatomy in Relation to Clinical Medicine*. New York: Oxford Univ. Press.

Bullock, T. H. (1967) Signals and neuronal coding. In *The Neurosciences*, ed. Quarton, G. C., Melnechuk, T. and Schmitt, F. O., pp. 347–352. New York: Rockefeller Univ. Press.

Bullock, T. H. (1970) Operations analysis of nervous functions. In *The Neurosciences Second Study Program*, ed. Schmitt, F. O., Quarton, G. C., Melnechuk, T. and Adelman, G., pp. 375–383. New York: Rockefeller Univ. Press.

Byers, M. R., Fink, B. R., Kish, S. J. and Aasheim, G. M. (1975) Arrest of rapid axoplasmic transport in a sensory nerve *in vivo* by ligature or lidocaine treatment. In *Progress in Anesthesiology*, ed. Fink, B. R., pp. 25–38. New York: Raven Press.

Craik, K. J. W. (1959) Theory of the human operator in control systems. II. Man as an example in a control system. In *Cybernetics*, ed. Evans, C. R. and Robinson, A. D. J., pp. 131–139. London: Butterworths.

Darian-Smith, I. (1966) Neural mechanisms of facial sensation. *Int. Rev. Neurobiol.*, **9**, 301–395.

Darian-Smith, I. and Johnson, K. O. (1977) Temperature sense in the primate. *Brit. med. Bull.*, **33**, 143–148.

Eccles, J. C. (1967) Postsynaptic inhibition in the central nervous system. In *The Neurosciences*, ed. Quarton, G. C., Melnechuk, T. and Schmitt, F. O., pp. 408–427. New York: Rockefeller Univ. Press.
Eccles, J. C. (1973) *The Understanding of the Brain*. New York: McGraw-Hill.
Elias, P. (1967) Personal communication. 30 Nov. 1967.
Funakoshi, M. and Zotterman, Y. (1963) A study in the excitation of dental pulp fibres. In *Sensory Mechanisms in Dentine*, ed. Anderson, D. J., pp. 60–72. Oxford: Pergamon.
Gray, J. A. B. (1966a) Part of a general discussion in *Touch, Heat and Pain*, p. 84, cited below.
Gray, J. A. B. (1966b) The representation of information about rapid changes in a population of receptor units signalling mechanical events. In *Touch, Heat and Pain*, ed. De Reuck, A. V. S. and Knight, J., pp. 299–324. London: Churchill.
Hodgkin, A. C. (1967) *The Conduction of the Nervous Impulse*. Liverpool: Liverpool Univ. Press.
Hubel, D. H. (1979) The brain. *Scient. Amer.*, **241**, 39–47.
Iversen, L. L. (1979) The chemistry of the brain. *Scient. Amer.*, **241**, 118–129.
Katz, B. (1966) *Nerve, Muscle and Synapse*. New York: McGraw-Hill.
Katz, B. (1967) How cells communicate. In *Psychobiology. The Biological Bases of Behaviour*, ed. McGraw, J. L., Wienberger, N. M. and Whaken, R. E., pp. 215–224. San Francisco: Freeman.
Lele, P. P., Sinclair, D. C. and Weddell, G. (1954) The reaction time to touch. *J. Physiol. (Lond.)*, **123**, 187–203.
Milsum, J. H. (1966) *Biological Control Systems Analysis*. New York: McGraw-Hill.
Mountcastle, V. B. (1967) The problems of sensing and the neural coding of sensory events. In *The Neurosciences*, ed. Quarton, G. C., Melnechuk, T. and Schmitt, F. O., pp. 393–408. New York: Rockefeller Univ. Press.
Mountcastle, V. B. and Powell, T. P. S. (1969). Neural mechanisms subserving cutaneous sensibility, with special reference to the role of afferent inhibition in sensory perception and discrimination. In *Readings in Physiological Psychology. Neurophysiology Sensory Processes*, pp. 147–179. New York: Harper and Row.
Naylor, M. N. (1963) Studies on the mechanism of sensation to cold stimulation of human dentine. In *Sensory Mechanisms in Dentine*, ed. Anderson, D. J., pp. 80–87. Oxford: Pergamon.
Sato, M. and Ozeki, M. (1966) Initiation of impulses by mechanosensory nerve terminals. In *Touch, Heat and Pain*, ed. De Reuck, A. V. S. and Knight, J., pp. 203–231. London: Churchill.
Stevens, C. F. (1979) The neuron. *Scient. Amer.*, **241**, 49–59.
Szentàgothai, J. (1970) Glomerular synapses, complex synaptic arrangements, and their operational significance. In the *Neurosciences Second Study Program*, ed. Schmitt, F. O. *et al.*, pp. 427–443. New York: Rockefeller Univ. Press.
Valois, R. L. de (1966) Neural processing of visual information. In *Frontiers in Physiological Psychology*, ed. Russell, R. W., pp. 51–91. New York: Academic Press.
Walter, W. G. (1963) *Introduction to Electroencephalography. A Symposium on its Various Aspects*, ed. Hill, D. and Parr, G., pp. 9–24. London: Macdonald.
Young, J. Z. (1966) *The Memory System of the Brain*. London: Oxford Univ. Press.

# 3

# Transmission of trigeminal nerve impulses in the central nervous system

When the sensory root of the trigeminal nerve enters the brain its fibres pass to three sensory nuclei, the mesencephalic nucleus (upper-most), the principal nucleus, and the spinal nucleus (lowest), the latter two being continuous with each other.

The mesencephalic nucleus receives fibres carrying proprioceptive impulses from the muscles of mastication, the tongue, the facial muscles, the orbital muscles (Hitchcock and Forrester, 1968), and also from the periodontal membrane (Smith and Marcarian, 1968). Many fibres, from all three divisions (Hassler and Walker, 1970), dichotomise to form ascending and descending branches. The former go to the principal nucleus carrying impulses mediating touch and pressure.

The descending branches, also carrying impulses mediating touch and pressure, run with fibres which have not dichotomised, some of which carry impulses mediating pain and temperature. Together they form a distinct bundle called the spinal tract of the trigeminal nerve which extends to the lower end of the medulla oblongata (Brodal, 1969). Fibres derived from all three divisions, in man as well as lower animals, descend as far as the second and often the third cervical segment (Torvik, 1956; Denny-Brown and Yanagisawa, 1973). As it descends, its fibres pass to the spinal nucleus which lies medial to it, the fibres mediating touch and pressure terminating in the upper part of the nucleus (Kawamura and Nishiyama, 1966).

In the spinal tract, nerve fibres derived from the mandibular division of the trigeminal nerve run postero-medially, fibres from the ophthalmic division run laterally, and the maxillary division fibres lie in between (Fig. 3.1, 3.2). According to Kunc (1966) this arrangement is absolutely constant, and allows selective cutting in patients suffering from facial neuralgias. The ophthalmic fibres terminate lower than the others (Fig. 3.2). Kunc also stated, as did Hitchcock and Forrester (1968), that fibres from the middle part of the face terminate at the highest levels (Fig. 3.3).

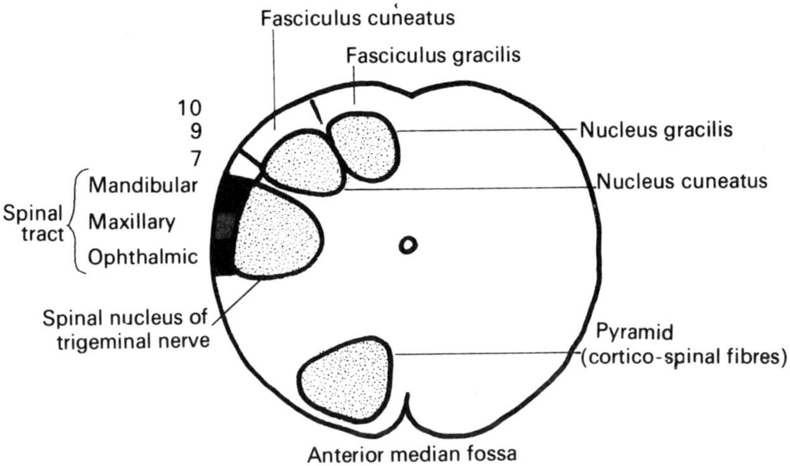


**Fig. 3.1.** Spinal tract of the trigeminal nerve in the medulla oblongata showing the position of fibres from the three divisions. Fibres of the facial, glossopharyngeal and vagus nerves travel in the zone indicated 7, 9, 10. (After Kunc, 1966.)

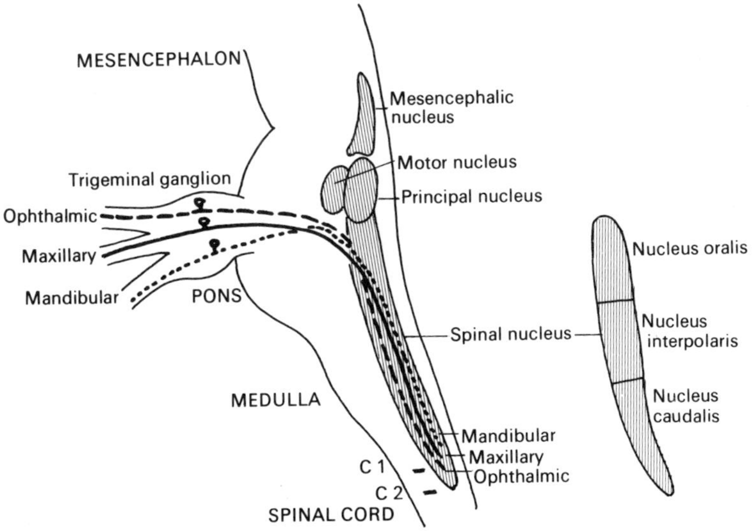


**Fig. 3.2.** The spinal tract showing how nerve fibres from the ophthalmic and mandibular divisions change positions before ending in the spinal nucleus. At the right side of the illustration are shown the subnuclei of the spinal nucleus. (After Kunc, 1966; Brodal, 1969).

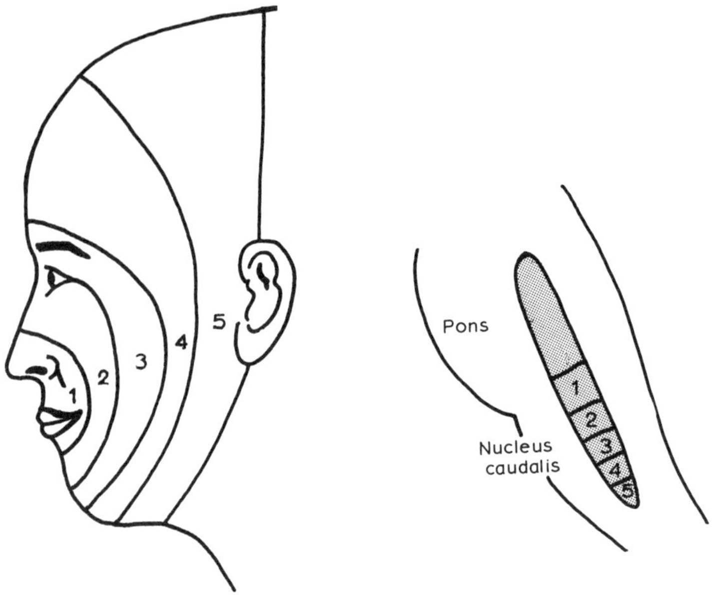


**Fig. 3.3.** Fibres mediating pain terminate as shown. The fibres nearest to the lips terminate highest in the nucleus caudalis, and this applies to all three divisions of the trigeminal nerve. (Modified from Kunc, 1966).

This 'onion-peel' distribution was accepted by Darian-Smith (1966) but he thought that all three divisions terminated at about the same level (the second cervical segment).

The spinal nucleus is further divided into three zones (Figs. 3.2, 3.3), the nucleus oralis being uppermost (rostrally), the nucleus caudalis being lowest (caudally) and the nucleus interpolaris between, the nucleus caudalis being the most significant part for the arrival of impulses mediating pain. There is no clear segregation within the trigeminal nuclei regarding transmission of tactile and pain impulses but it seems equally clear from clinical experience that the lowest part of the spinal nucleus together with the upper cervical segments of the spinal cord dorsal horn are especially important in the conduction of impulses mediating pain in the teeth, jaws and face (Brodal, 1969). This clinical experience follows the introduction of trigeminal spinal tractotomy for the relief of pain by Sjöqvist (1938). Since then it has been supposed that trigeminal fibres mediating pain have ended in the nucleus caudalis. However, following nociceptive stimulation of teeth in the cat, less neural activity was recorded in the nucleus caudalis than in the nucleus oralis and main sensory nucleus (Greenwood, 1972; 1973). Indeed, in some cases there was no response in the nucleus caudalis (Davies *et al.*, 1971; Vyklicky and Keller, 1973). As Vyklicky and Keller (1974) remark, the clinical and neurophysiological findings are hard to reconcile. Since then Vyklicky *et al* (1977) have sectioned the trigeminal spinal tract in cats and found that both reflex jaw opening and escape behaviour persisted on noxious tooth pulp stimulation, which suggests that information about pain from tooth pulp stimulation passes not only through the nucleus caudalis but also through the more rostral divisions.

The interpretation of some earlier investigations was somewhat bedevilled by the then prevailing view that pain was the only sensation experienced on stimulating human teeth. Another factor that might be confusing is that neural activity recorded (in animal experiments) in the main sensory nucleus and the nucleus oralis need not be due to a direct input from the trigeminal nerve but could be relayed from activity in the nucleus caudalis (Hu and Sessle, 1979). A further factor to be considered is that recording neural input to the trigeminal nuclei on one side of the midline reveals neural input from teeth on both sides of the mouth (Nord, 1976; Anderson *et al.*, 1977; Westrum and Canfield, 1977; Yokota, 1979). This is presumed to be because the trigeminal nerve fibres from anterior teeth cross the midline of the face and jaws; cross-over in the brainstem has not been conclusively demonstrated. These results of animal experiments are compatible with those obtained with human experimental subjects (Mumford and Newton, 1974a and b). At present it is supposed that such overlap only extends as far as canines in animals and lateral incisors in man.

In general the larger nerve fibres of the trigeminal nerve go to the principal sensory nucleus and the nucleus oralis, the smaller nerve fibres going to nucleus caudalis, and this seems to apply also to the fibres from the dental pulp (Nord, 1978; Hu *et al.*, 1978). In the nucleus caudalis fibres end in the substantia gelatinosa and in the more superficial marginal layer. The marginal layer contains projection neurones. The substantia gelatinosa contains two kinds of interneurone, one of which is excitatory and the other inhibitory (Gobel, 1977, 1979). In other words, the morphology is similar to that of the dorsal horn of the spinal cord.

Although it is now accepted that the principal nucleus is homologous with the dorsal column nuclei, and the nucleus caudalis with the spinal cord dorsal horn, the functional position of the nuclei oralis and interpolaris are not fully established (Kruger, 1979).

## SECONDARY PATHWAYS

The second order neurones of the trigeminal system form three secondary pathways which ascend in the brain.

Fibres from the principal sensory nucleus form the trigeminal lemniscus which crosses the midline to travel with the medial lemniscus which has already crossed at a lower level (Fig. 3.4). This means that the trigeminal nerve second order fibres are now travelling with comparable input from the spinal nerves. Together

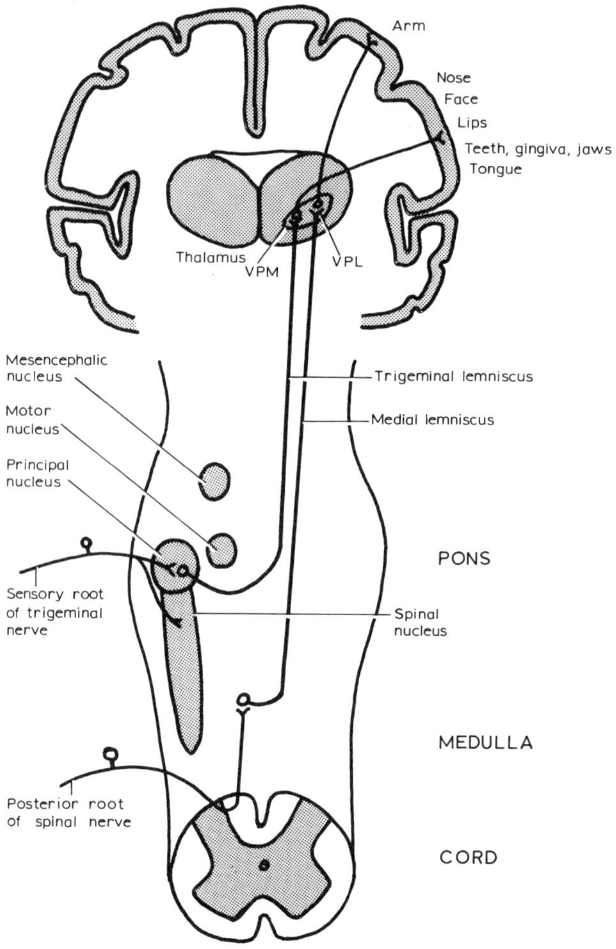


**Fig. 3.4.** Secondary and tertiary paths of the trigeminal system carrying impulses mediating mechanoreceptive information. The cortical areas indicated are from Penfield and Jasper (1954). VPM, VPL; medial and lateral parts of the ventroposterior thalamic nucleus.

they go to the thalamus where they end somatotopically in the ventroposterior nucleus, the trigeminal relay being in the medial part of the nucleus (Fig. 3.4). The trigeminal lemniscus and medial lemniscus are in every way homologous.

From animal experiments it seems possible that there is also a small number of fibres which ascend without crossing the midline (Torvik, 1957).

The other two secondary pathways take origin in the spinal trigeminal nucleus (Fig. 3.5). One of them, analogous with the neo-spinothalamic tract, must be assumed to arise from the cells which receive the descending branches of the dichotomised primary trigeminal axons; the ascending branches terminate in the principal nucleus as described earlier (Fig. 3.4). It follows that the

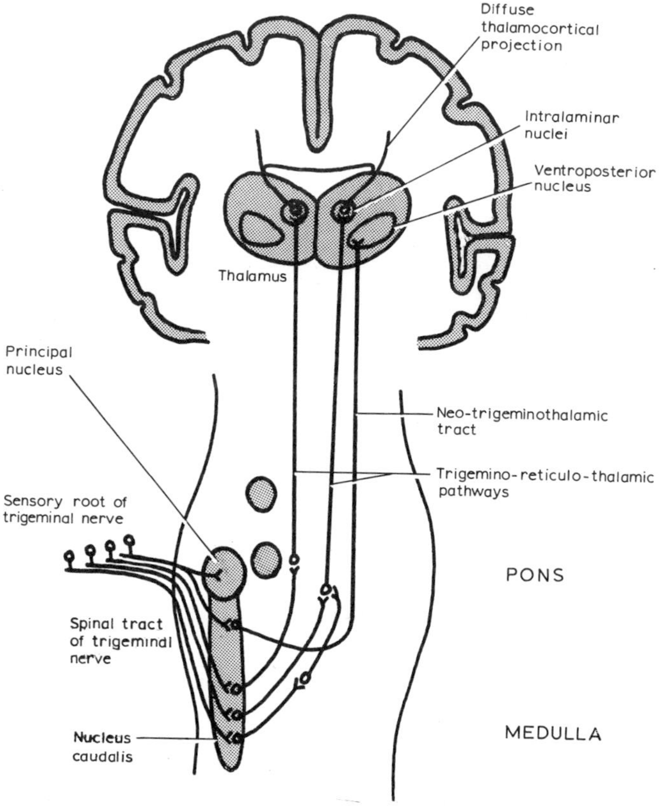


**Fig. 3.5.** Secondary paths of the trigeminal system carrying impulses which are eventually interpreted as pain. Notice the multisynaptic character of the trigemino-reticulo-thalamic paths. The neo-trigemino-thalamic tract, as drawn, is presumed to carry mechanoreceptive information (but see text).

cells of origin of this neo-trigeminothalamic tract receive mechanoreceptive information; in addition, they receive, from unbranched primary trigeminal axons discriminative (i.e. localised) information from thermal and pricking pain receptors, both travelling in small myelinated axons. The neo-trigeminothalamic tract joins the trigeminal lemniscus and medial lemniscus and conveys its information in a point-to-point fashion to the medial part of the ventroposterior thalamic nucleus (Bowsher, 1971).

The third secondary pathway, which also originates in the spinal trigeminal nucleus, arises from cells whose input consists of small myelinated and unmyelinated fibres in the trigeminal nerve coming from high threshold mechanoreceptors and thermoreceptors, whose messages are consciously translated as poorly-localised sensations ranging from 'unpleasantness' to 'pain'. Their output is to the reticular formation which may be thought of as two zones, one being the lateral reticular formation lying immediately subjacent to the nucleus caudalis. The other zone, deeper still, is the medial reticular formation which receives convergent high intensity input from all over the body, and part of this information is transmitted to the intralaminar nucleii in the thalamus. In other words, this is the trigemino-reticulo-thalamic pathway, analogous to the spino-reticulo-thalamic pathway. Some of the fibres cross the midline but others are uncrossed (Fig. 3.5). The fact that input to this area is widely spread (Albe-Fessard *et al.*, 1970; Hassler, 1970, 1972; Bowsher, 1974; Woda et al, 1975) is of tremendous importance in the treatment of pain for it means that impulses mediating pain can, in the diencephalon, find a way around any localised destruction that the surgeon might produce.

An important point made earlier by Bowsher (1965) was that to evoke activity in this system stimuli do not necessarily need to be noxious, but they must be brusque, and require summation.

It seems possible that the multisynaptic nature of this secondary pathway at least partly accounts for the wide range of sensations reported by human subjects on having their teeth stimulated (see Chapter 5).

From the lower part of the spinal nucleus there are connections with the nucleus of the facial nerve and also fibres which eventually convey impulses to the superior cervical ganglion; in this way reactions to noxious stimuli reach peripheral effectors (Hassler and Walker, 1970).

The spinal nucleus also receives connecting fibres from the facial, glossopharyngeal and vagus nerves, as well as from the reticular system and cortex (Brodal, 1969).

## TERTIARY PATHWAYS

Neural impulses mediating touch and pressure are conveyed from the thalamus via the posterior limb of the internal capsule, where they occupy a very compact area, to the post central gyrus of the cerebral cortex (Fig. 3.4).

It is not so certain what happens to impulses mediating pain, and efforts to trace nervous traffic related to pain alone beyond the thalamus have proved difficult. However, as described earlier, one of the secondary trigeminal pathways reaches the intralaminar nuclei in the thalamus on both sides of the midline. The intralaminar thalamic nuclei are at the origin of the diffuse thalamocortical projection, which serves to activate (desynchronise) the whole cortex (except the primary sensory and motor areas).

## REPRESENTATION AT THE CORTEX

The structures of the mouth and face, including teeth, are represented at the cortex for touch and pressure in the post central gyrus, the primary somatic sensory area, (area SI) in the well defined manner described by Penfield and Jasper (1954), as in Figs. 3.4, 3.6, and representation of the face area is not inverted as often supposed. Since the amount of cortex allotted to any part of the body depends on the richness of the nerve supply, rather than size, the lips have a large representation but it should not be supposed that this large sensory representation is for pain; it is the

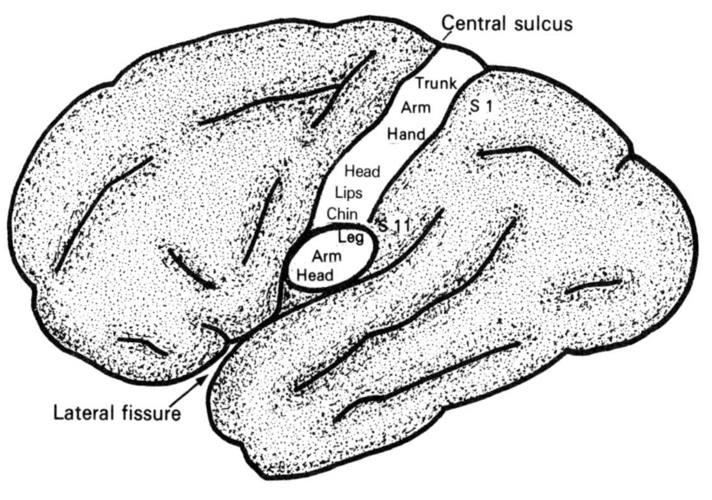


**Fig. 3.6.** Representation at the cortex.

sensory input needed for muscular control. Moreover, the somatotopic representation of body surface is only real on a gross scale. In finer detail the same spot on the periphery is represented in many different ways, often over different routes and relay mechanisms (Szentàgothai and Arbib, 1974).

There is representation for the teeth in the cortex of cats (Anderson, Keller and Vyklicky, 1973; Anderson *et al*, 1977), rats (Shigena *et al*, 1974; Richardson and Cody, 1977) and rhesus monkeys and baboons (Biedenbach, van Hassel and Brown, 1979). The latter investigators found a tooth pulp projection area within the face area of the primary somatosensory cortex. Neurones activated by pulp stimulation were located in deep cortex in the base of the central sulcus whereas soft tissue adjacent to the tooth, when stimulated, activated neurones which were located in the superficial cortex of the post central gyrus. Amongst the pulp-activated cells there were three kinds; some were activated from one pulp only; some from more than one pulp; and some from one pulp and its adjacent soft tissue.

These observations are compatible with existing knowledge of the innervation of the teeth and their surrounding structures (Chapter 1). The observation that some cortical cells could be activated from one pulp only means that, in principle, it should be possible to localise pulpal pain to one tooth. Biedenbach, van Hassel and Brown (1979) also point out that it is possible that tooth pulp projections also occur to other deep but as yet unidentified cortical sites.

The fibres carrying sensory information terminate mainly within the fourth layer of the primary sensory cortex (Chow and Leiman, 1970), the cortex being regarded as six layers, starting with the outer surface as number one. Messages to this area are relayed from the thalamus in a faithful manner to give the person information affecting the part concerned (Brodal, 1969).

There is also representation at the lower end of the post central gyrus and central sulcus along the superior border of the lateral sulcus or fissure, area SII (Fig. 3.6). The area SI has unilateral representation of sensation, whereas the area SII has bilateral representation which is less precise. It also appears, from animal experiments, that a third area (SIII) may be present (Darian-Smith *et al.*, 1966) but this is not yet well understood.

Electrical stimulation of the cortex in conscious humans does not often lead to them reporting a feeling of pain (Albe-Fessard, 1968). Penfield and Boldrey (1937) found only 11 out of more than 800 responses were described as pain; no patients experi-

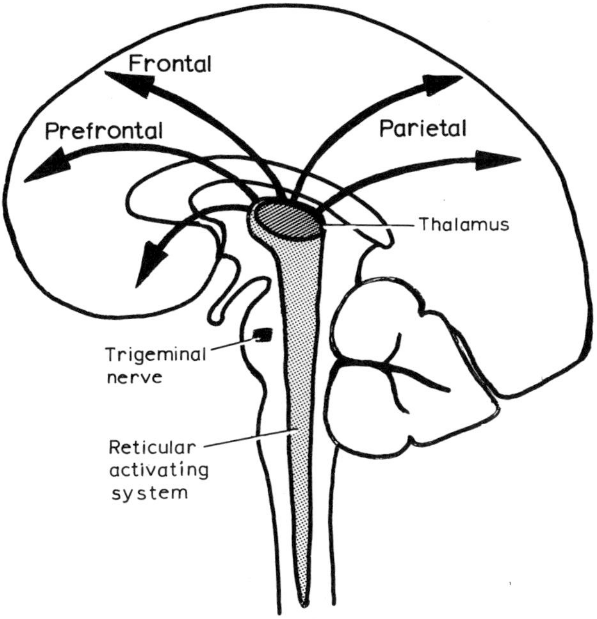


**Fig. 3.7.** The reticular activating system and diffuse thalamocortical projection (arrows).

enced pain in the jaws or teeth. They concluded that there was little, if any, true cortical representation for pain.

Following cortical ablations in man most authors have observed that the patient has retained his sensibility to painful stimuli, although others have found a reduction of pain sensibility (Brodal, 1969).

Cassinari and Pagni (1969) concluded that there was scant anatomical and physiological evidence for a cortical area specifically serving for the reception of impulses mediating pain. It is now considered (Bowsher and Albe-Fessard, 1962) that an essential requirement for regarding impulses as painful is that they involve the diffuse thalamocortical projection (Figs. 3.5, 3.7) which reaches a large area of the non-primary cortex (the association areas). This projection has been definitely shown to exist but it is not yet certain if the fibres terminate in superficial or deep cortical layers (Bowsher, 1976). What happens at the cortex is complex and not well understood but it is presumably here where the subject evaluates the sensations perceived in terms of his past experience. Moreover, there are return fibres — corticothalamic fibres (see below) — and these influence the manner in which the thalamic cell stations handle the cortically-directed information. There are also interhemispheric connections linking the area SII and the corresponding area of the opposite side (Bowsher, 1981), and this has been demonstrated for the incisors of rats (Shigenaga *et al*, 1974).

Following suitable stimulation it is possible to record an evoked potential when nerve impulses reach the cortex, and it may be tempting to regard this as indicating the moment when the subject becomes aware of the stimulus, but this does not necessarily follow, for such potentials can occur as a result of stimuli which fail to produce a conscious sensation (Libet *et al.*, 1967). It is not yet possible to say at what anatomical level impulses from painful stimuli reach consciousness.

**Descending nerve fibres**

In addition to the thalamocortical fibres there are corticothalamic (feedback) fibres passing from the somatomotor cortex to the thalamus.

Corticotrigeminal fibres have also been described (in the cat) as passing from widespread regions of the cortex to the principal nucleus and all subdivisions of the spinal nucleus, the connections being both crossed and uncrossed (Brodal, Szabo and Torvik, 1956).

Electrical stimulation of the cortex at the precentral gyrus results in muscle activity on the opposite side of the body. This includes activity in the facial muscles, but the muscles of mastication are involved bilaterally, presumably because they are normally active in a bilateral manner (Brodal, 1969).

The older idea that descending fibres acted only on efferent mechanisms is too simple, for they also convey impulses which regulate the transmission of sensory impulses passing from the periphery towards the brain including those which mediate pain sensations. This is enormously important in pain control and there may be more than one mechanism. In one of them periaqueductal gray stimulation might affect the 'gain' of transmission of nociceptive messages by a synaptic mechanism which need not be serotoninergic (Carstens, Yokota and Zimmermann, 1979). In the other mechanism control is via a descending inhibitory pathway which is part of the serotoninergic system, i.e. which uses the transmitter substance serotonin (5-hydroxytryptamine) (Bowsher, 1980). This pathway projects to the trigeminal spinal nucleus from the medullary nucleus raphe magnus, itself acting as a relay from the periaqueductal gray matter (Lovick, West and Wolstencroft, 1977; Oliveras, Guilbaud and Besson, 1977). The significance of the periaqueductal gray matter depends on the neuropeptides enkephalin and endorphin.

## THE NEUROPEPTIDES

Reynolds (1969) and Liebeskind (1974) found that electrical stimulation of the periaqueductal and periventricular gray matter greatly reduced or even abolished responsiveness of rats to all noxious stimuli employed, the effect being equivalent to 10 mg/kg of morphine. They suggested that the electrical stimulation might activate a pain suppressive system in these regions which acted, at least in part, by blocking nociceptive information through the spinal cord. The search for naturally occurring morphine-like substances bore fruit when Hughes *et al* (1975) discovered the two closely related pentapeptides leucine-enkephalin and metenkephalin. These have analgesic activity which is brief because they are rapidly broken down, but Hughes (1975) regarded the work as supporting the views of Mayer and Liebeskind.

A vast amount of work has already been done on these peptides and it is expected that they will be important in many ways so the interested reader should consult books, e.g. Hughes (1978), Beers and Bassett (1979). For the moment, however, it has been shown by Hökfelt *et al* (1977) that enkephalin is present in many parts of the nervous system, including the periaqueductal gray and periventricular gray matter, and also the substantia gelatinosa of the trigeminal nucleus caudalis, as well as the spinal cord dorsal horns.

## MOTOR PATHWAYS

Most afferent fibres of the mesencephalic nucleus travel in the motor root of the trigeminal nerve but fibres also reach it by each of the three divisions. They are thought to pass straight through the trigeminal ganglion without contacting any cell body (Warwick and Williams, 1973). Thus, the mesencephalic nucleus receives neural impulses from the muscles of mastication, the tongue, the facial muscles and the periodontal membranes. The cells are pseudo-unipolar cells and their central processes are presumed to go to the trigeminal motor nucleus to complete the two neurone arc for the jaw reflex (Fig. 3.8), homologous with the reflexes of the spinal cord. The neurones of the motor nucleus leave peripherally to form the motor root of the trigeminal nerve, and eventually supply the muscles of mastication, etc. (Chapter 1).

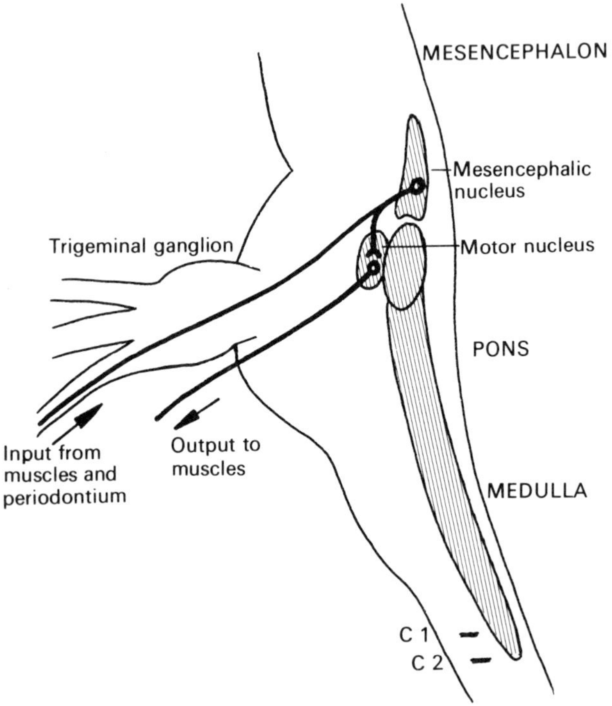


**Fig. 3.8.** Two neurone arc for the jaw reflex.

The motor root also conveys proprioceptive fibres from these muscles (Pelletier, Poulos and Lende, 1974).

It is possible, though not proved, that impulses which pass through the mesencephalic nucleus and reach consciousness are relayed in the principal nucleus (Brodal, 1969). Also, some proprioceptive impulses are possibly relayed from the mesencephalic nucleus to the cerebellum (Hitchcock and Forrester, 1968). The cerebellum is involved in the gradual alteration of muscle tensions needed to maintain posture, and the smooth orderly changes in muscles required for skilled movements.

## RETICULAR ACTIVATING SYSTEM

The reticular activating system is situated in the central core of the brain stem and spinal cord (Fig. 3.7), though it is essentially a crossed pathway since it responds preferentially to contralateral stimuli (Bowsher, 1976). As it ascends its fibres are distributed to the thalamus, especially the intralaminar nuclei, and also the hypothalamus, mainly the posterior part. Those going to the intralaminar nuclei may send collaterals to other thalamic nuclei but this is not yet well understood.

The system was named as the reticular formation because its neurones were scattered amongst a network or reticule of criss-crossing nerve fibres. Later its function was recognised by Moruzzi and Magoun (1949) and it became known as the reticular activating system. It should be noted that reticular system is an anatomical description whereas activating is a functional description, and the two do not exactly correspond (Brodal, 1969).

In the central nervous system messages from peripheral receptors are distributed, not only to long through pathways which relay through the thalamus to the cortex, but also through more primitive fibre systems to the reticular formation. Similarly the trigeminal nerve nuclei send branches to it and receive branches from it, as do the other cranial nerve nuclei. There may even be some trigeminal nerve fibres which pass directly into the reticular system (Clarke and Bowsher, 1962).

Its function is to arouse the cortex, not just with any signal, but acting on information significant to the individual such as a burning smell, a baby crying or pain; non-significant information such as a clock ticking or usual traffic noise is disregarded. Imagine the situation if this were not the case; the great sensory inflow would be tremendously distracting and the ability to concentrate seriously prejudiced.

The facility to discriminate requires time to develop for the system has to acquire experience. The reticular system is in effect a control centre, monitoring and integrating hosts of stimuli, sorting out what matters, focusing attention on it, and rejecting what does not matter. Its role in mediating and modulating impulses is obviously important in relation to pain experience.

## LIMBIC SYSTEM

The limbic system is a collection of richly interconnected structures around the upper brain stem, including the hypothalamus, rhinencephalon, thalamic nuclei and forebrain. It is largely responsible for the affective components of pain, including fear and aversion, but it would be wrong to say that it is the 'pain centre'.

It receives input mainly from the reticular formation and also from the frontal lobes. Its output is back into the reticular formation (Livingston, 1967).

## NEURONAL CONVERGENCE

When nerve impulses are conveyed from the periphery into the central nervous system the fibres conveying them become fewer at each synapse. This is neuronal convergence, and in some cases the reduction is as much as a hundred to one. For the trigeminal system there are 3 to 30 fibres in the trigeminal nerve converging on one fibre in the secondary pathway (as determined for the spinal nucleus of cats by Darian-Smith, Rowe and Sessle, 1968). These authors suggested that each primary afferent fibre had less effective excitatory action on second order neurones in the nucleus caudalis than in the nucleus oralis. However, convergence can occur at an earlier stage, namely in the trigeminal ganglion, for it has been shown that single ganglion cells can respond to stimulation of more than one tooth (in cats) and this presumably means that collateral branches go to separate teeth (Rosing and Anderson, 1978). This is compatible with research described in Chapter 1.

Yokota (1976) found brain stem cells activated by stimulation of the ipsilateral upper canine in 41 cases, the ipsilateral lower canine in 24 cases and both in 28 cases. Many cells were activated from a canine and also by tactile stimulation of its adjacent soft tissues; this was also found by Shigenaga, Sakai and Okada, 1976). Moreover, cells may be activated by stimulation of both ipsilateral and contralateral canines, and this is presumably explained by sensory overlap in the midline of the mouth (Chapter 1).

This convergence is of considerable importance in toothache and presumably accounts for the clinical observation that toothache is often poorly localised by the patient. From the investigations of Mumford and Newton (1971, 1974a, b) it seems that convergence in human subjects is such as to involve one tooth and two other teeth on each side.

Kawamura and Nishiyama (1966) assumed that one nerve fibre was related to a small number of periodontal receptors, and that a number of these fibres converge to one secondary neurone in the trigeminal nuclei.

From recordings made at the sensory cortex (also of cats) it appears that there is a high degree of convergence there from the teeth as well as of other afferents (Anderson, Keller and Vyklicky, 1973).

## SUMMARY

This is a difficult subject, not yet fully elucidated, and the chapter itself is only a summary. To summarise further means over simplification so the following is only a simple concept.

Impulses in the trigeminal nerves are relayed in the trigeminal nuclei which lie within the brain stem.

Impulses mediating touch and pressure are relayed higher in the nuclei and go to the thalamus by two routes, the trigeminal lemniscus and the neo-trigeminothalamic tract. They reach the ventroposterior nucleus where they are again relayed to the sensory areas of the cortex. Both in the thalamus and in the cortex the neurones are arranged in a somatotopic manner which allows the origin of the impulses to be accurately localised.

Impulses which may eventually give rise to pain are relayed lower in the nuclei and enter the central core of the brain stem which is a network of nerves — the reticular system. Neural impulses reach this network from all over the body and this intermingling prevents accurate localisation of their origin, though limited crude localisation may still be possible. Having passed through this network impulses are further relayed within several areas of the diencephalon, and these may also relay impulses to each other. By routes which are not yet understood the impulses reach various other parts of the brain where they are recognised as pain with its various states of sensation, emotion and motivation.

There is also some control over the sensory input, this being exercised via systems descending mainly from the cortex.

## REFERENCES


Albe-Fessard, D. (1968) Central nervous mechanisms involved in pain and analgesia. In *Pharmacology of Pain*, ed. Lim, R. K. S., Armstrong, D. and Pardo, E. G., pp. 131–168. Oxford: Pergamon.

Albe-Fessard, D., Arfel, G., Derome, P. and Dondey, M. (1970) Electrophysiology of the human thalamus with special reference to trigeminal pain. In *Trigeminal Neuralgia Pathogenesis and Pathophysiology*, ed. Hassler, R. and Walker, A. E., pp. 139–148. Stuttgart: Thieme.

Anderson, S. A., Keller, O., Roos, A. and Rydenhäg, B. (1977) Cortical projection of tooth pulp afferents in the cat. In *Pain in the Trigeminal Region*, ed. Anderson, D. J. and Matthews, B., pp. 355–364. Amsterdam: Elsevier/North Holland.

Anderson, S. A., Keller, O. and Vyklicky, L. (1973) Cortical activity evoked from tooth pulp afferents. *Brain Res.*, **50**, 473–475.

Beers, R. F., Jr. and Bassett, E. G. (eds.) (1979) *Mechanisms of Pain and Analgesic Compounds*. New York: Raven Press.

Biedenbach, M. A., Van Hassel, H. J. and Brown, A. C. (1979) Tooth pulp-driven neurons in somatosensory cortex of primates: role in pain mechanisms including a review of the literature. *Pain*, **7**, 31–50.

Bowsher, D. (1965) The anatomophysiological basis of somatosensory discrimination. *Int. Rev. Neurobiol.*, **8**, 35–75.
Bowsher, D. (1971) Personal communication. 1 June 1971.
Bowsher, D. (1974) Thalamic convergence and divergence of information generated by noxious stimulation. In International Symposium on Pain, ed. Bonica, J. J., pp. 223–232. *Advances in Neurology*. Vol. 4. New York: Raven Press.
Bowsher, D. (1976) Role of the reticular formation in noxious stimulation. *Pain*, **2**, 361–378.
Bowsher, D. (1979) Central mechanisms of orofacial pain. *Brit. J. oral. Surg.*, **17**, 185–197.
Bowsher, D. (1980) Peptides and pain. In *Persistent Pain*, ed. Lipton, S. pp. 189–202. London: Academic Press.
Bowsher, D. and Albe-Fessard, D. (1962) Patterns of somatosensory organisation within the central nervous system. In *The Assessment of Pain in Man and Animals*, ed. Keele, C. A. and Smith, R., pp. 107–122. Edinburgh: Livingstone.
Brodal, A. (1969) *Neurological Anatomy in Relation to Clinical Medicine*, 2nd edition. London: Oxford Univ. Press.
Brodal, A., Szabo, T. and Torvik, A. (1956) Corticofugal fibres to sensory trigeminal nuclei and nucleus of solitary tract. An experimental study in the cat. *J. comp. Neurol.*, **106**, 527–555.
Carstens, E., Yokota, T. and Zimmermann, M. (1979) Inhibition of spinal neuronal responses to noxious skin heating by stimulation of mesencephalic periaqueductal gray in the cat. *J. Neurophysiol.*, **42**, 558–568.
Cassinari, V. and Pagni, C. A. (1969) *Central Pain*. Cambridge, Mass.: Harvard Univ. Press.
Chow, K. L. and Leiman, A. L. (1970) Aspects of the structural and functional organization of the neocortex. *Neurosci. Res. Prog. Bull.*, **8**, 157–220.
Clarke, W. B. and Bowsher, D. (1962) Terminal distribution of primary afferent trigeminal fibers in the rat. *Exptl. Neurol.*, **6**, 372–383.
Darian-Smith, I. (1966) Neural mechanisms of facial sensation. *Neurobiol.*, **9**, 301–395.
Darian-Smith, I., Isbister, J., Mok, H. and Yokota, T. (1966) Somatic sensory cortical projection areas excited by tactile stimulation of the cat; a triple representation. *J. Physiol. (Lond.)*, **182**, 671–689.
Darian-Smith, I., Rowe, M. J. and Sessle, B. J. (1968) 'Tactile' stimulus intensity: information transmission by relay neurons in different trigeminal nuclei. *Science*, **160**, 791–794.
Davies, W. I. R., Scott, D. Jr., Vesterstrom, K. and Vyklicky, L. (1971) Depolarization of the tooth pulp afferent terminals in the brain stem of the cat. *J. Physiol. (Lond)*., **28**, 515–532.
Denny-Brown, D. and Yanagisawa, N. (1975) The function of the descending root of the fifth nerve. *Brain*, **96**, 783–814.
Gobel, S. (1979) Neural circuitry in the substantia gelatinosa of Rolando: anatomical insights. In *Proceedings of the Second World Congress on Pain*, eds. Bonica, J. J., Liebeskind, J. C. and Albe-Fessard, D. G., pp. 175–195. *Adv. Pain Res. Therap.*, Vol. 3. New York: Raven Press.
Gobel, S. and Hockfield, S. (1977) An anatomical analysis of the synaptic circuitry of layers I, II and III of trigeminal nucleus caudalis in the cat. In *Pain in the Trigeminal Region*. ed. Anderson. D. J. and Matthews, B., pp. 203–211. Amsterdam: Elsevier/North Holland.
Greenwood, F. (1972) Site of termination of nerve fibres from the dental pulp. In *Oral Physiology*, ed. Emmelin, N. and Zotterman, Y., pp. 259–262. Oxford: Pergamon.

Greenwood, F. (1973) An electrophysiological study of the central connections of primary afferent nerve fibres from the dental pulp in the cat. *Archs. oral Biol.*, **18**, 771–785.

Hassler, R. (1970) Dichotomy of facial pain conduction in the diencephalon. In *Trigeminal Neuralgia Pathogenesis and Pathophysiology*, ed. Hassler, R. and Walker, A. E., pp. 122–138. Stuttgart: Thieme.

Hassler, R. (1972) The division of pain conduction into systems of pain sensation and awareness. In *Pain*, ed. Janzen, R. *et al.*, pp. 98–112. Stuttgart: Thieme.

Hassler, R. and Walker, A. E. (1970) *Trigeminal Neuralgia Pathogenesis and Pathophysiology*. Introduction. Stuttgart: Thieme.

Hitchcock, E. R. and Forrester, J. M. (1968) The nervous system. In *A Companion to Medical Studies*, ed. Passmore, R. and Robson, J. S., Vol. 1. Oxford: Blackwell.

Hökfelt, T., Elde, R., Johansson, O., Terenius, L. and Stein, L. (1977) The distribution of enkephalin immunoreactive cell bodies in the rat central nervous system. *Neurosci. Letters*, **5**, 25–31.

Hughes, J. (1975) Isolation of an endogenous compound from the brain with pharmacological properties similar to morphine. *Brain Res.*, **88**, 295–308.

Hughes, J. (1978) (ed.) *Centrally Acting Peptides*. London: Macmillan.

Hughes, J., Smith, T. W. and Kosterlitz, H. W. (1975) Identification of two related pentapeptides from the brain with potent opiate, agonist activity, *Nature (Lond.)*, **258**, 577–579.

Hu, J. W., Lucier, G. E. and Sessle, B. J. (1978) Presynaptic modulation of tooth pulp afferents: a compound action potential analysis. Second World Congress on Pain. *Pain Abstracts*, **1**, 65.

Hu, J. W. and Sessle, B. J. (1979) Trigeminal nociceptive and non-nociceptive neurones: brain stem intranuclear projections and modulation by orofacial, periaqueductal gray and nucleus raphe magnus stimuli. *Brain Res.*, **170**, 547–552.

Kawamura, Y. and Nishiyama, T. (1966) Projection of dental afferent impulses to the trigeminal nuclei of the cat. *Japanese J. Physiol.*, **16**, 584–597.

Kruger, L. (1979) Functional sub-division of the brainstem sensory trigeminal nuclear complex. In *Proceedings of the Second World Congress on Pain*. ed. Bonica, J. J. Liebeskind, J. C. and Albe-Fessard, D. G., pp. 197–209. *Adv. Pain Res. Therap.*, Vol. 3. New York: Raven Press.

Kunc, Z. (1966) Significance of fresh anatomic data on spinal trigeminal tract for possibility of selective tractotomies. In *Pain*, ed. Knighton, R. S. and Dumke, P. R., pp. 351–363. London: Churchill.

Libet, B., Alberts, W. W., Wright, E. J. and Feinstein, B. (1967) Responses of human somatosensory cortex to stimuli below threshold for conscious sensation. *Science*, **158**, 1597–1600.

Livingston, R. B. (1967) Brain circuitry relating to complex behaviour. In *The Neurosciences*, ed. Quarton, G. C., Melnechuck, T. and Schmitt, F. O., pp. 499–515. New York: Rockefeller Univ. Press.

Lovick, T. A., West, D. C. and Wolstencroft, J. H. (1977) Interactions between brain stem raphe nuclei and the trigeminal nuclei. In *Pain in the Trigeminal Region*. ed. Anderson, D. J. and Matthews, B. pp. 307–317. Amsterdam: Elsevier/North Holland.

Mayer, D. J. and Liebeskind, J. C. (1974) Pain reduction by focal electrical stimulation of the brain: an anatomical and behavioural analysis. *Brain Res.*, **68**, 73–93.

Moruzzi, G. and Magoun, H.W. (1949) Brain stem reticular formation and activation of the EEG. *Electroenceph. clin. Neurophysiol.*, **1**, 455–473.

Mumford, J. M. and Newton, A. V. (1971) Convergence in the trigeminal system on stimulating human teeth. *Archs. oral Biol.*, **16**, 1089–1097.

Mumford, J. M. and Newton, A. V. (1974a) Trigeminal convergence from human teeth: influence of contralateral stimulation and stimulus frequency on the pain perception threshold. *Archs. oral Biol.*, **19**, 145–149.

Mumford, J. M. and Newton, A. V. (1974b) Electrical stimulation of human teeth and convergence in the trigeminal system. In *International Symposium on Pain*, ed. Bonica, J. J., pp. 357–363. *Advances in Neurology*. Vol. 4. New York: Raven Press.

Nord, S. G. (1976) Bilateral projections of the canine tooth pulp to bulbar trigeminal neurons. *Brain Res.*, **113**, 517–525.

Nord, S. G. (1978) Behavioural and neuronal responses evoked by stimulation of the monkey tooth pulp. Second World Congress on Pain. *Pain Abstracts*, **1**, 64.

Oliveras, J. L., Guilbaud, G. and Besson, J. M. (1977) The use of tooth pulp stimulation to evaluate the analgesia induced by stimulation of raphe nuclei in the cat. In *Pain in the Trigeminal Region*. ed. Anderson, D. J. and Matthews, B., pp. 319–330. Amsterdam: Elsevier/North Holland.

Pelletier, V. A., Poulos, D. A. and Lende, R. A. (1974) Functional localization in the trigeminal root. *J. Neurosurg.*, **40**, 504–513.

Penfield, W. and Boldrey, R. (1937) Somatic motor and sensory representation in the cerebral cortex of man as studied by electrical stimulation. *Brain*, **60**, 389–443.

Penfield, W. and Jasper, H. (1954) *Epilepsy and the Functional Anatomy of the Human Brain*. London: Churchill.

Reynolds, D. V. (1969) Surgery in the rat during electrical analgesia induced by focal brain stimulation. *Science*, **164**, 444–445.

Richardson, H. C. and Cody, F. W. J. (1977) Responses of cerebral cortical neurones to trigeminal inputs in the rat. In *Pain in the Trigeminal Region*. ed. Anderson, D. J. and Matthews, B., pp. 343–354. Amsterdam: Elsevier/North Holland.

Rosing, H. S. and Anderson, K. V. (1978) An analysis of the physiological properties of primary afferent cells that innervate the teeth of cats. Second World Congress on Pain. *Pain Abstracts*, **1**, 64.

Shigenaga, Y., Matano, S., Kusuyama, M. and Sakai, A. (1974) Cortical neurones responding to electrical stimulation of the rats incisor pulp. *Brain Res.*, **67**, 153–156.

Shigenaga, Y., Sakai, A. and Okada, K. (1976) Effects of tooth pulp stimulation in trigeminal nucleus caudalis and adjacent reticular formation in rat. *Brain Res.*, **103**, 400–406.

Sjöqvist, O. (1938) Studies of pain conduction in the trigeminal nerve. *Acta. Psychiat. Scand., Suppl.* **17**, 1–139.

Smith, R. D. and Marcarian, H. W. (1968) Centripetal localization of tooth and tongue tension receptors. *J. dent. Res.*, **47**, 616–621.

Szentágothai, J. and Arbib, M. A. (1974) Conceptual models of neural organisation. *Neurosci. Res. Prog. Bull.*, **12**, 307–510.

Torvik, A. (1956) Afferent connections to the sensory trigeminal nuclei, the nucleus of the solitary tract and adjacent structures. *J. comp. Neurol.*, **106**, 51–141.

Torvik, A. (1957) The ascending fibres from the main trigeminal sensory nucleus. An experimental study in the cat. *Amer. J. Anat.*, **100**, 1–16.

Vyklicky, L. and Keller, O. (1973) Central projection of tooth pulp primary afferents in the cat. *Acta Neurobiol. Exp.* (*Warsz.*), **33**, 803–809.

Vyklicky, L. and Keller, O. (1974) Cortical representation of **A**δ tooth pulp primary afferents in the cat. In *International Symposium on Pain. Advances in Neurology*, Vol. 4, ed. Bonica, J. J., pp. 233–240. New York: Raven Press.

Vyklicky, L., Keller, O., Jastreboff, P., Vyklicky, L. Jr, and Butkhuzy. S. M. (1977) Spinal trigeminal tractotomy and nociceptive reactions evoked by tooth pulp stimulation in the cat. *J. Physiol.* (*Paris*), **73**, 379–386.

Warwick, R. and Williams, P. L. (1973) (ed.) *Gray's Anatomy*. Edinburgh: Longman.

Westrum, L. E. and Canfield, R. C. (1977) Light and electron microscopy of degeneration in the brain stem spinal trigeminal nucleus following tooth pulp removal in adult cats. In *Pain in the Trigeminal Region*. ed. Anderson, D.J. and Matthews, B., pp. 171–179. Amsterdam: Elsevier/North Holland.

Woda, A., Azerad, J., Guilbaud, G. and Besson, J. M. (1975) Etude microphysiologique des projections thalamiques de la pulpe dentaire chez le chat. *Brain Res.*, **89**, 193–213.

Yokota, T. (1976) Two types of tooth pulp units in the bulbar lateral reticular formation. *Brain Res.*, **104**, 325–329.

Yokota, T., Nishikawa, N. and Nishikawa, Y. (1979) Trigeminal nociceptive neurons in the trigeminal nucleus caudalis and bulbar lateral reticular formation. In *Proceedings of the Second World Congress on Pain*. ed. Bonica, J. J., Liebeskind, J. C. and Albe-Fessard, D. G., pp. 211–217. *Adv. Pain Res. Therap.*, Vol. 3. New York: Raven Press.

# 4

# Theories of pain

It is often assumed that pain is a warning that damage has occurred whereas no pain means that everything is all right. Yet a moment's thought indicates that this is not strictly true. Pain may occur when there is no obvious disease as in the primary neuralgias, and many diseases do not cause pain, at least in the early stages. Early tuberculosis and neoplasia are obvious examples, as are dental caries and chronic gingivitis. It is a pity that there is no pain warning in these conditions, perhaps until too late to prevent extensive damage, but when pain does occur it is reasonable to say that it is essentially the sense of injury having been done. Moreover, pain is also a state of awareness that repair and recuperation are necessary, and heralds a period of withdrawal and rest (Wall, 1979; Bolles and Fanselow, 1980). In those conditions where pain occurs without obvious disease it is probably only a matter of time before fuller recognition occurs of what is really involved.

To account for those diseases where pain does not arise, it has been suggested (Hardy, 1962) that pain occurs only when the rate of tissue damage is sufficiently rapid, the damage being done particularly to the pain nerve endings. However, traumatically-caused damage is usually very rapid but does not necessarily evoke pain, at least until some considerable time afterwards. This is partly because the immediate excitement or danger has passed and the injured person or animal has time to think about it (Wall, 1979), and/or because of chemical changes (Keele and Armstrong, 1964). The latter authors attributed pain in many cases to destructive changes in non-nervous cells and in body fluids enveloping the pain nerve endings rather than to changes within the nerve endings themselves. They stressed the primary importance of biochemical changes in the tissues, and these will be described in Chapter 10.

It is against this background of damage and pain that one should consider the various theories that have been put forward on how nerve impulses give rise to the sensation of pain, and it should be understood at the outset that there is not yet a generally accepted theory. Moreover, each of these theories is not a fixed entity but is the subject of various modifications so that a theory as at first proposed may be different from the modern form of the same theory.

## INTENSITY THEORY

According to this view pain is produced when any sensory nerve is stimulated beyond a certain level. This is true of nerves mediating the sensation of touch when stimulated to an excessive degree. It is also possible to experience pain (unpleasantness?) from too much light or too much sound. In other words pain is supposed to be a non-specific sensation, and depends only on high intensity stimulation. At first sight this is an attractive view because it is common knowledge that pain occurs in association with damage, and also that damage is due to tissue being subjected to excessive stimulation. Thus, application of heat is pleasant but excessive heat causes burning. The theory does not take into account that the more intense thermal stimulus excites additional high threshold fibres as well as those mediating the sensation of warmth.

If human teeth are stimulated by an electric current threshold sensation is variously described as hot, cold, tingling or slightly painful, but increasing the intensity of the same stimulus leads to a sensation which is more definitely painful in a larger percentage of cases. However, the more intense stimulus is supposed to involve additional pulpal nerve fibres (Mumford and Newton, 1971), and the pattern of neural impulses reaching the brain may also be modified. The trigeminal system also provides another example against the theory. In cases of trigeminal neuralgia the patient can suffer excruciating pain from a stimulus no greater than a gentle touch provided it is applied to a trigger zone.

Although the Intensity Theory is not accepted, it remains true to say that intensity of stimulation is a factor in causing pain.

## SPECIFICITY THEORY

According to this view pain is a specific modality equivalent to vision and hearing, etc. Just as there are Meissner corpuscles for the sensation of touch, Ruffini end organs supposedly for warmth, and Krause end organs supposedly for cold, so also is pain mediated by free nerve endings. Associated with these peripheral pain receptors there are pain nerves and even supposed to be a specific central apparatus, the pain centre in the thalamus. However, the theory applies essentially to the periphery. In a way, it could be described as the opposite of the Intensity Theory.

The nerves concerned are small fibres of the A-delta and C groups (Bishop, 1946) which pass into the spinal cord where their impulses are relayed, many going to the spinothalamic tract via which they are conveyed to the thalamus. In terms of this theory there is a direct line from the receptor to the brain and the requisite stimulus at the receptor is necessarily followed by the pain sensation. In its simplest form (Fig. 4.1) it has been related to pulling on one end of a rope causing a bell at the other end to ring (Descartes, 1664). This is equivalent to a labelled line in engineering, even if the line happens to have one or two connections, as for synapses.

It is accepted that C fibres convey impulses mediating pain, but some C fibres will respond to mechanical stimuli of only a few

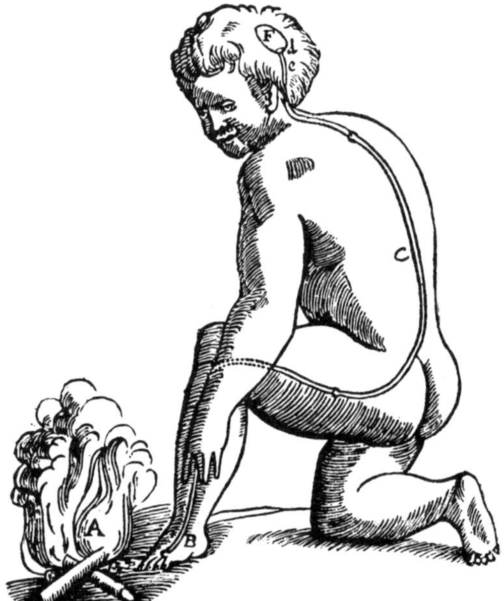

**Fig. 4.1.** Fire (A) approaches the foot (B) affecting the skin, pulling on the little filet (C) which opens at the same instant the pore (d), just like pulling on the end of a rope makes a bell at the other end ring at the same time. Opening the pore releases animal spirits from the space (F) which go to the muscles of the leg to pull the foot away from the fire, to the eye muscles to watch, and also to those of the hands. (Free translation of Descartes, 1909. Original edition, 1664.)

milligrams of skin pressure which does not cause pain (Iggo, 1960). In other words they are not specific for nociceptive stimuli.

Certain psychophysical studies have been regarded as supporting the Specificity Theory because of the mathematical relationship shown to exist between the strength of the stimulus and intensity of pain. In this field the investigations of Hardy, Wolff and Goodell over a number of years (1952) are perhaps the most impressive (though it is not suggested that these investigators supported the Specificity Theory). However, there is no doubt that these experiments require the subject to concentrate in a way he might not do with naturally occurring pain, and that this could be expected to alter the psychological state of the subject and his attitude to the pain sensations. Moreover, as Beecher (1959) has pointed out, the characteristics of experimentally produced pain are different from pain caused by disease. Beecher's view is supported by investigations on human teeth which revealed a considerable difference in the quality of sensation as described by subjects experiencing experimental pain and patients suffering from pathological pain (Mumford, 1969).

Specialisation is known to exist in the nervous system and there are well known tracts in the central nervous system. Nevertheless, it is possible to accept physiological specialisation without accepting the psychological assumption that pain is determined entirely by impulses in a straight-through transmission system from the skin to a pain centre in the brain (Melzack and Wall, 1965). This comment can be readily appreciated by anyone who has suffered injury during an exciting game, and not noticed it until later. For the Specificity Theory to have been correct he would have had to feel considerable pain even though sufficiently interested in the game to carry on playing. This also militates against the Intensity Theory.

Also, the concept of a pain centre in the brain is incorrect (Melzack and Wall, 1968; Zimmermann, 1979). Moreover, surgical disruption of nerves, such as by trigeminal tractotomy, may fail to abolish pain in the area; indeed, pain can even become worse. This is because the direct line implied by the Specificity Theory can be by-passed, impulses mediating pain being conveyed to higher levels via the reticular activating system (see Chapter 3).

Finally, even the concept of specific nerve endings is no longer tenable. The Krause and Ruffini endings are absent from the dermis of almost all hairy skin and also from both glabrous and hairy skin of the foot and leg, so it is certain that these structures cannot be the receptors of cold and warmth (Miller, Ralston and

Kasahara, 1960). In fact, these two structures are mechanoreceptors (Iggo, 1977). No cutaneous receptors have an absolute specificity though they have a high degree of selective sensitivity; that is, a much reduced threshold to one form of stimulation, e.g. mechanical indentation, in contrast to their thresholds for all others, e.g. temperature change (Iggo, 1977). In a modified form, then, the organisation of peripheral receptors and their response is compatible with the Specificity Theory.

## PROTOPATHIC AND EPICRITIC THEORY

Head and Rivers (1908) postulated the existence of two groups of cutaneous sensory nerves extending from the periphery to the central nervous system, the protopathic and the epicritic systems. The protopathic system is primitive, yielding diffuse impressions of pain, including extremes of temperature, and is ungraded. The epicritic system is concerned with touch, discrimination and small changes in temperature, and is phylogenetically a more recent acquisition.

Walshe (1948) regarded the theory as fatally handicapped by a fallacious notion of the structure of peripheral machanisms of cutaneous sensibility. Nevertheless, he thought there was material for more realistic interpretation. Mountcastle (1966) found the words valuable, and Iggo (1966) thought the old idea might be right even though based on wrong evidence. Stanley-Jones (1967) regretted that the theory had become disreputable and that the words protopathic and epicritic were almost *verba non grata* in present-day physiology. Whilst pointing out the difficulties of the theory Sinclair (1967) thought the attributes of the spinothalamic and lemniscal systems irresistibly suggested the sort of distinction made by Head between protopathic and epicritic sensibility. Bowsher and Albe-Fessard (1962) concluded that there are only two basic types of somatic sensation, the discriminative and non-discriminative, the former being phylogenetically recent. Mumford and Bowsher (1976) thought it useful to retain the term 'protopathic for the ill-defined sensory experiences evoked by the activation of small primary afferent fibres in the absence of activity in the Aα and Aβ fibres.

## PATTERN THEORY

Essentially, this theory is that pain sensation depends upon the spatio-temporal pattern of nerve impulses reaching the brain.

According to Weddell (1962) warmth, cold and pain are words used to describe reproducible spatio-temporal patterns or codes of neural activity evoked from the skin by changes in its environment. The precise pattern of nerve impulses entering the central nervous system will be different for different regions and will vary from person to person because of normal anatomical variations. Nevertheless, in an individual person a given stimulus will evoke a certain pattern of activity and no other; this will be learned and will be recognisable. It is also generally meaningful despite the fact that each individual is probably decoding a different pattern; only thus can one individual communicate with another in a manner which is significant.

As support for the theory, Weddell points out the falseness of the common view that corneal stimulation leads to reports only of pain. Lele and Weddell (1956) found that reports of touch, warmth and cold can all be evoked from the cornea in addition to pain provided that suitable stimuli are used. It is interesting to note that pain is similarly reputed to be the only sensation reported from the dental pulp but this is also not the case (Mumford, 1965).

One form of the Pattern Theory of pain is based on a view of all or nearly all receptors being essentially non-specialised (Weddell, 1955) but their qualities are important, including the thresholds of excitation, adaptation rates, response ranges, and the distribution of branches of nerve fibres. These qualities differ considerably. Some are more sensitive to heat, some to pressure; they have different adaptation rates, different stimulus strength — response curves; different sizes and shapes of receptor field, etc. All these factors mean that any individual receptor is specialised to what Melzack (1973) called an 'astonishing degree'. (It will not have escaped the readers' notice that in this one paragraph the words specialised and non-specialised are used to describe the same state. The essential point is that they are not specialised as in the Specificity Theory but there is nevertheless a wide range within the one continuum).

The Pattern Theory is not the whole story, and Weddell (1966) does not completely deny the Specificity Theory, having himself found some specific thermal fibres. However, he stresses the danger of correlating the evocation of a particular sensation with the activity produced in cutaneous nerve fibres by stimuli having specific physical attributes.

Melzack and Wall (1965) also point out the risks of premature attempts at correlating anatomical, physiological and psychological observations. Both as regards teeth and other tissues it is obvious on reflection that the designation of sensation as hot, cold, tingling, etc., is somewhat arbitrary since there are many grades between. This is reflected in the multiplicity of words and phrases used by patients and human experimental subjects to whom the same stimulus is applied (Mumford, 1969).

## GATE CONTROL THEORY

Without accepting the simplistic view of the original Specificity Theory there seems no doubt that the smaller nerves fibres, being of high threshold, are important in the mediation of impulses which play a part in producing the sensation of pain. These smaller fibres conduct more slowly than do large fibres so impulses in the latter reach the spinal cord (or brain stem) first. Here, Noordenbos (1959) postulated, the 'fast fibres exert an inhibiting influence on the slowly conducting fibres'. Loss of large fibres, as in post-herpetic neuralgia, would then lead to diminished inhibition of small fibre activity, thereby causing pain.

Melzack and Wall (1965) took this further with the concept of a Gate Control. This theory of pain takes into account the relative input of neural impulses along large and small fibres, the modulating activity of the former on the latter, and additional modulation by impulses descending from higher centres.

The small nerve fibres reach the dorsal horn of the spinal cord and relay impulses to further cells which transmit them to higher levels (Fig. 4.2). The large nerve fibres have collateral branches which carry impulses to the substantia gelatinosa where they stimulate secondary neurones (Fig. 4.2). These substantia gelatinosa cells (SG) terminate on the smaller nerve fibres just as the latter are about to synapse, thus reducing their activity; i.e. causing presynaptic inhibition. The result is that ongoing activity is reduced or stopped altogether — the 'gate' is closed. If, for any reason, the large nerve fibres carry fewer impulses their modulating activity is reduced and the 'gate' opens again. A great deal depends upon their being many more small fibres than large fibres; this means that an intense stimulus will create a barrage of neural impulses and this breaks through the gate.

As the large nerve fibres reach the cord they bifurcate, one branch going to the substantia gelatinosa, as described above. The other branch passes into the dorsal columns on the same side conveying impulses to the dorsal column nuclei (nucleus gracilis and nucleus cuneatus). From here they are relayed to the thalamus and

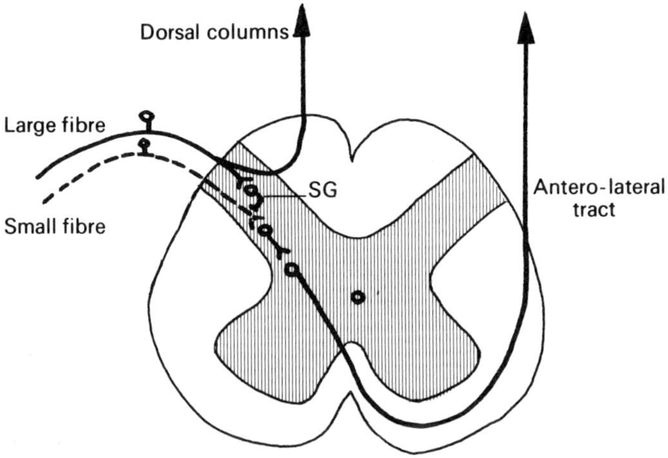


**Fig. 4.2.** The 'gate' which allows modulation of small fibre activity by large fibre activity.

thence to the cerebral cortex. From the cortex efferent fibres descend to the substantia gelatinosa where they, too, exert a modulating activity. This also controls onward transmission by closing the gate. This descending control is via two systems. One is by corticospinal fibres in the pyramidal tracts; the other is by corticoreticular followed by reticulo-spinal fibres (Melzack, 1973).

Melzack and Wall represented these various activities by the diagram in Fig. 4.3. This illustrates further features of the gate control theory; neural impulses arriving along the small fibres can inhibit the substantia gelatinosa cells thus preventing them from closing the gate. The central control trigger in the diagram is the input to the brain via the dorsal columns, and is effectively a feed-forward loop. The fibres descending from the brain to the gate are a feed-back loop.

The output of the T cells is into the anterolateral tract which conveys impulses to the thalamus (VPL nucleus) and into the reticular formation which conveys impulses to the thalamus (intralaminar nuclei) and to the limbic system. Although the substantia gelatinosa cells are shown in this diagram as inhibiting by presynaptic control, postsynaptic mechanisms are also present (Melzack, 1973). Melzack also pointed out a further possibility for modulation of input to occur at higher levels. The dorsal column fibres and the more slowly conducting spinothalamic fibres project to overlapping areas of the thalamus (VPL nucleus) so modulation of neural inputs could occur there.

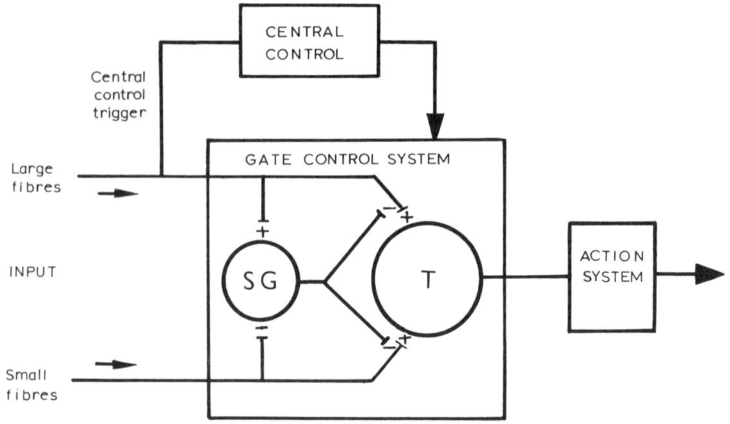


**Fig. 4.3** Cells of the substantia gelatinosa (SG) exert an inhibitory effect on the afferent fibre input. These cells are themselves affected by the afferent fibres in such a way that their influence is increased by activity in the large fibres and decreased by activity in the small fibres (+ is excitatory; — is inhibitory). (Melzack and Wall, 1965, 1968.)

The effect of stimulating peripheral nerves depends upon the total number of active fibres, the nerve impulse frequency, and the balance of activity in large and small fibres. Consequently the output of the transmission cells may differ from the total input that converges on them from the peripheral fibres. The signal that triggers the action system responsible for pain experience and response occurs when the output of the transmission cells reaches or exceeds a critical level. There is no evidence, they say, that activity in the small number of high threshold fibres is more important for pain perception and response than that in the low threshold fibres (Melzack and Wall, 1968).

The brain is able to exert control over the sensory input by means of its descending fibres, the gate control system being set and reset as the temporal and spatial patterns of the input are analysed. This analysis depends on attention, emotion, memories of past experience, anticipation, anxiety, suggestion, hypnosis, conditioning and culture (Casey and Melzack, 1967). Reducing central influence opens the gate whereas increasing it closes the gate. The presence or absence of pain therefore depends upon the balance between the peripheral and central inputs to the gate control system.

It may thus be appreciated how the above psychological factors can have a profound effect on pain experienced by patients with orofacial pain or subjected to operative treatment, and they will be considered in the next chapter.

The Gate Control Theory explains how people suffering from toothache may obtain relief by the application of heat to the face. The well known soothing effect would result from excitation of additional large nerve fibres, activity of which would close the gate mechanism, thereby reducing the through-put of the noxious impulses. Fig. 4.4 represents the arrangement in the trigeminal system, comparable with that in the spinal cord (Fig. 4.2).

The Gate Control Theory has been supported by some investigations (e.g. Besson *et al.*, 1972), and has also been the subject of adverse criticism (Franz and Iggo, 1968; Zimmerman, 1968) some of which has been rebutted (Dawson, Merrill and Wall, 1970). Though the cutaneous input arriving in the dorsal horn is subjected to modification this cannot be attributed simply to an effect of large fibres on small ones (Dykes, 1975). In particular, the small fibre input was found to be also capable of producing inhibition rather than facilitation (Zimmermann, 1979). The debate continues but the theory is not now accepted in the form as originally proposed. Nevertheless, it has been of great value in provoking argument and stimulating research. It has also been

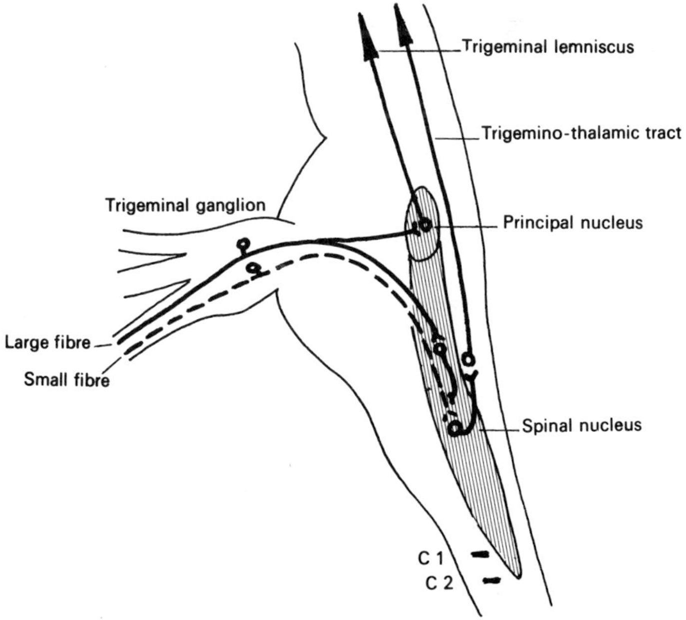


**Fig. 4.4** The 'gate' in the trigeminal spinal nucleus.

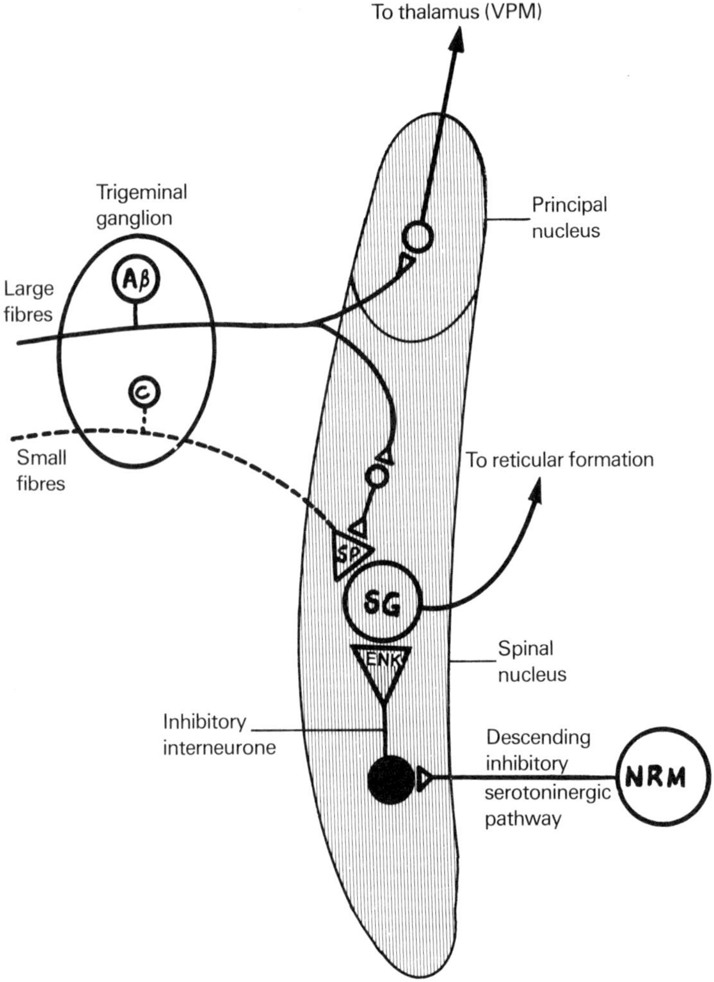


**Fig. 4.5.** The small unmyelinated nerve fibres (C) are now thought to have terminals containing substance P as a neurotransmitter (SP). This excites cells of the substantia gelatinosa (SG) which project to the reticular formation and towards the thalamus. The large myelinated fibres (Aβ) have axon collaterals which can exert presynaptic inhibition either directly or via an inhibitory interneurone. The enkephalinergic interneurone (ENK) exerts postsynaptic inhibition, and is itself subjected to descending control from the nucleus raphe magnus which in turn is affected by events in the periaqueductal gray matter. (Based on Bowsher, 1980a, b.)

found possible to modify the theory as new knowledge becomes available, and clinicians and scientists seem to think in terms of some updated form of the Gate Control Theory. One major advance that the theory has been able to accommodate is the discovery and deeper understanding of the various peptides in the nervous system (Fig. 4.5, and see also descending control pathways in Chapter 3). The theory has encouraged a fresh look at the methods available for dealing with pain, especially intractable pain, and some of these methods will now be mentioned since they illustrate not only how therapeutic advantage can be taken of the theory but also how the control systems seem to work.

*Dorsal column stimulation*

By a surgical operation a plastic disc holding electrodes is placed within the vertebral canal alongside the dorsal columns of the spinal cord. The lead from these electrodes is placed beneath the skin and terminates in a convenient accessible place. Externally, a radiofrequency generator is provided with a lead to a ring antenna which is placed over the terminal of the internal electrodes. The skin, of course, intervenes but the externally generated impulses are transferred to the internal circuit by induction (similar to the system with the cardiac pacemaker). The result is that the dorsal columns are subjected to stimulation and the dorsal column fibres conduct neural impulses both up and down the spinal cord. The patient adjusts the frequency of stimulation, etc., to give the desired pain relief.

It is supposed that the neural impulses descending (antidromic) in the dorsal column fibres pass into the collateral branches to stimulate the substantia gelatinosa cells which then modulate the

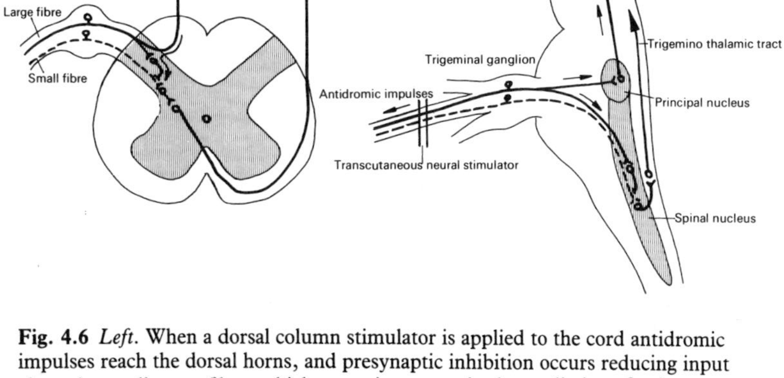


**Fig. 4.6** *Left.* When a dorsal column stimulator is applied to the cord antidromic impulses reach the dorsal horns, and presynaptic inhibition occurs reducing input along the small nerve fibres which are so important in the mediation of pain. *Right.* With a transcutaneous neural stimulator applied to (say) the cheek orthodromic impulses cause presynaptic inhibition in the trigeminal spinal nucleus, thus reducing input along the small nerve fibres.

input along the smaller fibres (Fig. 4.6 left). It would not be expected that such activity could modulate input within the trigeminal system, but the ascending impulses (orthodromic) in the dorsal column fibres are conveyed to higher centres and might have an influence on the trigeminal system in this way. Moreover, the situation is much more complex than the simple version just given and a great deal still needs to be learned.

*Transcutaneous nerve stimulation*

This is a much simpler method using electrodes (usually moistened pads) which are placed on the skin, one being over the painful area, and the other elsewhere. The stimulus intensity, frequency and duration are adjusted by the patient to obtain relief from pain, the rationale being that the electrical stimulation generates synchronous activity in the large fibres and their collaterals; these neural impulses go to the substantia gelatinosa allowing reduction of impulses in the smaller nerve fibres. This method can also be used in the trigeminal area (Fig. 4.6 right), and has been shown to raise the pain perception threshold of human teeth (Mumford, 1976), though this method of treating orofacial pain has been found to have only limited value. For intra-oral pain it may be necessary to incorporate an electrode in a denture-type appliance (Mumford, 1980b).

*Cerebral stimulation*

Not many people are prepared to have electrodes placed in their brains but, for those who are desperate, where all the more conventional methods have been tried, this may be done. Using stereotaxic methods the electrodes are applied to the periaqueductal gray matter and stimulation results in reduction or relief of pain (Richardson and Akil, 1977; Hosibuchi, Adams and Linchitz, 1977). This is supposed to be by activation of enkephalinergic neurones which descend to the raphe nuclei in the brain stem reticular formation (Bowsher, 1980b). Here fibres arise which descend in the dorsolateral funiculus of the spinal cord to end in the substantia gelatinosa where they activate enkephalinergic interneurones and these postsynaptically block transmission in the small primary afferents. Comparable descending fibres go to the trigeminal oralis and caudalis nuclei (Lovick, West and Wolstencroft, 1977; Bowsher, 1980a) (Fig. 4.5), where it has been shown, in cats, that suppression occurs of responses evoked by tooth pulp stimulation (Sessle et al, 1976; Lovick and Wolstencroft, 1979).

## CONCLUSION

The Intensity Theory and Specificity Theory as simply stated do not give a satisfactory explanation of pain, but it is accepted that high intensity stimulation is a factor, and some measure of specificity exists in so far as receptors have selective sensitivity and some have higher thresholds of excitation than others and may be called nociceptors. The present concept of specificity may be stated in the words of Mountcastle (1967), 'when active, different sets of nerve fibres elicit different sensations by virtue of their central connections, and a given set therefore elicits an identical sensation no matter how activated'. In modern terms it seems desirable to retain at least a part of the concept of protopathic and epicritic sensibility, provided the concept is restricted to the central nervous system, and it might be better to use the words non-discriminative and discriminative. The pattern of impulses reaching the central nervous system is important, as are the modulating effect and central control suggested in the Gate Control Theory. The author therefore thinks of these different theories of pain as being partial contributions to the whole rather than as mutually exclusive, and ventures the following statement of his own interpretation of the various theories.

When a part of the body is stimulated the physical character of the stimulus is first modified by the tissue which intervenes between the stimulus and the nerve receptors, the extent of this modification depending upon the nature and condition of the intervening tissue. Cornified skin has a greater influence than non-cornified areas, and dentine and enamel have an even greater effect (Mumford, 1980a).

The physiological properties of the receptors are of great importance for they vary in their thresholds to thermal change, chemical concentrations, mechanical distortion, peak sensitivity, adaptation rates, size of receptive field, etc. Considering the density and overlap of free nerve endings in the skin (and in the dental pulp or cornea) there is therefore an enormous range in the way in which neural impulses are generated; e.g. the number, frequency, and distribution in different fibres. These neural impulses reach the dorsal horn in the spinal cord (or the trigeminal spinal nucleus in the brain stem) in a staggered manner, depending on conducting rates in the various nerves fibres. Here the neural impulses are modulated at the various synapses before being transmitted to higher levels; the integration being complex as suggested by the

Gate Control Theory. Pain occurs when the impulses arrive in the brain in a particular pattern and intensity.

Some neural impulses pass rapidly to the brain via the dorsal column nuclei (or the principal nucleus of the trigeminal system) where they are relayed to the thalamus (ventroposterior nucleus) where they are again relayed to the sensory areas of the cerebral cortex. Here somatotopic representation permits recognition of the site of stimulation. This is a discriminative feature of pain.

Other neural impulses ascend more slowly via the neo-spinothalamic tract (or neo-trigeminothalamic tract) to the ventro-posterior nucleus of the thalamus where they are relayed to the sensory cortex, and this system also permits localisation.

Further neural impulses are conveyed even more slowly via the multisynaptic paths of the reticular fomation to the hypothalamus and the thalamic intralaminar nuclei, etc. (see Chapter 3). From here impulses are conveyed to various parts of the brain. Because of the diffuse and primitive nature of the reticular formation and the large amount of converging neural traffic these impulses do not convey discrete spatial or temporal information though a limited and rather vague degree of localisation may be possible.

The neural impulses conveyed to the hypothalamus generate emotional responses, the feeling state being quantity dependent. If the neural frequency and spatial pattern warrant it there may be fear, with hyperadrenalinaemia and its concomitants of increased pulse rate, altered respiration and 'butterflies in the stomach', etc. This emotional feature of pain is primitive and may demand imperative action, ordinary on-going behaviour being disrupted until something is done to get back to normal. In other words, this is the motivational aspect of pain (do something!). However, the disruption of ongoing activity can be regarded as the appropriate action in itself, rest being desirable for healing (Wall, 1979).

From the thalamic intralaminar nuclei neural impulses reach the cortex via the diffuse thalamocortical projection, thus allowing them to be analysed in the cortex, not just by themselves but in relation to information from other parts of the body including the eyes and ears. It is also related to previous experience to evaluate its significance. Does it indicate a threat or not? Does something have to be done? If so, can action be delayed until a more convenient time? If action is necessary the appropriate neural signals for this are initiated via the motor areas of the cortex. (Reflex action will already have dealt with any essential withdrawal). This cognitive and evaluative feature of pain depends on such factors as culture which will be considered in Chapter 5.

The above statement suggests a vast number of possible arrangements of neural impulses spread over a wide continuum so it is evident that the author does not regard pain as a sensation strictly separated from all others. Finally, not enough is known about chronic pain or the emotional and cultural components of pain (to be discussed in Chapter 5). In particular, the influence of higher brain functions on the periaqueductal gray matter needs to be elucidated, thereby testing the speculative hypothesis that brain stem inhibiting systems can be influenced by psychological variables (Zimmermann, 1979).

## REFERENCES

Beecher, H.K. (1959) *Measurement of Subjective Responses.* New York: Oxford Univ. Press.

Besson, J. M., Conseiller, C., Hamann, K. F. and Maillard, M. C. (1972) Modification of dorsal horn activities in the spinal cord, after intra-arterial injection of bradykinin. *J. Physiol. (Lond.)*, **221**, 189–205.

Bishop, G. H. (1946) Neural mechanisms of cutaneous sense. *Physiol. Rev.*, **26**, 77–102.

Bolles, R. C. and Fanselow, M. S. (1980) A perceptual-defensive-recuperative model of fear and pain. *Behavioural and Brain Sci.*, **3**, 291–323.

Bowsher, D. (1980a) Central mechanisms of orofacial pain. *Brit. J. oral Surg.*, **17**, 185–197.

Bowsher, D. (1980b) Peptides and pain. In *Persistent Pain. Modern Methods of Treatment*, Vol. 2, ed. Lipton, S., pp. 189–202. London: Academic Press.

Bowsher, D. and Albe-Fessard, D. (1962) Patterns of somatosensory organization within the central nervous system. In *The Assessment of Pain in Man and Animals*, ed. Keele, C. A. and Smith, R., pp. 107–122. Edinburgh: Livingstone.

Casey, K. and Melzack, R. (1967) Neural mechanisms of pain; a conceptual model. In *New Concepts in Pain and its Clinical Management*, ed. Way, E. L. Philadelphia: Davis.

Dawson, G. D., Merrill, E. G. and Wall, P. D. (1970) Dorsal root potentials produced by stimulation of fine afferents. *Science*, **167**, 1385–1387.

Descartes, R. (1664) L'Homme. In *Œuvres de Descartes*, pp. 119–215. Published 1909. Paris: Adam and Tannery.

Dykes, R. W. (1975) Nociception. *Brain Res.*, **99**, 229–245.

Franz, D. N. and Iggo, A. (1968) Dorsal root potentials and ventral root reflexes evoked by nonmyelinated fibres. *Science*, **162**, 1140–1142.

Hardy, J. D. (1962) The pain threshold and the nature of pain sensation. In *The Assessment of Pain in Man and Animals*, ed. Keele, C.A. and Smith, R., pp. 170–201. Edinburgh: Livingstone.

Hardy, J., Wolff, H. and Goodell, H. (1952) *Pain Sensations and Reactions.* Baltimore: Williams and Wilkins.

Head, H. and Rivers, W. R. H. (1908) A human experiment in nerve division. *Brain*, **31**, 323–450.

Hosibuchi, Y., Adams, J. E. and Linchitz, R. (1977) Pain relief by electrical stimulation of the central gray matter in humans and its reversal by naloxone. *Science, N. Y.*, **197**, 183–185.

Iggo, A. (1960) Cutaneous mechanoreceptors with afferent C fibres. *J. Physiol. (Lond.)*, **152**, 337–353.

Iggo, A. (1966) Part of a general discussion in *Touch, Heat and Pain*, ed. de Reuck, A. V. S. and Knight, J., p. 144. London: Churchill.

Iggo, A. (1977) Cutaneous and subcutaneous sense organs. *Brit. Med. Bull.*, **33**, 97–102.

Keele, C. A. and Armstrong, D. (1964) *Substances producing Pain and Itch.* London: Arnold.

Lele, P. P. and Weddell, G. (1956) The relationship between neurohistology and corneal sensibility. *Brain*, **79**, 119–154.

Lovick, T. A., West, D. C. and Wolstencroft, J. H. (1977) Interactions between brain stem raphe nuclei and the trigeminal nuclei. In *Pain in the Trigeminal Region*, ed. Anderson, D. J. and Matthews, B., pp. 307–318. Amsterdam: Elsevier/ North-Holland.

Lovick, T. A. and Wolstencroft, J. H. (1979) Inhibitory effects of nucleus raphe magnus on neuronal responses in the spinal trigeminal nucleus to nociceptive compared with non-nociceptive inputs. *Pain*, **7**, 135–145.

Melzack, R. (1973) *The Puzzle of Pain.* Harmondsworth, Middlesex. Penguin.

Melzack, R. and Wall, P. D. (1965) Pain mechanisms; a new theory. *Science*, **150**, 971–979.

Melzack, R. and Wall, P. D. (1968) Gate control theory of pain. In *Pain*, ed. Soulairac, A., Cahn, J. and Charpentier, J., pp. 11–31. London: Academic Press.

Miller, M. R., Ralston, H. J. and Kasahara, M. (1960) The pattern of cutaneous innervation of the human hand, foot and breast. In *Cutaneous Innervation*, ed. Montagua, W., pp. 1–47. *Advances in Biology of Skin*, Vol. 1. Oxford: Pergamon.

Mountcastle, V. B. (1966) Part of a general discussion in *Touch, Heat and Pain*, ed. de Reuck, A. V. S. and Knight, J., p. 144. London: Churchill.

Mountcastle, V. B. (1967) The problem of sensing and the neural coding of sensory events. In *The Neurosciences*, ed. Quarton, G.C., Melnechuk, T. and Schmitt, F. O., pp. 393–408. New York: Rockefeller Univ. Press.

Mumford, J. M. (1965) Pain perception threshold and adaptation of normal human teeth. *Archs. oral Biol.*, **10**, 959–968.

Mumford, J .M. (1969) Measurement of toothache. *J. Brit. Endo. Soc.*, **3**, 48–51.

Mumford, J. M. (1976) Influence of transcutaneous neural stimulation on the pain threshold of human teeth. In *Proceedings of the First World Congress on Pain*, ed. Bonica, J. J. and Albe-Fessard, D. G., pp. 415–419. *Adv. Pain Res. Therap.*, Vol. 1. New York: Raven Press.

Mumford, J. M. (1980a) Transmission mechanisms in dental pain. *Brit. J. oral Surg.*, **17**, 198–217.

Mumford, J. M. (1980b) Atypical facial pain. In *Persistent Pain. Modern Methods of Treatment*, ed, Lipton, S. pp. 249–281. London: Academic Press.

Mumford, J. M. and Bowsher, D. (1976) Pain and protopathic sensibility. A review with particular reference to the teeth. *Pain*, 223–243.

Mumford, J. M. and Newton, A. V. (1971) Convergence in the trigeminal system following stimulation of human teeth. *Archs. oral Biol.*, **16**, 1089–1097.

Noordenbos. W. (1959) *Pain: Problems Pertaining to the Transmission of Impulses which give rise to pain.* Amsterdam: Elsevier.

Richardson, D. E. and Akil, H. (1977) Pain reduction by electrical brain stimulation in man. *J. Neurosurg.*, **47**, 178–183, 184–194.

Sessle, B. J., Dubner, R., Greenwood, L. F. and Lucier, G. E. (1976) Descending influences of periaqueductal gray matter and somatosensory cerebral cortex on neurones in trigeminal brain stem nuclei. *Canad. J. Physiol. Pharmacol.*, **54**, 66–69.

Sinclair, D. (1967) The major theories. In *Cutaneous Sensation.* Sinclair, D. pp. 362–382. Oxford: Oxford University Press.

Stanley-Jones, D. (1967) Protopathy, paraesthesia and sensory suppressor zones. In *Progress in Brain Research*, 23. *Sensory Mechanisms*, ed. Zotterman, Y., pp. 200–218. Armsterdam: Elsevier.

Wall, P. D. (1979) On the relation of injury to pain. *Pain*, **6**, **253–264**.

Zimmerman, M. (1979) Peripheral and central nervous mechanisms of nociception, pain and pain therapy: facts and hypotheses. In *Proceedings of the Second World Congress on Pain*. ed. Bonica, J. J., Liebeskind, J.C. and Albe-Fessard, D. G., pp. 3–32. *Adv. Pain Res. and Therap.*, Vol. 3. New York: Raven Press.

Walshe, F. M. R. (1948) *Critical Studies in Neurology*. Edinburgh: Livingstone.

Weddell, A. G. M. (1962) Observations on the anatomy of pain sensibility. In *The Assessment of Pain in Man and Animals*, ed. Keele, C. A. and Smith, R., pp. 47–59. Edinburgh: Livingstone.

Weddell, A. G. M. (1966) Concluding discussion in *Touch, Heat and Pain*, ed. de Reuck, A. V.S. and Knight, J., pp. 359–360. London: Churchill.

Weddel, G. (1955) Somesthesis and the chemical senses. *Ann. Rev. Psychol.*, **6**. 119–136.

Zimmerman, M. (1968) Dorsal root potentials after C-fibre stimulation. *Science*, **160**, 896–898.

# 5

# Pain threshold and reaction to pain

When people talk of the pain threshold it is not always clear what they mean because at least two thresholds can be defined — the pain perception threshold and the pain reaction threshold. The former is the least possible pain sensation that can be perceived and is fairly stable from person to person and from time to time. The pain reaction threshold is the level at which a person or an animal reacts to pain, as shown by moaning or pulling away from the source of pain. This is much more variable, depending to a large extent on psychological and other factors which will be described later.

## PAIN PERCEPTION THRESHOLD

The pain perception threshold is the lowest intensity of pain just perceived by a person under given conditions. It applies only to human beings since animals are obviously unable to communicate the fact that they have just perceived pain at this minimal intensity. It is important to note the given conditions because the pain perception threshold depends on many factors including the part of the body being investigated, the nature of the stimulus and the area of contact made between the body and the stimulating object.

The person whose pain perception threshold is being measured may be a subject who has volunteered for scientific investigation or a patient undergoing a clinical test. In either case the procedure to be used is first explained to him and he is then required to pay attention as the stimulus is gradually increased. When he observes the slightest perceivable pain he indicates this in some way such as by raising his arm, pressing a button or moving a lever. It is essentially a method of determining the excitability of the sensory receptors at the site being tested under carefully defined conditions, sufficient nerve impulses being generated for the effect to be conveyed to consciousness in the attentive subject.

For clinical tests on teeth, as when pulp testing, it is most convenient if the patient indicates that the threshold has been reached by simply saying 'ah' at which point the intensity of the stimulus is noted, and is called the threshold value.

**Relationship to animal experiments**

Although animals cannot tell an investigator that they have just perceived minimal pain, physiological experiments can be made to record the nerve impulses produced as a result of stimuli which are presumed to cause pain. This involves dissection to reach the nerve fibres concerned and such a procedure is not usually possible on human beings, but an elegant investigation by Hensel and Boman (1960) deserves mention. Under carefully controlled conditions human volunteers were each given an ultra-short anaesthetic while the superficial branch of the radial nerve was dissected free from connective tissue. With the subject recovered and conscious, various stimuli were applied while recordings of nerve impulses were made. At the same time the human subject was able to give an account of his sensations. Perhaps the most remarkable thing about the experiments was that for hair receptors the mechanical stimulus required for a threshold sensation was of the same order as that for setting up a single impulse in a single nerve fibre! In contrast, thermal sensations were aroused only from a stream of nerve impulses. (However, it appears that each hair may be associated with several nerve fibres so some neural impulses may not have been recorded.) It might be expected that a stream of impulses would also be needed for pain to be perceived, and this view is supported by investigations on human teeth (Mumford and Newton, 1971).

More recently, Torebjörk and Hallin (1974a, b) have been able to insert fine electrodes intradermally in awake human subjects, applying them to the radial nerves. Subjects spontaneously reported increased pain when C fibres were recruited.

**Lowest intensity of pain**

Determination of the pain perception threshold usually requires that the stimulus be increased so that pain is perceived in every case, but for experimental rather than clinical purposes it is possible to determine an even lower threshold in the following way. A subthreshold stimulus is applied a number of times and of course there is no response from the subject. The stimulus intensity is increased until the subject responds to one of the stimuli. The stim-

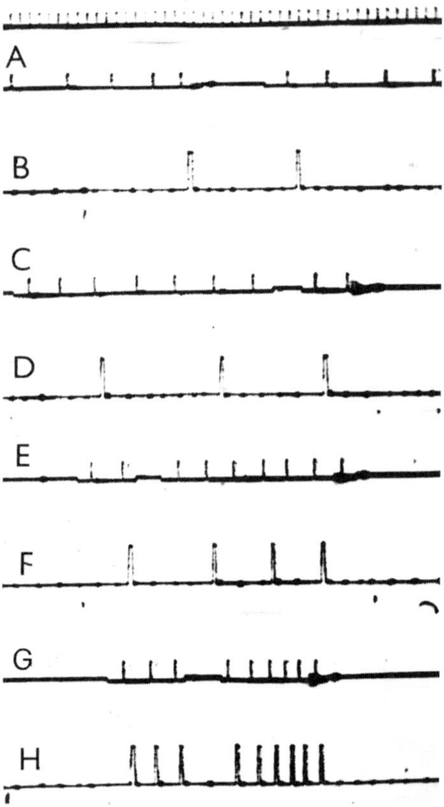


**Fig. 5.1.** The number of responses increased as the stimulus intensity increased. The first line is a time scale with one second intervals.

A Stimuli were applied to the tooth and recorded as shown.

B The human subject indicated that he felt the stimulus on only 2 occasions.

C and D. There were 3 responses.

E and F. There were 4 responses.

G and H. There was a response to each stimulus.

The delay in responding is the reaction time. In no case was there a false response in the absence of a stimulus.

ulus is increased further until the subject responds to two of the stimuli, and so on until the subject responds to all of them (Fig. 5.1). It is this last result which is equivalent to the usually accepted single clinical test because in the latter case the stimulus is increased for each patient as much as may be necessary to produce a response. However, a purist could reasonably argue that the strict threshold was one out of ten, or one out of a hundred, or one out of an even larger number. To say the least this would be an inconvenient experimental criterion. A more usual method, especially used in testing drugs, is to determine the stimulus needed to give 50 per cent responses.

Notice that with experiments such as those just described it is necessary to use 'blind testing'; in other words the subject is not allowed to know when the stimulus is being applied.

## Quality of sensation

For a long time it was usually thought that pain was the only sensation elicited by stimulation of pulpal nerves (Brashear, 1937; Goetzl, Bien and Lu, 1951; Brookhart, Livingston and Haugen, 1953; Boréus and Sandberg, 1955; Anderson and Howard, 1958; Heng Chin and Domino, 1961; Scott and Tempel, 1963; Kawamura and Nishiyama, 1966; Greenwood, 1973; Olgart, Haegerstam and Edwall, 1974; Horiuchi and Matthews, 1974). However, the quality of sensation has been assessed by questioning subjects who had had their teeth subjected to electrical stimulation to determine the pain perception threshold (Mumford, 1965). Some subjects found difficulty in expressing themselves, and some used more than one word, but in 229 tests the following words were used. Tingling (104 times), pain or slight pain (62), cold (44), sharp (31), warm or hot (24), toothache (13), pressure or pulp swelling (8), dull twinge (4), electric or galvanic (4), non-painful twinge (1), vibration (1). Since then numerous subjects have stated quite firmly that the sensation was not necessarily pain. They have said that when they reported cold sensation they did not mean a cold pain; and similarly for the hot sensation. Hannam, Siu and Tom (1974) also found sensations other than pain, as did Martin and Chapman (1979).

Sometimes, when the margin of a filling is defective it is possible to press the teeth together in such a way as to set up a feeling of tension within the crown and this lasts for several seconds after the pressure is released. This may be related to the suggestion of Lowenstein and Rathkamp (1955) that there might be pressure receptors in dentine (as well as in the periodontium). They thought that tactile sensibility might be at least partly mediated by pulpal nerves.

It could therefore be argued that pain is not the only sensation arising from stimulation of dental nerves, and why should the teeth only have 'pain' fibres?

It used to be said that the free nerve endings in skin mediated only pain, leaving the Krause and Ruffini end organs to mediate cold and warmth, but this is no longer accepted (Specificity Theory, Chapter 4). Similarly, nerve fibres in the cornea were supposed only to mediate pain until Lele and Weddell (1956) obtained reports of touch, cold, and heat as well as pain.

Leaving the periphery and considering more central factors further doubt is expressed. Greenwood (1972) remarks that 'if pain is the only sensation evoked in man when the dentine or pulp is stimulated, whatever the nature of the stimulus, it is surprising to find activity evoked by stimulation of the tooth pulp in parts of the trigeminal nuclei other than the nucleus caudalis'. In 1973, she went further, 'the pattern of activity evoked in the (spinal) nucleus by tooth pulp stimulation . . . is difficult to reconcile with the notion of specific nociceptive neurons'.

Having recorded from cells within the nucleus oralis Davies *et al.* (1971) also found this a surprising localisation if it is assumed that pain is the only sensation from the pulp.

The sensations reported by patients are important in pain investigation and have been subjected to analysis as in the McGill Pain Questionnaire (Dubuisson and Melzack, 1976). This consists of three classes of word descriptors — for sensory quality, affective quality, and evaluative. Although some words are synonymous others indicate different intensities and there are also sub-classes, e.g., the sensory qualities include temporal, spatial, thermal etc. This pain questionnaire has been found to be a reliable multidimensional measure of immediate pain rather than pain over some defined period of time (Godham *et al*, 1980). Also, memory for pain, assessed by using this questionnaire has been found to be more accurate than expected (Hunter, Phillips and Rachman (1979); recall was over a 5 day period, and this observation is obviously important in clinical practice.

The relationship between word descriptors and stimulus intensity has been investigated by Mumford and Stanley (1981). For experimental subjects, at the threshold of sensation the highest electrical stimulus was needed for pain, followed in descending order by burning, hot, tingling, sharp, 'other', cold and warm. The position of burning is important in relationship to the difficult clinical problem of patients who complain of burning pain.

### Metaesthesia

The discrepancy between the different views is perhaps less than appears because, to some extent, a semantic difficulty is involved. Variability of sensation appears to be a feature of low-intensity pain and, to take this into account, Smith (1962) has suggested that the weaker 'non-painful' sensations be termed metaesthetic and stronger painful sensations termed algaesthetic. This is a useful division.

Related to this Shimizu (1964) reported that 'pre-pain' sensation became painful when the stimulus intensity was increased by amounts ranging from 5 per cent to as much as 165 per cent.

It could be that in scientific investigations of the pain perception threshold the stimulus should be raised until the effect is frankly painful (though volunteers might be harder to find!). For clinical tests, however, such as in dental pulp testing the object is essentially to find if the pulpal nerves are functioning, indicating a vital pulp, and for this purpose the very earliest sensation is sufficient. There is no reason why patients should be made to suffer unnecessarily.

**Strength-duration relationship**

As stated above the conditions must be carefully defined since many factors influence the result. Those affecting determinations on teeth will be considered later but one fundamental effect common to all stimuli will be considered here. It is the strength-

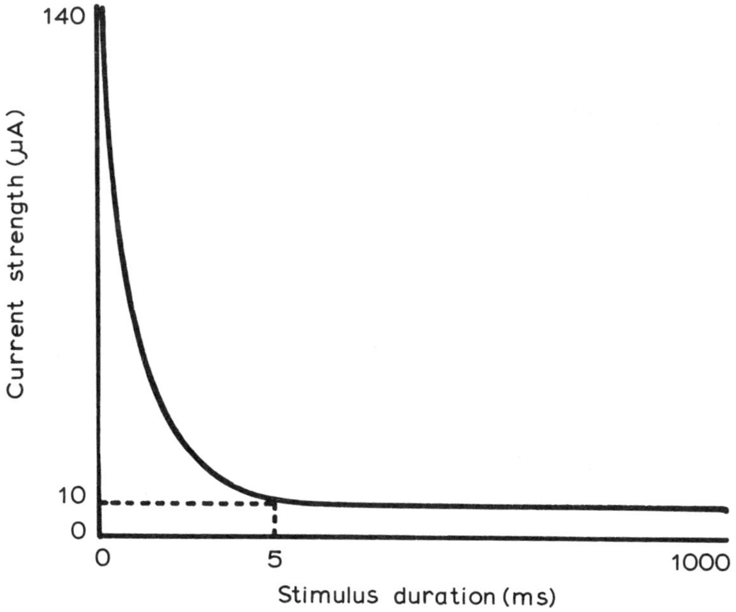


**Fig. 5.2.** Strength-duration curve obtained by stimulating a human tooth to determine the pain perception threshold. In this example 10 $\mu$A is the rheobase, i.e. the lowest current intensity which, continued for an infinite time, will just cause pain perception. Notice that the abscissa is logarithmic.

duration relationship. The strength (intensity or amplitude) of a stimulus required to produce perception of pain depends upon the duration of the stimulus. If the pain perception threshold is determined using stimuli of different durations the results can be plotted to give a strength-duration curve. This has been done for normal human teeth (Mumford, 1965) and a representative result is shown in Fig. 5.2. The stimulus used was a repetitive square wave electrical stimulus because this can be accurately defined and measured. A comparable result obtained by exposing the skin of the forehead to heat showed a lowest intensity of 45 m cal/sec/$cm^2$ and this required 90 seconds of exposure to the heat (Hardy, Jacobs and Meixner, 1953).

## THRESHOLD VALUES FOR TEETH

Provided that the appropriate conditions are maintained the pain perception threshold is fairly reproducible. The best known work on this topic is that of the Hardy, Wolff and Goodell group (1940) who, then and subsequently, used a thermal dolorimeter on human skin. It is more appropriate here, however, to review the threshold values published for human teeth subjected to thermal, osmotic, pressure and electrical stimuli.

### Thermal thresholds

Hensel and Mann (1956) found that the threshold of pain was reached when the dentino-enamel junction cooled to 26·4°C, at which stage the temperature of the pulp had undergone no significant change. This suggested to them that pain due to temperature change originates in dentine. On stimulating with heat the corresponding temperature was 47·7°C. This is similar to the threshold on applying heat to undamaged skin (Lynn, 1980).

Naylor (1961) found the threshold of sensation to cold stimuli to be in the range of 26·1°C–31·4°C.

It is interesting to note that raising the temperature of the pulpodentinal junction to 45°C in dogs has been shown to produce many nerve impulses (Funakoshi and Zotterman, 1963).

### Osmotic thresholds

The main investigations have been carried out by Anderson and his co-workers who applied various materials to the teeth including ethanol, glycerol and solutions of sugars and calcium chloride. Analysis of these (Anderson and Matthews, 1967) has shown that the lowest threshold value was 25 atmospheres, obtained when using dextrose, with a mean threshold value for all solutions of 380 atmospheres.

## Pressure thresholds

By applying hydrostatic pressures to bare dentine Brännström (1961) was able to cause pain in some cases. The lowest pressure to do this was 2 kg/cm$^2$ (0.196 MN/m$^2$), which is thus the threshold value. It is interesting that such a pressure has been shown to produce an electrical potential across the dentine, and this might be part of the mechanism by which pain is perceived (Mumford and Newton, 1969).

## Electrical thresholds

Pain perception threshold values for normal teeth are given in Table 5.1 (Mumford, 1965). The considerable range that exists is presumably at least partly due to experimental variations but there appears to be a definite tendency towards lower threshold values for teeth at the front of the mouth. The threshold values rise as teeth are situated more posteriorly, and this has also been demonstrated by Björn (1946).

Notice that these values and the ones that follow were obtained with a stimulus duration of 30 milliseconds repeated 20 times per second (20 Hz). Similar values have been obtained using a stimulus duration of 10 ms at 50 Hz which is a more convenient stimulus to use where it is the mains supply frequency.

**Table 5.1.** Pain Perception Threshold Values for Normal Teeth. The stimulus duration was 30 ms with a frequency of 20 Hz and an electrode area of 9.5 mm$^2$ (Mumford, 1965)

| Upper teeth | Number tested | Mean threshold value ($\mu$A) | Range of threshold values ($\mu$A) | Standard deviation |
|---|---|---|---|---|
| Central incisors | 40 | 6·4 | 2·4–14·5 | 2·53 |
| Lateral incisors | 40 | 6·3 | 2·9–12·3 | 2·50 |
| Canines | 40 | 8·9 | 2·6–19·1 | 2·96 |
| First Premolars | 20 | 7·5 | 2·2–14·5 | 3·37 |
| Second premolars | 20 | 7·9 | 2·5–17·0 | 3·35 |
| First molars | 10 | 14·0 | 6·8–20·5 | 4·95 |
| Second molars | 9 | 13·8 | 8·8–18·0 | 3·99 |
| *Lower teeth* | | | | |
| Central incisors | 20 | 5·6 | 2·2–10·5 | 2·36 |
| Lateral incisors | 20 | 7·0 | 3·1–11·0 | 2·31 |
| Canines | 20 | 8·3 | 3·1–15·0 | 3·24 |
| First premolars | 20 | 8·8 | 3·8–15·2 | 3·48 |
| Second premolars | 20 | 8·7 | 3·2–14·0 | 3·01 |
| First molars | 6 | 10·1 | 6·5–15·2 | 3·33 |
| Second molars | 12 | 11·8 | 8·5–17·0 | 2·68 |

*Influence of age on the threshold value*

The values given in Table 5.1 were for subjects aged 18–28 years, but similar values were obtained for patients aged 58–73 years and for children aged 10–15 years. This does not support the usual view that teeth in children of this age are less sensitive. Harkins and Chapman (1976) obtained similar results for old people, and it seems that there is no obvious change in sensitivity to electrical stimulation from the age of 10 years to 73 years. Moreover, this also applies to retained deciduous teeth in this age group (Mumford, 1971).

For children aged 6–9 years inclusive it was not found possible to obtain adequate results by the methods of the author. Although the children were intelligent and co-operative they gave false results, such as by indicating the pain threshold even when the stimulator was not connected to the power supply! It seems possible that the state of innervation of the teeth at that age is a factor (Mumford, 1965).

*Influence of sex on the threshold value*

The first 120 teeth of Table 5.1 were divided equally between male and female subjects. Statistical analysis revealed the mean values of the pain perception thresholds to be 7·8 microamps for males and 6·5 microamps for females. The range for males was 3·7–19·1 microamps compared with 2·4–18·6 microamps for females, the standard deviations being 3·31 and 3·12. Further analysis gave a variance ratio of 5·98 which is significant at the 5 per cent level but not at the 1 per cent level. This suggests that females have a lower pain perception threshold than males. However, earlier work (Mumford, 1963) suggested that the pain perception threshold for females was higher. It is therefore considered that, with this form of stimulation, any difference that may exist between the pain perception thresholds of males and females has not been clearly demonstrated.

*Influence of ongoing activity on the threshold value*

There is a constant barrage of neural impulses reaching the central nervous system from all over the body and this input plays a role in determining the threshold of sensation (Nathan, Noordenbos and Wall, 1973).

Neural input from adjacent areas has a more important influence than that from farther afield because of neuronal convergence which allows spatial summation to occur. The influence of this on the pain perception threshold has been demonstrated by stimulating adjacent teeth in human subjects; when one incisor is subjected to a subthreshold electrical stimulus the adjacent incisor needs less than the normal stimulus for perception to occur (Mumford and Newton, 1974a, b).

**Adaptation**

One of the sources of variability when making pain measurements on teeth is adaptation. This occurs after excitation and means, in psychophysical terms, that the subject ceases to feel sensation even though the stimulus is continued. In neurological terms it is the diminution in frequency of nerve impulses and their eventual cessation, even though the stimulus is continued (Chapter 2). It is not the same as accommodation, which develops before nerve excitation occurs, and is the gradual raising of the threshold level caused by a stimulus which rises too slowly to cause early excitation.

When teeth are stimulated electrically so that threshold pain occurs, after a while pain is no longer observed, i.e. adaptation occurs. This is illustrated by Fig. 5.3 which represents the traces made on a polygraph to indicate the stimulus amplitude and also the subject's indication of his pain experience. The basis of this is presumed to be reduction of neural activity due to fatigue.

The adaptation time has been measured and ranged from 3–34 seconds with a mean value of 11·6 seconds (Mumford, 1965), but see below. In this investigation nerve impulses were not recorded,

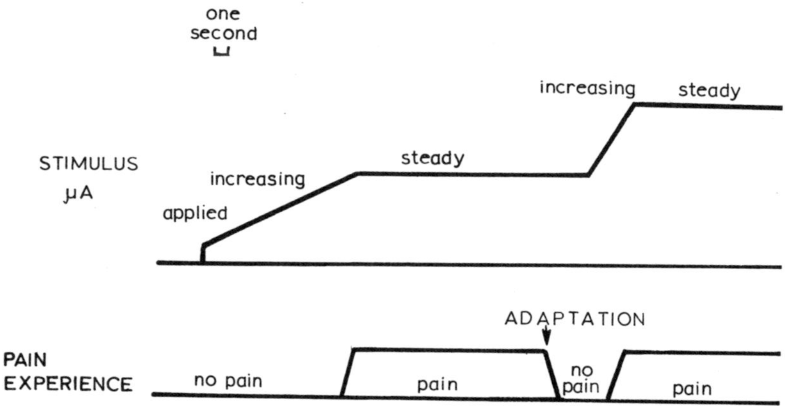


**Fig. 5.3.** Polygraph traces showing adaptation to a repetitive stimulus. The upper trace indicates the peak current value of an electrical stimulus applied to a tooth of a human subject. When he experienced pain he moved a lever which formed the lower trace on the polygraph.

but Yamada and Sakada (1961) have done so working on dogs. After applying threshold concentrations of various chemicals to the teeth, impulses in the inferior dental nerve gradually ceased. Such adaptation is in agreement with adaptation to threshold pain in skin due to thermal stimuli (Stone and Dallenback, 1934; Hardy and Stolwijk, 1966).

It may be supposed that adaptation does not occur for supra threshold stimuli because Hensel (1960) found complete adaptation of skin receptors only within the range 19–40°C, and Kenshalo and Scott (1966) obtained similar results. Indeed, Hardy (1966) pointed out that, although adaptation occurs in skin on being heated to temperatures up to 45°C, beyond that temperature there is no adaptation and pain even becomes worse. However, whilst investigating pain tolerance by stimulating teeth Mumford, Newton and Ley (1973) found some human subjects 'getting used to' repetitive electrical impulses at a strength several times the pain perception threshold value, but more intense stimuli seem to require longer times for adaptation to occur. Adaptation does require a longer time when stronger pressures are applied to periodontal nerves of a cat, as indicated by cessation of nerve impulses (Kawamura *et al.*, 1965).

When adaptation occurs in teeth the subjective effect is that the sensation gradually fades, although the stimulus intensity is maintained at the threshold value. Since the pain perception threshold is defined as the least discernible sensation it might reasonably be objected that the sensation could not then diminish, but this is what the subjects report and it is compatible with the facts given in the earlier section of this chapter on the *Lowest intensity of pain.* It should be noted that, throughout these investigations, the subjects were not able to indicate with precision the moment when the sensation came, and they usually found it even more difficult to be sure of when it ceased.

This adaptation may not be exactly what happens when the sensitivity of a cavity diminishes with a sequence of stimulations from osmotic agents (Anderson and Ronning, 1962). In such a case diminution of the fluid flow in dentine is a factor (Anderson, Matthews and Goretta, 1967), as it was in Brännström's investigations. He found that when the cavity in the test tooth was exposed to reduced pressure or a stream of air, pain lasted for the duration of the experiment when it lasted as long as 3 minutes, but not when the experiment lasted 5 minutes (Brännström, 1960a, b). After subjection to the air stream for 5 minutes the dentine was insensitive to scraping with a sharp probe. In four teeth tested for a further 20 minutes the insensitivity to scraping and to the air stream persisted.

Further work is needed on the subject of adaptation in human teeth before it is fully understood. Meanwhile it should be regarded as being due to more than one factor.

**Cortical evoked response**

If stimulation causes nerve impulses to be conveyed to the brain this produces at the cerebral cortex an electrical potential change called the cortical evoked response. This potential change cannot be recorded as a single response because it is too small to show up against the normal variability of the electroencephalogram (E.E.G.). However, if a considerable number (say 50 or more) of evoked responses are produced and the E.E.G. tracings are analysed by a suitable computer the average response becomes apparent. It is tempting to regard this evoked response as an indication that the neural impulses initiated by the stimulus have reached consciousness, and that it is a physical indication of perception, but the two factors are not necessarily co-incident. It has been shown (in cats) that changes in attention produce alterations in the evoked response (Hernández-Peón, 1966; Hernández-Peón *et al.*, 1957). Moreover, cortical evoked responses are detectable with sensory inputs below the adequate level of conscious sensation (Fig. 5.4) even when the human subject's attention is directed to the stimulus (Libet *et al.*, 1967). Perception presumably requires awareness but this problem is a very difficult one and still controversial. As described in Chapter 3 the reticular activating system is considered to play an important part in determining which incoming information (in the form of neural impulses) is worthy of attention.

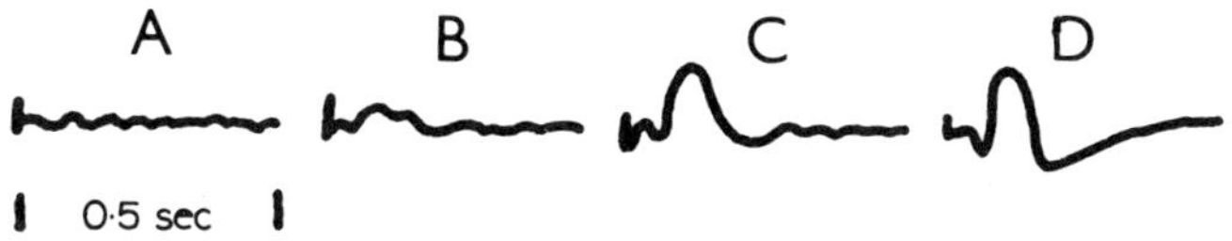


**Fig.5.4.** Average evoked potentials at the somatosensory cortex following stimulation of skin, each trace the average of 500. (Derived from Libet *et al.*, 1967.)

**A.** No evoked potential.
**B.** Small evoked potential but the human subject did not experience a sensation.
**C.** Greater evoked potential, but the subject did not feel all of the 500 stimuli.
**D.** Evoked potential greatest. The stimulating current was twice that used for C, and all the stimuli were felt distinctly.

### Differential threshold

Once the pain perception threshold has been reached the differential threshold is the smallest change in stimulus intensity which the subject can detect. It produces a difference in sensation which is just noticeable, and which is called the just noticeable difference (jnd). According to Hardy, Wolff and Goodell (1947, 1952) there were 21 jnds between perception and the highest intensity of pain. They also made 2 jnds equal to 1 'dol' which was then supposed to be a unit of pain. On this basis pain of moderate intensity would be 3–5 dols. However, despite the high reputation of these investigators, their view in this respect is not generally accepted. In the author's investigations on teeth the higher intensities of pain, at the pain tolerance level, seemed to rise and fall and rise again in a wave (subjects' description). How could this sensation be placed on such a scale?

Keele and Armstrong (1964) and others use a much simpler scale of pain intensity ranging from nil to mild, moderate, severe and very severe. The author uses a similar scale which is illustrated in later chapters. It is only an ordinal scale and the intervals are not regarded as being equal. In other words, the difference between mild and moderate does not equal that between moderate and severe.

## PAIN TOLERANCE

It is common knowledge that pain can be better tolerated by some people than by others, but Wolff (1968) has defined pain tolerance more specifically. It is the largest stimulus that can be tolerated by a subject under given experimental conditions, and it is the same as the severe pain threshold (Merskey and Spear, 1967). If the pain perception threshold has also been determined the difference between the two values is the pain sensitivity range (Wolff, 1968), or the reaction interval (Merskey and Spear, 1967).

Newton and Mumford (1972) have determined the pain tolerance of human subjects by stimulating their teeth electrically. The pain perception threshold of each tooth was first determined, after which each was again stimulated, the subject having been asked to allow pain to increase until it was too unpleasant to tolerate, whereupon he signalled, and the current amplitude was noted. For 144 anterior teeth in 24 subjects the mean pain perception threshold was 5·35 microamps whereas the mean pain tolerance was 15·52 microamps, giving a mean value for the pain sensitivity range of 10·17 microamps. The drawback of using the pain sensitivity range is that a simple physical change such as a crack that allowed a wider current path would result in a higher pain threshold value and a proportionately greater pain tolerance level, and hence a greater pain sensitivity range — which might be misleading. In comparison, this adverse factor would be compensated by using a ratio, so it is considered that the factor which might be most significant is the ratio between the perception and tolerance level. This is called the Pain Tolerance Ratio, expressed as pain tolerance/pain perception threshold. For the above 144 teeth the mean value of the pain tolerance ratio was 2·9.

It is thought that the pain tolerance is more likely to be affected by psychological factors than the pain perception threshold, and that it is likely to be lower in cases associated with anxiety or depression (Sternbach, 1976).

### Lateral dominance

Most people are right-handed, this side being dominant, and it has been suggested (Wolff, 1968) that this influences pain perception, the dominant side being less sensitive; i.e. it has a higher pain perception threshold. Moreover, it is suggested, the dominant side can withstand more pain; i.e. it has greater pain tolerance.

The subject was reviewed by Merskey and Watson (1979) who found that pain is more often lateralised on the left (except for idiopathic trigeminal neuralgia). They suggested that this might be because the right cerebral hemisphere is dominant for emotional experience, and is less well able to integrate sensory information. However, they also thought that few studies provided evidence that the right and left sides of the body have differential sensitivity. Using electrical stimulation on the upper anterior teeth of 24 subjects (Newton and Mumford, 1972) found that the pain perception thresholds were not significantly different on the right and left sides. Also there was no significant difference in pain tolerance.

## REACTION TO PAIN

Reaction to pain naturally depends at least partly on the intensity of pain but patients suffering from pain react in different ways. Some show no change in behaviour and, if questioned, admit only reluctantly that pain is present. Others have fixed expressions as though the slightest facial movement would make matters worse. Some nurse the affected part, such as by cradling the face in a bent arm or resting it in the hand. Some moan or complain to anyone who will listen. Some weep noisily, others silently, while in some cases the whole body is involved, the patient rocking to and fro in misery. This behaviour may make the situation worse especially if it affects onlookers, but it may be helpful to the affected individual because of the additional sensation it provides (Petrie, 1967). In this respect it is related to the pleasant stimulation afforded by a warm pack applied to the face of a toothache sufferer. It is recognised that the increased sensory input afforded by muscular and tactile activity might inhibit pain (Albe-Fessard, 1968).

**Significance of pain**

Perhaps the most important factor affecting reaction to pain is its significance or feared significance. A pain in the leg might well elicit less of a reaction than a pain of equal intensity in the chest because the latter might appear to the sufferer to signify heart disease. Pains in the head (including the face) are also regarded with greater apprehension since they might appear to threaten the innermost being. Some cases of toothache fall into this category, especially those that cannot be treated expeditiously and successfully. Less fortunate patients for whom investigation and treatment are more prolonged should be reassured about the outcome whenever possible. Perhaps it is true to say that reassurance in some form is always possible. Fear must be controlled for failure to do so leads to continued adrenalinaemia with raised blood pressure and increased pulse rate.

The significance of pain to the individual is not only considered in organic terms, for other factors are involved, one of the best examples being that given by Beecher (1956). He found that American soldiers wounded in battle, at the Anzio beach landings during World War II, needed to be given less pain killing drug than did civilians in the U.S.A. suffering from comparable injuries. The reason for this difference was apparently that for the soldiers the wound meant that they would be removed from the battle zone and able to return home, whereas the civilians were worried about the effect on their jobs and loss of income for their families.

The significance of pain is not the same for pathological pain and experimentally induced pain. With pain of pathological origin the patient is threatened, whereas with experimental pain there is no threat because the experiment can be terminated at any time. Beecher (1962) regards the two kinds of pain as differing from

**Table 5.2.** Subject's Description of the Quality of Sensation or Pain Felt in His Tooth

| Quality of pain | Patients complaining of toothache (110 cases) | Subjects stimulated electrically (290 teeth) |
|---|---|---|
| | *per cent* | *per cent* |
| No answer | 30 | 0 |
| Ache | 19 | 0 |
| Throbbing | 10 | 0 |
| Sharp | 7 | 12 |
| Hot | 2 | 10 |
| Cold | 2 | 23 |
| Tingling | 2 | 37 |
| Other words | 28 | 18 |

each other, and it is interesting that dental patients describe the two differently. Investigations on teeth gave the results shown in Table 5.2 (Mumford, 1969).

## Personality

Common experience suggests that personality is an important factor in determining pain reaction. It is obvious that some people complain about a mild level of pain which might be ignored by others. On the other hand stoical personalities appear to tolerate severe pain with little apparent reaction. To some extent this is a feature of environment and upbringing, boys in particular being encouraged to 'grin and bear it'.

According to Petrie (1967) persons with higher extraversion scores, as determined by the Maudsley Personality Inventory, are more tolerant of both experimental and pathological pain.

The emotional display of patients does not give a clear indication of painfulness or the amount of associated damage. Indeed, cases are sometimes seen when such a display is not the result of pain, but because pain has been successfully stopped and the patient is merely indicating his (perhaps more usual her) relief.

When examining objects by tactile sense some individuals appear to think the objects are larger than they really are whereas others consider them to be smaller. Petrie (1967) has called these people augmentors and reducers respectively. She demonstrated that augmentors will feel painful stimuli to be greater than they really are, thereby suffering greater pain, whereas reducers will feel less pain in similar circumstances. This subject is considered further in Chapter 19.

Mumford, Newton and Ley (1973) analysed the personalities of 39 clinical dental students using the Sixteen Factor Personality Questionnaire (Cattell and Eber, 1964; Cattell, 1967). The students then had electrical impulses applied to their teeth to determine the pain perception threshold and the pain tolerance level, each measured in microamps. It was found that there was no statistically significant correlation between personality and either of these factors, or with the interval between the two factors, or with the ratio between them. It could be that these intelligent, co-operative, non-apprehensive subjects, though not having a personality influence on experimentally induced pain, might have revealed an influence had pain been of pathological origin and therefore threatening.

**Psychological factors**

It is said that everybody is psychologically ill at some time in his life, so when a person suffers in this way he should recognise that in this respect he is like everybody else, and be unafraid of asking for help. Unfortunately, many people do not behave in this way and regard psychological illness as fundamentally different from other ills. They think that it is one thing to have a damaged leg or sick stomach but something quite different to have a sick mind which must be kept hidden. For this reason they may ask for help in an indirect manner, complaining about something which they regard as being socially more acceptable, and one way of doing so is to complain of pain in the face, mouth or teeth. They may in fact have such a pain, and dental disease is so common that there may be no difficulty in finding an apparent dental cause for the pain, in which case the teeth and the patient are treated in a routine manner and pain may cease. This is desirable as far as it goes for dental disease may contribute to the patient's stress, but the background neurosis may remain so that the patient continues to seek dental treatment at a time when the physician's help would be more appropriate. If the dentist asks a few pertinent questions the patient is likely to reveal a life situation which is, for the moment, too much for him, and he can then be referred to his medical adviser. Timely questioning in these cases can avoid numerous dental procedures which in themselves are likely to be stress producing.

Psychological aspects of pain are considered at greater length in Chapter 19.

## Cultural attitudes

There are wide differences in cultural attitudes to pain. Some people accept it as inevitable and bear it with fortitude, whereas others regard it as completely avoidable and do their best to achieve this end.

In some cultures pain is deliberately inflicted, perhaps self-inflicted, to attain a desired status, such as by filing the incisor teeth to make them sharp, or cutting large areas of skin. This is comparable with experimentally induced pain rather than pain of pathological origin and is significant, not of disease, but of achievement. In the one case bearing the pain soon removes the threat of failure, perhaps of not attaining adulthood, whereas with pain of pathological origin continuing to bear the pain means that the disease is still present.

In dental practice it is possible to improve a patient's reaction to pain by using the idea of success as opposed to failure, since we have a cultural pattern which respects achievement. This is likely to be especially suitable for children.

## Anticipation and apprehension

Anticipation of pain is an important part of pain experience and usually makes it seem worse. It is better for the patient not to see the hypodermic needle, and advisable not to talk about it unnecessarily. On the other hand the threat of pain from an operation may make pathological pain appear less and even disappear. The hoary old joke about toothache stopping in the dentist's waiting room is related to this; the threat of the drill or forceps makes the patient increasingly apprehensive until the existing toothache seems the lesser of two evils and he hastily departs. Such behavioural disturbance is fortunately less common nowadays, but fears in this category are still important, and dentists' waiting rooms should be carefully planned and situated to avoid any unpleasantness as well as providing quiet distraction.

## Attention and distraction

During periods of pleasant emotional stress, or of high interest, damage may occur but pain is not necessarily noticed until later. Pain can also be reduced by deliberately distracting the sufferer, and the opposite effect is at least partly the explanation of how toothache seems worse at night when distraction is not so readily available, the rest of the family being asleep and television programmes ended. The sufferer, lying restless and sleepless, dwells on the pain which seems to become worse (which means that it does become worse) and he grows afraid that it might become so much worse as to be intolerable. Moreover, help is not readily available, not before morning at the earliest, so the condition is more threatening, and some people 'break down'; in other words the entire personality is threatened. Under these conditions a child with toothache can and does disrupt the entire family.

Distraction is also effective in reducing pain caused by operative procedures, and this is partly the explanation of how audeoanalgesia works. Gardner and Licklider (1959) were able to carry out cavity preparation, scaling and even extractions without any local or general anaesthesia, simply using audeoanalgesia but some patients did experience moderate pain.

The patient is provided with recorded music together with a masking sound. The latter is sometimes called 'white sound' and is likened to the noise of a waterfall. To hear the music properly, against the background of white sound, the patient must concentrate, thus focusing his attention away from the potentially painful operative procedures. Another factor is probably the increased sensory input. As mentioned earlier, Albe-Fessard (1968) has pointed out that pain may be inhibited by intense muscular and tactile activity.

During operative procedures the patient should concentrate on relaxing and breathing regularly as this gives him something on which to focus his attention, and certainly seems to reduce pain experience. For those patients who request it, quiet background music is helpful, but white sound seems unnecessary, the noise of the air turbine being sufficient in itself.

It should be fully understood that one of the most important features of modern neurophysiology is enhanced recognition of brain control over the inflow of sensory impulses. The effect of this is to sort out sensory impressions so that some receive attention and others do not. It is highly desirable to educate patients to understand that each person can learn to exercise this control himself, at least to some extent. The most unpleasant sensations have been eliminated from modern dentistry already. The lesser ones can be controlled in the above manner so that treatment is often a pleasant relaxed experience.

**Biofeedback**

This involves a form of operant conditioning in which some physiological process is recorded and amplified so that the patient can see or hear it. The objective is to enable the patient to learn to control it and, in so doing, to control his symptoms; the electromyograph can be used to control muscle tension, or the skin temperature to reduce migraine. As usual, the non-specific effects of personal attention and care plus the distraction and satisfaction of 'doing something' are helpful, and relaxation can be expected to help, but a survey of the literature has revealed inadequate controls in many cases (Jessup, Neufeld and Merskey, 1979).

### Diurnal variation

There appears to be an influence on pain of circadian rhythm, the intensity of pain being greatest in the evening, but the effect is multifactorial, other factors being related to sex difference and whether or not patients go out to work (Glynn and Lloyd, 1976; Lloyd, 1977).

### Reassurance

A good way of reducing pain reaction is by reassuring the patient whenever possible, and this can be done at the diagnosis stage, during treatment and when treatment has been completed. For this to be effective there must have been a comprehensive investigation, with radiography, etc, and possibly a second opinion, so that reassurance can be given with authority. The reassurance offered during operative treatment is also a distraction, and patients treated in this way can be seen to relax; in some cases a patient can be 'ordered' to relax, with great success.

### Hypnosis and suggestion

There can be no doubt that hypnosis has a profound effect on a patient's reaction to what would otherwise have been painful stimulation. There appear to be two essential requisites for hypnosis to occur. Firstly, the subject's sensory input must be reduced. In addition to the room being quiet there must be bodily relaxation so as to reduce input from the body itself; i.e. muscular relaxation. Secondly, the subject must have such good rapport with the hypnotist to allow him to take over responsibility; to take his decisions. In other words, the subject must suppress his critical faculties allowing his conscious mind to be by-passed. The more this suppression is achieved the greater is the depth of hypnosis (Scott, 1974).

It is said that up to 90 per cent of people can attain the lightest level of hypnosis (Scott, 1971). Though not exactly the same, this state is akin to the state we pass through just before going to sleep and on waking. Furthermore, in about 20 per cent of people hypnoanalgesia can be sufficient to carry out surgical procedures without an anaesthetic.

In general a therapist hypnotises the patient using methods that depend on suggestion. These suggestions are made in the form of predictions about to be fulfilled — 'your eyelids are beginning to feel heavy' — and, as a rule, the patient must wish the hypnotic state to develop. Indeed, it is quite possible for a patient to hypnotise himself, although the author has treated only one patient who regularly used self-induction to achieve a hypnotic state sufficiently deep to allow routine operations on her teeth, and she was medically qualified. However, many patients are able to relax to a stage akin to light hypnosis. In these cases suggestion by the dentist is particularly successful, and it should be used routinely to help lessen pain reaction. It is really an early phase of hypnotic suggestion.

The mechanism of hypnosis is obscure but there is an altered state of consciousness associated with a trusting relationship with another person (Finer, 1980), and the subject's intelligence, personality and motivation are factors. It is thought that hypnotic analgesia is unlikely to involve the central pain inhibitory mechanism because it is not altered by the administration of naloxone hydrochloride, a specific narcotic antagonist (Barber and Mayer, 1977). In this respect it is different from acupuncture, and the two are also different in time. In some cases hypnosis can become effective in a second whereas acupuncture requires about 20 minutes. Similarly hypnosis can terminate almost instantly whereas the effects of acupuncture linger.

Barber and Mayer also found an increase in pain threshold, including that of the teeth.

**Body image**

A person has a concept of the boundaries of his body but this is not obvious unless part of it is lost. Thus, a severed limb may still seem to be 'there', almost as though there is a denial of loss and the person is trying to maintain his body boundary. However, it is not always the entire limb that seems to be present; often only the hand or foot is present, apparently attached to the remaining stump. This is distressing in itself but even worse is the fact that the phantom hand or foot can be painful, possibly very painful.

The above explanation is not accepted by many people who prefer a more neurophysiological explanation. Neural impulses still pass along the severed nerves within the stump and, reaching the central nervous system, may be interpreted as originating in what were the peripheral branches. This explanation is not yet adequate and will need additions to explain all the features of phantom limb.

Phantom teeth are considered in Chapter 13.

**Pain behaviour and pain games**

A sick person becomes the recipient of more attention than usual. When a man is sick at home his wife cooks his favourite food and keeps the children quiet. When a woman is sick her husband helps with the housework and does the shopping. In hospital a person receives gifts of fruit, flowers, chocolates and magazines. He is relieved of his everyday responsibilities to work etc., father-figure doctors listen to his troubles, attractive young nurses smooth the bed clothes and see that the pillows are comfortable, nursing sisters dispense drugs which make the patient feel good; he may even be paid by state or private insurance. There is a lot to be said for it.

Unfortunately, this treatment may be so pleasant that the patient may want it to continue; there is a powerful disincentive to getting better. It follows that hospital staff and family must realise that such cosy treatment must come to a halt as soon as possible, and this proper ending is normally achieved. Some patients, however, may seek to maintain the pleasant status of being a patient, claim that the pain (or other trouble) continues and thus throw responsibility on to the clinician to continue looking after him. The clinician then has a problem and may have to be rather firm; the pain games that may develop between clinician and patient are amusingly described by Sternbach (1974).

**Sex difference**

It is sometimes said that women react less to pain than do men, possibly because they suffer, or expect to suffer pain in childbirth, but this is difficult to evaluate. In our present society a woman is 'allowed' a few tears which might therefore be discounted, whereas a man in the same condition would be regarded as 'soft'. This view seems to extend to nurses who are much more likely to refuse a man's request for analgesics than a woman's request (Bond, 1978).

Generally speaking a man is the breadwinner, and pain associated with damage might make him fearful of the consequences to his family of disability; this could make him react more to pain, as mentioned in an earlier section.

**Effect of age**

As people grow older they experience pain in various ways and mostly get over it. Their enhanced knowledge often helps them to recognise pain of little or no significance, whereas younger people suffering for the first time might be more anxious and react accordingly. In this way pain reaction is probably diminished in older people. Pain perception is not necessarily affected, although operations on teeth in older patients can be less painful because dentinal tubules are probably narrower or blocked, and pulps might have receded, but in such circumstances the effective stimulus would be less anyway — pain reaction is not necessarily being measured.

**Acupuncture**

In classical Chinese medicine it is postulated that a vital force or life energy (ch'i) flows through the body in channels or meridians. Disease is associated with disturbance of this flow but, fortunately, the fault can be corrected by inserting one or more needles into the meridian concerned. The point of insertion is an acupuncture point (Acus — a needle) and there are approximately a thousand of these located along the meridians. The appropriate meridian is determined mainly by means of the pulse diagnosis; the radial pulse is taken at each wrist using three fingers, first with light pressure and then with heavy pressure. This procedure yields information about twelve pulses named after the twelve main meridians which are themselves named after the internal organs such as the stomach, heart and liver. The Chinese physician does not neglect the case history, nor does he omit appropriate inspection and palpation.

Tao, the ancient Chinese religion, has an influence for it is the way of maintaining harmony in this world as well as beyond (Veith, 1966; Rawson and Legeza, 1973). The complementary opposites, Yin and Yang, influence the flow of ch'i and should be taken into consideration, these being the mutual affinities as well as the mutual antipathies. Further factors which influence the choice of acupuncture point are the five elements, wood, fire, earth, metal and water. The time of day must also be considered since the life energy (ch'i) flows through the body in a 24-hour cycle. This is a very brief statement and even an entire textbook might not adequately cover the subject. Further reading does not guarantee a proper understanding and it can safely be said that a western-trained person finds the concepts involved to be difficult. One explanation could be that the concepts are wrong, and it would be fair to say that, despite the availability of so many methods of histological investigation, no satisfactory evidence has been seen which supports the existence of meridians and acupuncture points.

However, this may not matter. What does matter is that insertion of a needle stimulates peripheral nerves thus causing neural impulses to go to the central nervous system where they may produce various effects. One such effect is said to be the cure of disease provided this is functional rather than physical; e.g. headache or rheumatism might be cured whereas a fractured bone or a decayed tooth would not heal.

Though used for several centuries for treating disease, acupuncture was not used to produce analgesia until 1958. This followed closely on its use for treating post-operative pain but was not heard of in the west until about 1971. The delay was partly because China was more isolated at that time but also because it did not become popular in China itself until 1968 following the Cultural Revolution (Hoel, 1974; Kaada, 1974).

At first it took 40 needles in all four extremities and four acupuncturists and a kind of conductor to direct the whole thing but research reduced the number of needles to a few or sometimes even one (Geiger, 1973).

The earliest reports suggested that as many as 80 per cent of surgical cases were treated by acupuncture but this became approximately 50 per cent (Kerr, 1973); then 20–30 per cent (Geiger, 1973), 15–20 per cent (Kaada, 1974) and a team from the U.S.A. judged that it is probably used less than 10 per cent of the time and that total incidence of use may be as low as 1·3 per cent of all surgical operations (Ingle, 1973). Some part of this variation may be due to different use in different areas of such a large country.

It is claimed that acupuncture analgesia is successful in most hospitals in about 85 per cent of cases. However, Kaada (1974) draws attention to the fact that this success is graded; even with the top grade of analgesia there is still pain during a few of the surgical steps. Even at this grade pethidine is used in doses of 1–1·5 mg/kg in a 2-hour period.

Below this grade, grades 2 and 3 are also classified as successful. Also the operating field may be washed with a local anaesthetic solution (Brown, 1972; Geiger, 1973; Wall, 1974).

*Electro-acupuncture*

Partly to leave more space around the operating table, the Chinese have provided rhythmic stimulation via the acupuncture needles by using an electric current, and this electro-acupuncture has been used to produce analgesia. Power is derived from dry batteries giving approximately 7·5 volts and the frequency of stimulation is usually 2 Hz. Anderson *et al.* (1973) used a constant current stimulator to determine the pain perception threshold, and found that this was 2·5–3·0 times higher after stimulation than before, a result also obtained by Chapman, Chen and Bonica (1977). Using a similar method, also on teeth, Mumford and Bowsher (1973) did not find that the pain perception threshold was raised even after electro-acupuncture which lasted for 30 minutes at a current intensity as high as 60 mA, an amount of electricity which is not without risk. Neither did they find any convincing change in sensitivity to either light or heavy pinprick on the skin of the anterior part of the chest. Moreover, this intensity of stimulation produced jerking of the limbs which would certainly have disturbed any surgeon. However, intensity is an important factor. Experimental subjects reported lower pain estimates following high intensity acupuncture — sufficient to produce unpleasant sensation and muscle twitch — but not at low intensities (Mao *et al*, 1980). These authors found that only a small proportion of their chronic pain patients were helped by acupuncture. Their depressed and anxious patients were not helped.

Lynn and Perl (1977) were unable to find any localised change to pain producing stimuli at specified places, and this applied to all sensory tests used, for all subjects, for all acupuncture points, for both acupuncturists and for different levels of experimental pain.

Any differences between the results with teeth might be explained by technical difficulties of stimulating teeth electrically (Mumford and Björn, 1962; Mumford, 1963). Other differences might be due to placebo response, suggestion, culture, anxiety reduction, etc.

*Mechanism*

Acupuncture needles may be inserted so that they just penetrate the skin, and this does not hurt because they are fine and sharp. When rotated they drag on the skin causing it to twist in a spiral manner about the needle; this does hurt, presumably by exerting traction on the somatic afferents in the skin. The places most frequently chosen for insertion, as determined by the meridian theory, seem to correspond with areas known to have a rich sensory innervation.

The needles may also be inserted more deeply when they penetrate into muscle in which situation they might be effective by stimulating the muscle afferents. It is presumably by this that needle-less acupuncture is supposed to work. One of the points used in this way is the Ho-ku point (large intestine 4 which lies in the web between the thumb and forefinger) and the muscle is vigorously massaged by deep pressure, presumably sending impulses along the muscle afferents.

In either case neural impulses travel along the afferent nerves to the central nervous system. It has been suggested that acupuncture works to relieve pain by these neural impulses blocking the onward transmission of the impulses already mediating pain (A-delta and C fibres); in other words, by the mechanisms discussed in Chapter 4. However, though blocking is supposed to occur by impulses mediating the sensation of touch the impulses produced by acupuncture are painful in themselves. Moreover, although acupuncture can be applied in the same segment as the pain it is usually applied in some other segment, possibly far removed; for example, in one of our cases (Mann *et al.*, 1973) a man who had suffered right supraorbital post-herpetic neuralgia for 18 months had a single acupuncture needle placed in the skin about 3 cm below the lateral malleolus of the right foot (bladder 62). Pain relief was immediate and lasted 44 hours. At the time it was thought that this result could be explained by neural impulses being conveyed via the spinal cord to the spinal trigeminal nucleus, probably via the spino-reticulo-trigeminal route. Now, however, it seems that the neural input is conveyed to the brain causing release of endogenous opioid peptides from the periaqueductal gray matter with subsequent descending inhibition of pain (Chapter 3). This view is supported by work on rats (Toda, 1978; Takeshiga *et al*, 1979; Takeda *et al*, 1979).

Another suggestion is that the subject is in a hypnotic state, but this does not seem correct for the cases seen by the author. Also, the cases treated in China which have been shown on film and reported in various publications do not appear to have been hypnotised. Nevertheless, hypnosis seems to be a factor in some cases. Though many patients smile happily during operative procedures under acupuncture analgesia and even eat and drink, others, witnessed in China, lie sufficiently immobile to suggest a hypnotic state (Kerr, 1973). Moreover, people can be hypnotised and still have their eyes open (Wall, 1972; Kroger, 1973). It is well known that hypnosis can be induced by repetition of rhythmic stimulation, and acupuncture is certainly rhythmic whether by digital movement or electrical stimulation. It also seems possible that the most suitable subjects for acupuncture could be those who would also be the best subjects for hypnosis.

Conditioning is also a factor in some cases. Prior to operation under acupuncture analgesia in China the patient is in the hospital for several days so that he will understand how the method works.

The factor of attention is very important and seems to operate at two levels. At the cortical level, a person concentrating on some absorbing activity is less likely to notice a stimulus that would be presumed painful. Similarly, a person in pain can be distracted by something that excites his attention. At a lower level the reticular formation plays an important part in attention as described in Chapter 3 (Moruzzi and Magoun, 1949). Suggestibility is a possible factor but Anderson *et al.* (1973) did not find this.

Analysis of any method of treatment should include double blind investigations with inert drugs (or deceptive surgery), randomisation of the treatment given and statistical analysis of the results, but it is not easy to know how an inert or deceptive acupuncture needle could be used. It is certain, however, that the placebo response will be present and it is well known that in many therapeutic situations approximately a third of cases will show some success for this reason alone. Not the least factor in this placebo will the factor of the patient being given attention — that somebody cares. The placebo response is considered to be especially strong in people who have a burning faith, and this would appear to apply to many people in China at the present time.

Culture also has an important influence on a person's tolerance of pain and his reaction to it. Associated with this are ethnic, educational and propagandist factors, all of which could enhance the results of acupuncture. At least part of this effect would be by descending control from the cerebral cortex.

It seems reasonable to conclude that a number of different factors play a part in acupuncture which is further supported by the drugs mentioned earlier, and it will be some time before the method is properly understood.

## REFERENCES

Albe-Fessard, D. (1968) Central nervous mechanisms involved in pain and analgesia. In *Pharmacology of Pain*, ed. Lim, R. K. S., Armstrong, D. and Pardo, E. G., pp. 131–168. Oxford: Pergamon.

Anderson, D. J., Curwen, M. P. and Howard, L. V. (1958) The sensitivity of human dentine. *J. dent. Res.*, **37**, 669–677.

Anderson, D. J. and Matthews, B. (1967) Osmotic stimulation of human dentine and the distribution of dental pain thresholds. *Archs. oral Biol.*, **12**, 417–426.

Anderson, D. J., Matthews, B. and Goretta, C. (1967) Fluid flow through human dentine. *Archs. oral Biol.*, **12**, 209–216.
Anderson, D. J. and Ronning, G. A. (1962) Osmotic excitants of pain in human dentine. *Archs. oral Biol.*, **7**, 513–523.
Anderson, S. A., Ericson, J., Holmgren, E. and Lindqvist, G. (1973) Electro-acupuncture. Effect on pain threshold measured with electrical stimulation of teeth. *Brain. Res.*, **63**, 393–396.
Barber, J. and Mayer, D. (1977) Evaluation of the efficacy and neural mechanism of a hypnotic analgesia procedure in experimental and clinical dental pain. *Pain*, **4**, 41–48.
Beecher, H. K. (1956) Relationship of significance of wound to pain experienced. *J. Amer. med. Ass.*, **161**, 1609–1613.
Beecher, H. K. (1962) An inspection of our working hypotheses in the study of pain and other subjective responses. In *The Assessment of Pain in Man and Animals*, ed. Keele, C. A. and Smith, R., pp. 159–169. Edinburgh: Living-stone.
Björn, H. (1946) Electrical excitation of teeth. *Svensk tandl. Tidskr.*, **39**, Suppl.
Bond, M. R. (1978) *Pain, its Nature, Analysis and Treatment*. Edinburgh: Churchill Livingstone.
Boréus, L. O. and Sandberg, F. (1955) A comparative study of different algesimetric methods in animals and man. *Acta Pharm. Tox. Kbh.*, **11**, 198–214.
Bowsher, D. (1972) Personal communication. 4 May 1972.
Brännström, M. (1960a) Dentinal and pulpal response. I. Application of reduced pressure to exposed dentine. *Acta odont. Scand.*, **18**, 1–15.
Brännström, M. (1960b) Dentinal and pulpal response. II. Application of an air stream to exposed dentine. *Acta odont. Scand.*, **18**, 17–28.
Brännström, M. (1961) Dentinal and pulpal response. V. Application of pressure to exposed dentine. *J. dent. Res.*, **40**, 960–970.
Brashear, A. D. (1937) The controversy concerning the innervation of the teeth. *J. dent. Res.*, **16**, 5–17.
Brookhart, J. M., Livingston, W. K. and Haugen, F. P. (1953) Functional characteristics of afferent fibres from tooth pulp of cat. *J. Neurophysiol.*, **16**, 634–642.
Brown, P. E. (1972) Use of acupuncture in major surgery. *Lancet*, **1**, 1328–1330.
Cattell, R. B. (1967) *The Scientific Analysis of Personality*. Harmondsworth, England: Penguin.
Cattell, R. B. and Eber, H. W. (1964) *Handbook for the Sixteen Factor Personality Questionnaire*. Champaign, Illinois: The Institute for Personality and Ability Testing.
Chapman, C. R., Chen, A. C. and Bonica, J. J. (1977) Effects of intrasegmental electrical acupuncture on dental pain: evaluation by threshold estimation and sensory decision theory. *Pain*, **3**, 213–227.
Davies, W. I. R., Scott, D. Jr., Vesterstrøm, K. and Vyklicky, L. (1971) Depolarization of the tooth pulp afferent terminals in the brain stem of the cat. *J. Physiol. (Lond.)*, **218**, 515–532.
Dubuisson, D. and Melzack, R. (1976) Classification of clinical pain descriptions by multiple group discriminant analysis. *Exptl. Neurol.*, **51**, 480–487.
Finer, B. (1980) Hypnotherapy. In *Persistent Pain. Modern Methods of Treatment*. Vol. 2, ed. Lipton, S. pp. 27–57. London: Academic Press.
Funakoshi, M. and Zotterman, Y. (1963) A study in the excitation of dental pulp nerve fibres. In *Sensory Mechanisms in Dentine*, ed. Anderson, D. J., pp. 60–72. Oxford: Pergamon.
Gardner, W. G. and Licklider, J. C. R. (1959) Auditory analgesia in dental operations. *J. Amer. dent. Ass.*, **59**, 1144–1149.
Geiger, J. (1973) How acupuncture anaesthetizes: The Chinese explanation. *World Medicine*, Aug. 22, 15–22.

Glynn, C. J. and Lloyd. J. W. (1976) The diurnal variation in perception of pain. *Proc. Roy. Soc. B*, **69**, 369–372.

Graham, C., Bond, S.S., Gerkovich, M. M. and Cook, M. R. (1980) Use of the McGill Pain Questionnaire in the assessment of cancer pain: replicability and consistency. *Pain*, **8**, 377–387.

Greenwood, F. (1972) Site of termination of nerve fibres from the dental pulp. In *Oral Physiology*, ed. Emmelin, N. and Zotterman, Y., pp 259–262. Oxford: Pergamon.

Greenwood, F. (1973) An electrophysiological study of the central connections of the primary afferent nerve fibres from the dental pulp in the cat. *Archs. oral Biol.*, **18**, 771–785.

Hannam, A. G., Siu, W. and Tom, J. (1974) A comparison of monopolar and bipolar pulp-testing. *J. Canad. dent. Ass.*, **40**, 124–128.

Hardy, J. D. (1969) Personal communication. 16 Nov. 1966.

Hardy, J. D., Jacobs, I. and Meixner, M. D. (1953). Thresholds of pain and reflex contraction as related to noxious stimulation. *J. Appl. Physiol.*, **5**, 725–739.

Hardy, J. D. and Stolwijk, J. A. J. (1966) Tissue temperature and thermal pain. In *Touch, Heat and Pain*, ed. de Reuck, A. V. S. and Knight, J., pp. 27–56. London: Churchill.

Hardy, J. D., Wolff, H. G. and Goodell, H. (1940) Studies on pain. A new method of measuring pain threshold observations on spatial summation of pain. *J. clin. Invest.*, **19**, 649–657.

Hardy, J. D., Wolff, H. G. and Goodell, H. (1947) Studies on pain: discrimination of differences in intensity of pain stimulus as a basis of a scale of pain intensity. *J. clin. Invest.*, **26**, 1152–1158.

Hardy, J. D., Wolff, H. G. and Goodell, H. (1952) *Pain Sensations and Reactions*. Baltimore: Williams and Wilkins.

Harkins, S. W. and Chapman, C. R. (1976) Detection and decision factors in pain perception in young and elderly men. *Pain*, **2**, 253–264.

Heng Chin, J. and Domino, E. F. (1961) Effects of morphine on brain potentials evoked by stimulation of the tooth pulp of the dog. *J. Pharmacol.*, **132**, 74–86.

Hensel, H. (1960) *Arch. Ges. Physiol.*, **252**, 165. Quoted by Kenshalo and Scott, cited below.

Hensel, H. and Boman, K. K. A. (1960) Afferent impulses in cutaneous sensory nerves in human subjects. *J. Neurophysiol.*, **23**, 564–578.

Hensel, H. and Mann, G. (1956) Temperaturschmerz und Wärmleitung in menslichen Zahn., *Stoma*, **9**, 76–85.

Hernández-Peón, R. (1966) Physiological mechanisms in attention. In *Frontiers of Physiological Psychology*, ed. Russell, R. W., pp. 121–147. New York: Academic Press.

Hernández-Peón, R. C., Guzman-Flores, C., Alcaraz, M. and Fernandez-Guardiola, A. (1957) Sensory transmission in visual pathway during 'attention' in unanaesthetized cats. *Acta Neurol. Latinoamer.*, **3**, 1–8. Quoted by Gross, C. G. and Zeigler, H. P., ed. *Readings in Physiological Psychology. Neurophysiology Sensory Processes*. New York: Harper and Row.

Hoel, E. (1974) A brief history of acupuncture. *T. norske Laegeforen.* **94**, 418.

Horiuchi, H. and Matthews, B. (1974) Evidence on the origin of impulses recorded from dentine in the cat. *J. Physiol.* (*Lond.*), **243**, 797–829.

Hunter, M., Phillips, C. and Rachman, S. (1979) Memory for pain. *Pain*, **6**, 35–46.

Ingel, J. I. (1973) Acupuncture today. *Amer. dent. Ass. News*, Dec. 3, 4.

Jessup, B.A., Neufeld, R. W. J. and Merskey, H. (1979) Biofeedback therapy for headache and other pain. *Pain*, **7**, 225–270.

Kaada, B. (1974a) Acupuncture analgesia. General considerations. *T. norske Laegeforen.*, **94**, 419–422.

Kaada, B. (1974b) Mechanisms of acupuncture analgesia. *T. norske Laegeforen*, **94**, 422–431.

Kawamura, Y. and Nishiyama, T. (1966) Projection of dental afferent impulses to the trigeminal nuclei of the cat. *Japan, J. Physiol*, **16**, 584–597.

Kawamura, Y., Nishiyama, T., Funakoshi, M. and Majima, T. (1965) Dental nerve response of the cat induced by pressure on the incisor. *J. Osaka Univ. Dent. Sch.*, **5**, 1–9.

Keele, C. A. and Armstrong, D. (1964) *Substances Producing Pain and Itch.* London: Arnold.

Kenshalo, D. R. and Scott, H. A. (1966) Temporal course of thermal adaptation. *Science.*, **151**, 1095–1096.

Kerr, N. W. (1973) Personal communication.

Kroger, W. S. (1973) Acupunctural analgesia: Its explanation by conditioning theory, autogenic training and hypnosis. *Amer, J. Psychiat.*, **130**, 855–860.

Lele, P. P. and Weddell, G. (1956) The relationship between neurohistology and corneal sensibility. *Brain*, **79**, 119–154.

Libet, B., Alberts, W. W., Wright, E. W. and Feinstein, B. (1967) Responses of human somatosensory cortex to stimuli below threshold for conscious sensation. *Science*, **158**, 1597–1600.

Lloyd, J. W. (1977) Experiences in a pain relief unit 1970–1976. In *Pain; New Perspectives in Measurement and Management*, ed. Harcus, A. W., Smith, R. and Whittle, B., pp. 119–128.

Loewenstein, W. R. and Rathkamp. R. (1955) A study on the pressoreceptive sensibility of the teeth. *J. dent. Res.*, **34**, 287–294.

Lynn, B. (1980) Heat pain sensitivity of human skin after mild heat injury and its lack of dependence on the local blood flow. *Pain*, **8**, 189–196.

Lynn, B. and Perl, E. R. (1977) Failure of acupuncture to produce localized analgesia. *Pain*, **3**, 339–351.

Mann, F. (1966) Atlas of acupuncture. Points and meridians in relation to surface anatomy. London: Heinemann.

Mann, F., Bowsher, D., Mumford, J., Lipton, S. and Miles, J. (1973) Treatment of intractable pain by acupuncture. *The Lancet*, July 14, 57–60.

Mao, W., Ghia, J. N., Scott, D. S., Duncan, G. H. and Gregg, J. M. (1980) High versus low intensity acupuncture analgesia for treatment of chronic pain: effects on platelet serotonin. *Pain*, **8**, 331–342.

Martin, R. W. and Chapman, C. R. (1979) Dental dolorimetry for human pain research: methods and apparatus. *Pain*, **6**, 349–364.

Merskey, H. and Spear, F. G. (1967) *Pain, Psychological and Psychiatric Aspects.* London: Baillière, Tindall and Cassell.

Merskey, H. and Watson, G. D. (1979) The lateralisation of pain. *Pain*, **7**, 271–280.

Moruzzi, G. and Magoun, N. W. (1949) Brain stem reticular formation and activation of the E. E. G. *Electroenceph. clin. Neurophysiol*, **1**, 455–473.

Mumford, J. M. (1963) Pain threshold of normal human anterior teeth. *Archs. oral Biol.*, **8**, 493–501.

Mumford, J. M. (1965) Pain perception threshold and adaptation of normal human teeth. *Archs. oral Biol.*, **10**, 957–968.

Mumford, J. M. (1969) Measurement of toothache. *J. Brit. Endo. Soc.*, **3**, 48–51.

Mumford, J. M. (1971) Pain perception threshold of retained decidous teeth. *J. dent. Res.*, **50**, 506.

Mumford, J. M. and Björn, H. (1962) Problems in electric pulp testing and dental algesimetry. *Int. dent. J.* (*Lond.*), **12**, 161–179.

Mumford, J. and Bowsher, D. (1973) Electro-acupuncture and pain threshold. *The Lancet*, Sept. 22, 667.

Mumford, J.M. and Newton, A. V. (1969) Transduction of hydrostatic pressure to electric potential in human dentin. *J. dent. Res.*, **48**, 226–229.

Mumford, J. M. and Newton, A. V. (1971) Convergence in the trigeminal system following stimulation of human teeth. *Archs. oral Biol.*, **16**, 1089–1097.

Mumford. J. M. and Newton, A. V. (1974a) Trigeminal convergence from human teeth: influence of contralateral stimulation and stimulus frequency on the pain perception threshold. *Archs. oral Biol.*, **19**, 145–149.
Mumford, J. M. and Newton, A. V. (1974b) Electrical stimulation of human teeth and convergence in the trigeminal system. In *Pain*, ed. Bonica, J. J., pp. 357–363. *Advances in Neurology*, Vol. 4, New York: Raven Press.
Mumford, J. M., Newton, A. V. and Ley, P. (1973) Personality, pain perception and pain tolerance. *Brit. J. Psychol.*, **64**, 105–107.
Mumford, J. M. and Stanley, S. J. (1981) Sensations on stimulating the pulps of human teeth, thresholds and tolerance ratio. *Pain*, **10**, 391–398.
Nathan, P. W., Noordenbos, W. and Wall, P. D. (1973) Ongoing activity in peripheral nerve: interactions between electrical stimulation and ongoing activity. *Exptl. Neurol.*, **38**, 90–98.
Naylor, M. N. (1961) A thermo-electric tooth stimulator. *Brit. dent. J.*, **110**, 228–230.
Newton, A. V. and Mumford, J. M. (1972) Lateral dominance, pain perception, and pain tolerance. *J. dent. Res.*, **51**, 940–942.
Olgart, L., Haegerstam, G. and Edwall, L. (1974) The effect of extracellular calcium on thermal excitability of the sensory units in the tooth of the cat. *Acta. Physiol. Scand.*, **91**, 116–122.
Petrie, A. (1967) *Individuality in Pain and Suffering*. Chicago: Univ. Chicago Press.
Rawson, P. and Legeza, L. (1973) *Tao. The Chinese Philosophy of Time and Change*. London: Thames and Hudson.
Scott, D. and Tempel, T. R. (1963) Receptor potentials in response to thermal and other excitation. In *Sensory Mechanisms in Dentine*, ed. Anderson, D. J., pp. 27–46. London: Pergamon.
Scott, D. L. (1971) Personal communication. 11 March 1971.
Scott, D. L. (1974) *Modern Hospital Hypnosis*. London: Lloyd-Luke.
Serafetinides, E. A. (1968) Neuropsychiatric aspects of pain. In *Pain*, ed. Soulairac, A., Cahn, J. and Charpentier, J., pp. 61–92. London: Academic Press.
Shimizu, T. (1964) Tooth pre-pain sensation elicited by electrical stimulation. *J. dent. Res.*, **43**, 467–475.
Smith, R. (1962) The vocabulary of pain. In *The Assessment of Pain in Man and Animals*, ed. Keele, C. A. and Smith, R., pp. 32–40. Edinburgh: Livingstone.
Spear, F. G. (1964) A study of pain as a symptom in psychiatric illness. M. D. Thesis, Bristol University. Quoted by Merskey, H. and Spear, F. G. cited above.
Sternbach, R. A. (1974) Varieties of pain games. In *Pain*, ed. Bonica, J. J., pp 423–430. *Advances in Neurology*, Vol. 4. New York: Raven Press.
Sternbach, R. A. (1976) Psychological factors in pain. In *Proceedings of the First World Congress on Pain*, ed. Bonica, J. J. and Albe-Fessard, D. G., pp. 293–299. *Advances in Pain Research and Therapy*, Vol. 3. New York: Raven Press.
Stone, L. J. and Dallenback, K. M. (1934) Adaptation to the pain of radiant heat. *Amer. J. Psychol.*, **46**, 229–242.
Takeda, K, Taniguchi, N., Kuriyama, H. and Matsushita, A. (1979) Experimental study on the mechanism of acupuncture anesthesia. In *Proceedings of the Second World Congress on Pain*, ed. Bonica, J. J., Liebeskind, J. C. and Albe-Fessard, D. G., pp. 623–628. *Advances in Pain Research and Therapy*, Vol. 3. New York: Raven Press.
Takeshige, C., Luo, C. P., Kamada, Y., Oka, K., Murai, M. and Hisamitsu, T. (1979) Relationship between midbrain neurons (periaqueductal central gray and midbrain reticular formation) and acupuncture analgesia, animal hypnosis. In *Proceedings of the Second World Congress on Pain*, ed. Bonica, J. J., Liebeskind, J. C. and Albe-Fessard, D. G. pp. 615–621. *Advances in Pain Research and Therapy*, Vol. 3. New York: Raven Press.

Toda, K. (1978) Effects of electro-acupuncture on rat jaw opening reflex elicited by tooth pulp stimulation. *Jap. J. Physiol.*, **28**, 485–497.

Torebjörk, H. E. and Hallin, R. G. (1974a) Responses in human A and C fibres to repeated electrical stimulation. *J. Neurol. Neurosurg. Psychiat.*, **37**, 653–664.

Torebjörk, H. E. and Hallin, R. G. (1974b) Identification of afferent C units in intact human skin nerves. *Brain Res.*, **67**, 387–404.

Uchizono, K. and Homma, K. (1959) Electron microscope studies on nerves of human tooth pulp. *J. dent. Res.*, **38**, 1133–1141.

Veith, I. (1966) *Huang Ti Nei Ching Su Wên. The Yellow Emperor's Classic of Internal Medicine*, new edition. Berkeley: Univ. California Press.

Wall, P. (1972) An eye on the needle. *New Scientist*, 20 July, 129–131.

Wall, P. (1974) Acupunture revisited. *New Scientist*, Oct. 3, 31–34.

Wolff, B. B. (1968) Some behavioural mechanisms of human pain. In *Pharmacology of Pain*, ed. Lim, R. K. S., Armstrong, D. and Pardo, E. G., pp. 121–130. Oxford: Pergamon.

Yamada, M. and Sakada, S. (1961) The effects of some chemicals on cervix dentis. *J. dent. Res.*, **40**, 975–987.

# 6

# Investigation of toothache cases

Successful diagnosis demands a background of knowledge plus a systematic approach to elucidating information. To fulfill the latter requirement the diagnostic method is essentially standardised, although any one aspect is pursued to a greater or lesser extent, depending on the particular case being investigated. The amount of time available is also a factor and it is undesirable to waste both the patient's and the clinician's time with useless questions and tests. Thus, when a patient presents with toothache there may be obvious disease which can be treated in a straightforward manner; he might indicate a grossly carious tooth which obviously needs to be extracted. In a busy practice, such an expeditious approach is time-saving and economical. However, even for an apparently straightforward case it is obvious that a question about the possible use of anticoagulant drugs could avoid considerable trouble if the patient is found to be using them, and radiographic examination might reveal additional disease suggesting the need for a surgical removal rather than a simple extraction. In other words, though time should not be wasted, cases might not be so straightforward as they seem, and some difficult ones may require the clinician to use all appropriate diagnostic methods that are available. Lengthy questioning is not then a waste of time but it should be remembered that patients who have been suffering pain may become further distressed by extended questioning or by being subjected to numerous tests, so these should not be prolonged more than necessary.

The point about this preamble is that although the diagnostic method is essentially the same for all patients it is necessary to treat each case individually, selecting the most appropriate line of investigation for every one.

In what follows no attempt is made to cover the entire field of diagnosis, but only to deal with questions which should be asked and tests which need to be done when a patient complains of 'toothache'. The standard procedures of history taking, inspection, palpation, radiography, etc., are omitted to avoid needless repetition of material which is generally understood. Some further procedures appear later in the book.

## HISTORY AND DESCRIPTION OF THE PAIN

### Complaint

The patient complains of pain and may describe it in a clear manner while the clinician makes notes in the case history. However, even if the patient's description is poor he should still be allowed to have his say before a history and description are obtained by systematic questioning. Questions should be carefully formulated to avoid confusing the patient because apparently sensible questions may have more than one meaning. For example, if asked about the duration of pain the patient may think it means how long an attack lasts rather than the overall period of time during which he has experienced symptoms. To obtain the answer to the latter question it is better to ask when the pain first occurred.

### Site of pain

The patient, having complained of pain and stated in words where it is, is asked to indicate the site, using one finger to do so. If he uses his entire hand it may be difficult to see where he is pointing to. Sometimes the finger rests on a well defined place whereas at other times it hovers in a more indefinite manner because the patient is uncertain, the pain being more diffuse than localised. Even when the finger rests on a definite place it may be on the outside of the face although the patient means to indicate the underlying tooth; this may be because he wants to talk at the same time or is fastidous about putting his finger inside his mouth. He should be asked to 'show me where the pain is, using just one finger, pointing inside the mouth if necessary'. At this time he can indicate the direction in which pain radiates if it does so, and the clinician may prefer to make a note of this on a drawing of the face rather than simply in words. As well as being asked to indicate the site of pain the patient should be asked does he think it is localised or not. Naturally, there can be pain in more than one place and this must be considered.

At this early stage of the investigation the clinician might have heard and seen enough to be able to decide what to do, as suggested earlier. If not the diagnostic procedure continues.

### When pain was first noted

The patient is asked when pain first occurred. The more recently it started the more helpful is the information, especially if this can be related to a specific event such as some operative procedure. If, for instance, pain is first noticed at the end of local anaesthesia damage has been present since treatment, but nerve impulses have been blocked by the local anaesthetic agent. (Strictly, the correct expression is local analgesia, meaning no pain, rather than no feeling, but in this text the words local anaesthesia are used because they are so well established.) In the circumstances damage must be regarded as having been caused by the operation (iatrogenic), and the dentist who operated is the best person to deal with the problem because of his memory and the notes he has kept of the case. The cause may be overheating of the pulp or pulp exposure during cavity preparation, inadequate lining of the cavity or a leaking dressing, a high spot on the filling, galvanic activity, soreness following the local anaesthetic or a related chemical burn, and lip or tissue biting during anaesthesia.

*Some hours after treatment*

Local anaesthesia usually passes off uneventfully but in some cases pain occurs within a few hours. If this happens when the patient bites on a newly placed filling the dentist should look for a shiny 'high spot'. When this is reduced pain ceases, thus also confirming the diagnosis.

Also within a few hours the patient may suffer pain on eating or drinking hot or cold food, and this is probably because of an inadequate cavity lining.

*Two days after treatment*

After extraction of a tooth, especially under local anaesthesia, there may be apparently good recovery, but pain occurs in about 48 hours. In this case a dry socket should be suspected.

*Days or weeks*

Recurrent twinges of pain occurring within a variable period after operation suggest severe pulp damage which cannot be left untreated. Pulp exposure might not have been recognised under local anaesthesia because of the vasoconstrictor reducing the pulp's vascularity. On the other hand, the exposure might have been recognised and the pulp have been capped.

**What starts the pain**

The patient is asked what brings on the pain or if it just starts by itself. The latter is called spontaneously occurring pain although it is likely to be due to pulp disease. The word spontaneous simply means that no obvious external stimulus was applied.

If pain does start with external stimulation the patient is asked which stimuli cause the pain, and which stimulus is most effective in doing so.

## Duration of attack

The patient is asked how long an attack of pain lasts, and he should be encouraged to relate this to real time intervals even though these will be only approximate.

*Approximately one second*

Occasionally a brief pain of considerable severity occurs spontaneously but may not recur. This can be due to unknown factors and with a single episode the case is better watched than treated, but repeated episodes may indicate a moribund pulp.

A brief pain may be due to galvanic action in which case pain occurs on closing the mouth so that dissimilar metal restorations come together, or it may be due to a high spot on a filling.

*Several seconds*

The patient may describe toothache lasting several seconds associated with hot and cold foods, and this is even more likely if hot and cold foods are taken within a short time of each other, e.g. ice cream and hot coffee. Such pain often continues after the external stimulus has been removed because the temperature in the sensitive zone of the tooth is still altered, and thermal change might still be passing through the tooth (Chapter 7.)

Pain due to sweet foods such as chocolate lasts for several seconds by virtue of osmotic activity drawing fluids through dentine.

*Many minutes*

When pain continues long past the stimulus which provoked it this suggests a pathological condition. Such pain occasioned by thermal change suggests pulp disease, whereas continued pain following biting suggests disease of the periodontal tissues.

*Longer periods*

Toothache lasting for longer periods can be due to many different conditions, and differential diagnosis may be difficult.

## When the pain occurs

*On waking*

If the patient wakes up feeling stiffness and pain in the jaws which wears off in an hour or so, there may be temporomandibular joint or occlusal disturbance.

Pericoronitis of a partly erupted molar should also be considered since the pressure of inflammatory exudate may have built up during the night thus causing pain to be worse.

*When eating*

The teeth are subjected to a variety of stimuli on eating, including mechanical, thermal and chemical stimuli, the effects of which are considered in Chapter 7. The patient may be able to say which of these stimuli is responsible.

When pain occurs on biting it is correctly thought that this is likely to be due to periodontal disease, including acute periapical periodontitis, acute lateral periodontitis, and traumatic periodontitis due to a high, newly inserted restoration. However, pain on biting can also be due to soft caries with a pulp exposure, a loose inlay, food packing, ulceration or a buried root beneath a denture, a 'gum stripping' partial denture, an irregular alveolar ridge beneath a denture, and pericoronitis. It may also be due to biting of the tongue, lips and cheeks. When pain occurs in anticipation of eating, a blockage of the salivary ducts must be considered.

*After eating*

This may be after the first meal of the day, and may be associated with occlusal dysharmony. Remember that for some people the first meal of the day may be at lunch time.

*Late in the day and at night*

Fatigue is a factor here, either of the muscles of mastication or because the patient is generally tired. Pain due to occlusal dysharmony tends to become worse during the day.

If the patient is woken by pain in the face during the early hours of the morning and this occurs frequently for months , facial migraine (periodic migrainous neuralgia) should be considered.

During the night there are fewer distractions, the patient may feel alone, perhaps neglected, and pain seems to become worse (Chapter 5).

**Frequency of pain**

The patient is asked how often pain occurs, and if it is occurring more or less frequently or if the frequency remains constant.

*When a stimulus is applied*

If pain occurs when a stimulus is applied this is a useful piece of informatiom because it is so well defined. The various stimuli possible have already been considered.

*Paroxysms*

The main significance of paroxysmal pain relates to trigeminal neuralgia (Chapter 16), but paroxysms may also occur in more routine dental cases, a moribund pulp being the condition which should be considered.Occasionally, marked overclosure of the mandible can give rise to sharp paroxysmal pain which may simulate trigeminal neuralgia.

**Pain intensity**

An attempt is made to find how intense pain is, if it varies, and if there are well defined levels of pain. The classification of pain intensity is a difficult subject but it is considered that mild, moderate and severe are sufficient divisions for clinical use. Some examples will be illustrated in later chapters.

The patient should be asked if the intensity of pain is staying the same, becoming worse, or diminishing.

**Quality of pain**

It is difficult to ascribe a quality to pain, the vocabulary of the subject being limited, but the patient should be asked, if only because quality and intensity go together. Thus 'ache' may be regarded as a quality of pain but it is really a pain of long duration, perhaps with an intensity which is mild. Similarly 'throb' is usually described as a quality but it is really a variation in intensity with the pulse beat. It does not matter to the patient whether it is quality or intensity as long as the information is obtained, but the clinician should be clear in his own mind.

## VITALITY TESTS

**Mechanical stimulation**

If the dentine is already exposed as in a carious lesion or as a result of a fracture, a probe or excavator can be used by drawing it across the dentine. This method is also useful for demonstrating sensitivity at the neck of a tooth and at the defective margins of restorations. A jet of compressed air can also be used.

If dentine is not already exposed a bur can be used to cut through the enamel into dentine thereby demonstrating sensitivity or failing to do so. Its effect is thermal as well as mechanical, and the procedure is called 'making a test cavity'.

**Application of heat**

Heat may be applied as hot water or hot air, but the most commonly used method is by means of heated gutta percha. A stick of gutta percha is held with about 3 mm in the side of a flame for about two seconds, and applied to the labial or buccal surface of the tooth being investigated. Care is needed to avoid causing undue pain, so the gutta percha must be heated for only a brief period at first with the object of causing only the least possible sensation in the tooth. If this fails to produce sensation the gutta percha is heated for a longer period, but overheating should be avoided because it chars and bursts into flames. Application of the gutta percha causes its softened end to distort, so a fresh piece should be used each time in order to apply the heat to an approximately constant area. This is desirable because the area in contact with the tooth influences heat transfer. So much for the vitality test, but if the object is just to find out which tooth hurts when eating or drinking hot foods then the hot gutta percha is simply applied to the most vulnerable area, such as a metal filling.

An attempt has been made to control the thermal methods of stimulating teeth by Naylor (1961) who used a thermo-electric method. This allowed application of hot or cold stimuli via a thermode, the method depending on the Joule heating effect and the Peltier cooling effect, but when applied to enamel its thermal output or cooling effect were found inadequate (Reynolds, 1966).

Sorenson, Phatek and Everett (1962) used a thermal stimulator which delivered water to the tooth surface at temperatures between 0°–70°C, monitored by a thermistor.

It is possible to keep the source of applied heat constant within narrow limits, Heithersay and Brännström (1963) having kept such a source (thermode) at 150° ± 1°C. However, except in experimental situations, the temperature where excitation occurs is not known, and it is this that really matters (Chapter 7).

**Application of cold**

Cold may be applied as cold water, ice, cold air or frozen carbon dioxide, the latter being favoured by Ehrmann (1977), but the most commonly used method is by means of a pledget of cotton wool soaked in ethyl chloride. The pledget should be of standard size and excess ethyl chloride should be allowed to drip off before application to the tooth.

Sometimes a stream of ethyl chloride has been applied directly to a tooth, but this seems almost sadistic, not to mention the risk of the patient inhaling the vapour which is a general anaesthetic agent. There is also a risk of the glass vial shattering so it must be kept in a fabric sleeve. For this reason a refrigerant aerosol is now preferred (Eifinger, 1970).

## Comparative tests

Comparison is often made between corresponding teeth on opposite sides of the midline, the comparative tooth being supposedly normal. It is done in the mistaken belief that the pain perception threshold is being determined, but this is not the case. An approximately standard amount of heat or cold is applied, and the patient's reaction is noted. There is no satisfactory evidence that the extent of this reaction indicates the histological condition of the pulp, so only two pieces of information are required – is the pulp vital and does application of cold (or heat) provoke the pain complained of? This really means that comparative testing is unnecessary. It also means that there is no need to select an intact part of the tooth surface for applying the stimulus; on the contrary it would seem more reasonable to apply the thermal stimulus to the damaged or filled area since this is the zone which is presumably allowing hot and cold foods to cause pain.

Even when the thermal methods of pulp testing are used with care they do not give reproducible results in terms of the intensity of sensation (Mumford, 1964) and it is possible to obtain results which might be misleading. As an example, the results of testing one patient are given in Table 6.1. In this case the patient did not respond at any time to stimulation of the right lower central incisor, and surgical intervention revealed that the pulp was dead,

**Table 6.1** Results which might be misleading. + indicates a response whereas — indicates no response; the 1┐ was found to have a dead pulp

| Vitality test | 3┐ | 2┐ | 1┐ | ┌1 | ┌2 | ┌3 |
|---|---|---|---|---|---|---|
| Stimulation with hot gutta percha | + | + | — | — | — | — |
| Stimulation with ethyl chloride | — | — | — | — | + | + |
| Electrical stimulation; threshold value in microamps | 2 | 2 | — | 13 | 2 | 2 |

so all three tests were successful. On the other hand, stimulating the left lower central incisor evoked no response with heat and cold which would suggest that the pulp was dead, but there was a response with the electric test, so the pulp was vital. Moreover, the remaining four teeth shown in the table all gave opposite results on testing with heat and cold which might have been confusing. For this case electrical stimulation was obviously superior to the thermal tests, but it is not suitable for all cases, such as when a tooth is badly broken down or has large fillings. To obtain the best results from the thermal tests both heat and cold should be used, and this should prevent mistakes even in such extreme cases as that indicated in Table 6.1.

**Electrical tests**

The most convenient method of electrical pulp testing is to use a stimulator which provides a repetitive stimulus the amplitude of which is gradually increased until the patient perceives sensation. Such an instrument is illustrated in Fig. 6.1 and it has been designed to prevent harmful current reaching the patient. It also has a return spring on the potentiometer handle so that the current always returns to zero; this prevents painfully high current being inadvertently applied.

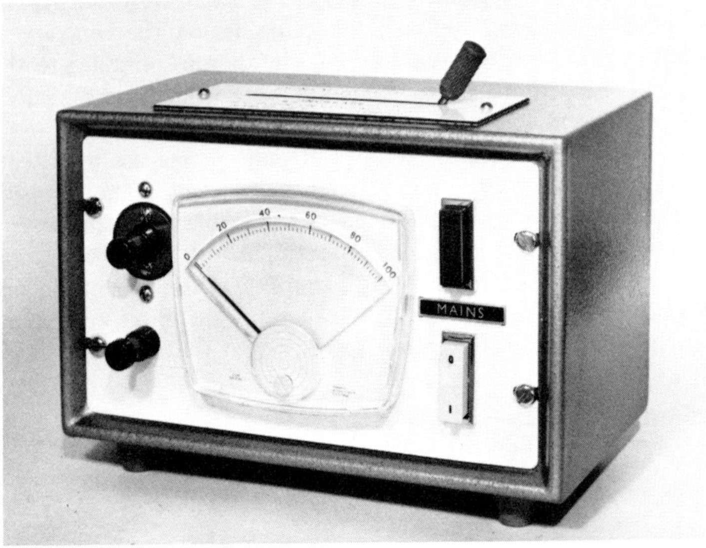


**Fig. 6.1.** Electric stimulator for testing pulp vitality. The lever on top allows increasing current to be applied. It has a spring return so that excessive current cannot be inadvertently applied to the next tooth to be tested, perhaps in the next patient!

Before making an electric pulp test the patient has the procedure explained to him and he is asked to say 'ah' when he notices a slight sensation. He holds one electrode in his hand while the other (the cathode) is placed on his tooth, and the current is slowly raised until he indicates that he feels a sensation in the tooth, when the microammeter reading is noted; this is the pain perception threshold value. It is an advantage to have the current increased automatically by electronic methods, and to give the patient control of the test by means of a microswitch built into the hand electrode (Mumford and Lewis, 1976). The stimulating electrode makes contact with the tooth via a tip of conducting rubber which adapts to the tooth surface. Alternatively, the tip may be a piece of orangewood stick or a piece of matchstick previously soaked in saline. Care must be taken that it does not dry out for this would raise its electrical resistance too high.

The tooth should be isolated, preferably by rubber dam, and the surface dried by application of a brief stream of air. This is necessary to prevent the electric current passing along the tooth surface direct to the gum margin, thus by-passing the pulp (Fig. 6.2). For the same reason the electrode should be kept well away

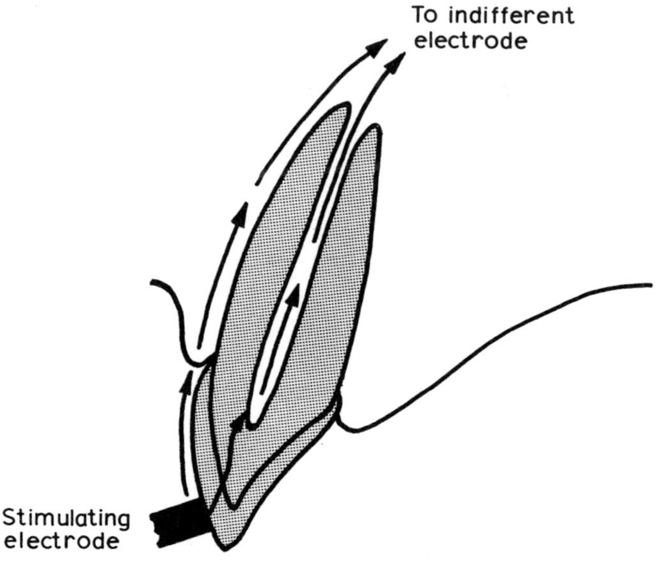


**Fig. 6.2.** The tooth being tested must have no saliva on its surface for this would allow surface conduction of part of the current direct to the gingival margin. This would give a falsely high current reading. The current is represented as going through the tooth towards the indifferent electrode (in the hand) but it could equally well be shown going in the opposite direction. The essential point to know is that the stimulating electrode is normally the cathode.

from the gum margin, being placed on the incisal edge or the labial surface near the incisal edge. For cheek teeth it is placed on the buccal aspect of a cusp near to the occlusal surface. The electrode must not be placed on a carious lesion or a filling if this would allow current to be conducted direct to the gingival margin (Fig. 6.3). On the other hand, it is all right to place the electrode on a metal filling or a carious lesion if this is separated from the gingiva by a reasonably large area of sound tooth.

Sometimes only a limited current will pass through the tooth and this is due to the dental tissues having too high an electrical resistance. This may be because the enamel surface has been dried too much, so a trace of moisture is added to the electrode tip and this enters the enamel, allowing more current to flow (Mumford, 1966). Even then there may still be only a limited current which indicates a high internal resistance such as occurs with a dry pulp or an empty pulp canal.

It is possible to use alternating current (A. C.) or direct current (D. C.) and there is no fundamental difference between the two forms. Indeed, one of the most commonly used methods is a

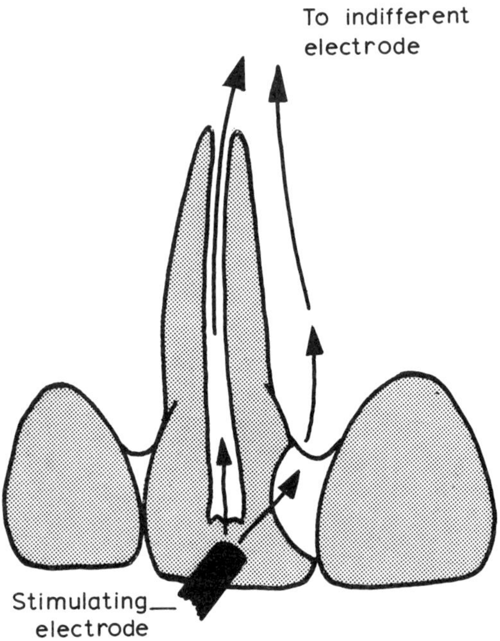


**Fig. 6.3.** A carious lesion or a metal filling may allow an unknown part of the current to go direct to the gingiva, thus by-passing the pulp.

direct current square wave pulse with a pulse duration of 10 milliseconds and an interval between the pulses of 10 milliseconds. The pulse is repeated 50 times per second, and since the square shape is modified as it passes through the tooth (Newton and Mumford, 1968) the D. C. square waves come to look like an A. C. sine wave (Figs. 6.4, 6.5).

Other times and frequencies of pulses are available but very brief durations of pulse should not be used since such a pulse does not have time to reach its full peak value (Fig. 6.6) because of the electrical characteristics of teeth (Newton and Mumford, 1968).

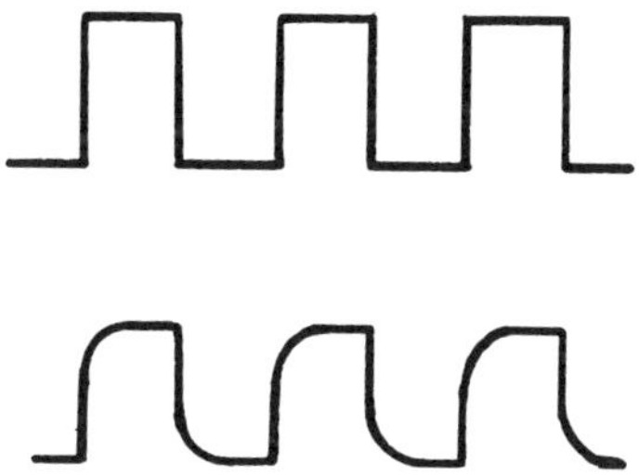

**Fig. 6.4**. A direct current square wave electrical pulse is modified as it passes through the tooth (integrated), and it begins to look more like an alternating current sine wave.

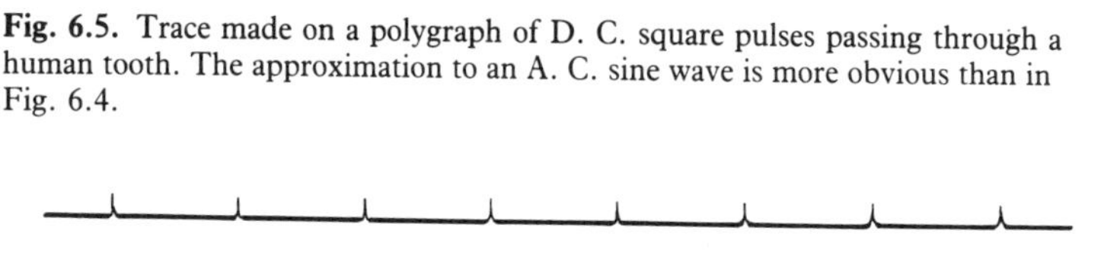

**Fig. 6.5.** Trace made on a polygraph of D. C. square pulses passing through a human tooth. The approximation to an A. C. sine wave is more obvious than in Fig. 6.4.

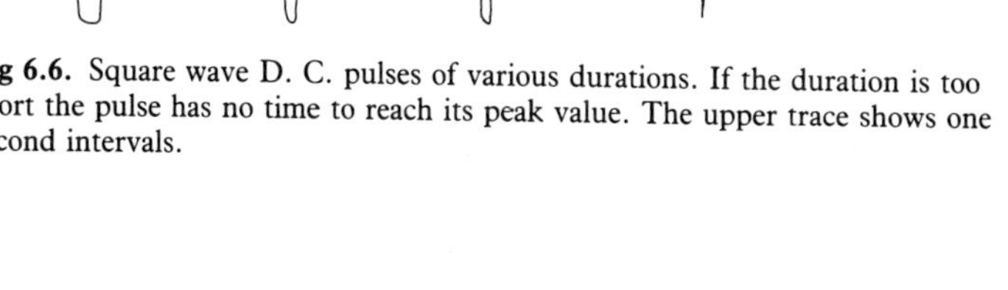

**Fig 6.6.** Square wave D. C. pulses of various durations. If the duration is too short the pulse has no time to reach its peak value. The upper trace shows one second intervals.

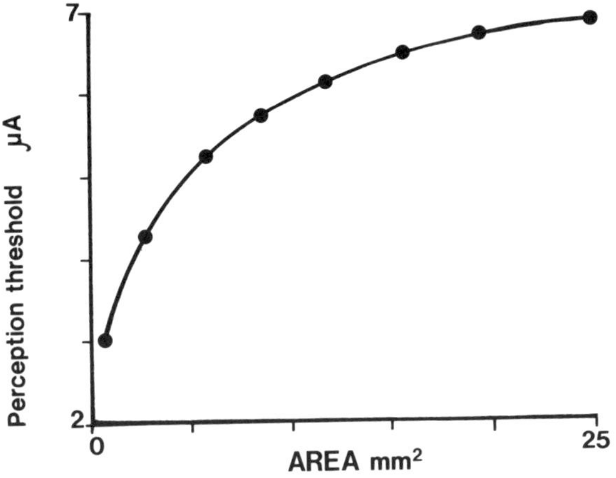


**Fig. 6.7.** When applying electrical stimuli to teeth the electrode contact is important, and larger contact areas necessitate passing greater current to reach the pain perception threshold (PPTh), though the rate of increase diminishes.

The area of electrode contact must be standardised because this directly influences the current density which is the essential factor in stimulating nerves (Mumford, 1963; Mumford and Newton, 1969). A larger electrode area requires a larger current (Fig. 6.7).

It is possible to place both electrodes on the tooth, one facially and the other lingually. The current is then confined to the coronal pulp (Mumford, 1959; Greenwood, Horiuchi and Matthews, 1972) and might give better diagnostic information than that obtained by passing current through the entire pulp. However, the threshold values obtained with both electrodes on the tooth were the same as with a single electrode (Matthews, Horiuchi and Greenwood, 1974; Hannam, Siu and Tom, 1974). Since a single electrode is more convenient this is the method of choice.

## Diagnostic significance of vitality tests

If the patient responds to mechanical stimulation this means that the pulp is vital, but care is needed with some patients who are nervous and may react without justification. An attempt should be made to disguise the moment of application of the stimulus and also the site at which it is applied, so that the patient will have to judge by sensation in the tooth rather than by observing the test being carried out.

Gentle palpation with a probe is the best method of determining the exact site of cervical sensitivity.

A response to hot stimuli almost always indicates a vital pulp, but pain may also be produced when the pulp has died with the production of gas. The heat causes this to expand greatly so that it presses onto nerves in the periapical area, and this can be very painful, so care is needed. The coefficient of thermal expansion of gas is approximately 10 times that of water (Weast, 1972).

When the patient responds to cold stimuli there is a vital pulp, but cold as well as hot stimuli may fail to produce a response even with a vital pulp, so lack of a response is not satisfactory evidence. The explanation of this is given in Chapter 7.

A response following electrical stimulation indicates a vital pulp whereas no response indicates a dead pulp, provided the method has been properly used. There is an exception to this for it has been found (Mumford, 1965) that children under the age of 10 years do not give reliable responses, perhaps because the permanent teeth are not fully innervated, or because children are unreliable reporters. It is wrong to think that the pulp in any one canal of a multirooted tooth can be preferentially stimulated, because the current passes through all canals.

Vitality tests do not indicate any more than whether the pulp is dead or vital, and a vital pulp can be moribund. They do not give an indication of the state of health of the pulp; such a level of diagnosis requires information from other diagnostic procedures, such as inspection of the tooth's colour.

**Pain on percussion**

Teeth are usually percussed using an instrument such as the reverse end of a mirror handle held as nearly as possible in the long axis of the tooth being tested. Care is needed to avoid tapping too hard because this can cause severe pain when there is acute periapical disease. Indeed, pain can be so severe as to leave the patient momentarily incapacitated, and further investigation or treatment must be delayed. A light tap should be applied in the first instance, and comparison should be made with other apparently normal teeth. It is also desirable to disguise, as far as possible, the tooth being percussed because this makes the patient's response more reliable.

For anterior teeth the author often uses his curved forefinger and finds that this is a gentler means of applying percussion, though other teeth are less accessible.

It is usually believed that pain on percussion indicates only acute periapical inflammation but this is not quite correct. Pain occurs normally if percussion is too strong. It also occurs if a loose restoration is percussed so that the restoration acts as a plunger forcing fluid through the dentinal tubules (Chapter 9). Pain also occurs when a lateral periodontal abscess (parodontal abscess) is present, and it is said that there may be a directional variation in intensity if the tooth is percussed from different angles. However, in the great majority of cases, if percussion is done with care, then pain indicates acute periapical periodontitis.

## Local anaesthetic test

When a patient presents in pain, or when pain can be provoked during examination, advantage of this can be taken by applying a local anaesthetic to the suspected area. When injecting the solution it is better to use infiltration anaesthesia if possible because its action is more confined, whereas a regional injection anaesthetises more teeth and is less definitive.

The local anaesthetic test also impresses the patient because, when applied successfully, pain ceases in about two minutes. This is particularly useful in cases of referred pain when it is possible to stop pain in one jaw by applying the local anaesthetic to a tooth in the other jaw.

A subdivision of the local anaesthetic test, not always considered, is the application of a surface anaesthetic to the mucosa for cases when it is suspected that the causative factor is superficial. A surface anaesthetic can also be used to spray the tonsillar area in cases of glossopharyngeal neuralgia, and mucosal trigger zones in trigeminal neuralgia.

## Pulp haemogram

When the pulp is exposed it is possible to take the first drop of blood that exudes and subject it to a differential white cell count. Prader (1949; 1962) suggested that this might be of help in diagnosing pulpal conditions, but no clear relationship was found between the haemogram and the pulp condition by Guthrie, McDonald and Mitchell (1965). Baume (1966) also found it of little help.

## REFERENCES

Baume, L. J. (1966) Clinical and pathological aspects of current endodontic therapy. *Int. dent. J. (Lond.)*, **16**, 30–54.

Ehrmann, E. H. (1977) Pulp testers and pulp testing with particular reference to the use of dry ice. *Austral. dent. J.*, **22**, 272–279.

Eifinger, F. F. (1970) Human tooth sensitivity test with cold aerosols. *Quintessence Int.*, **1**, 21–24. Abstracted from *Das Deutsche Zahnbl.*, **24**, 6.

Greenwood, F., Horiuchi, H. and Matthews, B. (1972) Electrophysiological evidence on the types of nerve fibres excited by electrical stimulation of teeth with a pulp tester . *Archs. oral Biol.*, **17**, 701–709.

Guthrie, T. J., McDonald, R. E. and Mitchell, D. F. (1965) Dental pulp haemogram. *J. dent. Res.*, **44**, 678–682.

Hannam, A. G., Siu, W. and Tom, J. (1974) A comparison of monopolar and bipolar pulp-testing. *J. Canad. dent. Ass.*, **40**, 124–128.

Heithersay, G. S. and Brännström, M. (1963) Observations on heat transmission experiments with dentine. I. Laboratory study. *J. dent. Res.*, **42**, 1140–1145.

Matthews, B. Horiuchi, H. and Greenwood, F. (1974) The effects of stimulus polarity and electrode area on the threshold to monopolar stimulation of teeth in human subjects, with some preliminary observations on the use of a bipolar pulp tester. *Archs. oral Biol.*, **19**, 35–42.

Mumford, J. M. (1959) Path of direct current in electric pulp testing using two coronal electrodes. *Brit. dent. J.*, **106**, 243–245.

Mumford, J. M. (1963) Pain threshold of normal human anterior teeth. *Archs. oral Biol.*, **8**, 493–501.

Mumford, J. M. (1964) Evaluation of gutta percha and ethyl chloride in pulp testing. *Brit. dent. J.*, **116**, 338–342.

Mumford, J. M. (1965) Pain perception threshold and adaptation of normal human teeth. *Archs. oral Biol.*, **10**, 957–968.

Mumford, J. M.(1966) Drying of enamel under rubber dam. *Brit. dent. J.*, **121**, 178–179.

Mumford, J. M. and Lewis, D. G. (1976) Electronic tooth stimulator for pain research. *Biomed. Eng.*, **2**, 22–23.

Mumford, J. M. and Newton, A. V. (1969) Zone of excitation when electrically stimulating human teeth. *Archs. oral Biol.*, **14**, 1383–1388.

Naylor, M. N. (1961) A thermo-electric tooth stimulator. *Brit. dent. J.*, **10**, 228–230.

Newton, A. V. and Mumford, J. M. (1968) Transduction of square wave stimuli through human teeth. *Archs. oral Biol.*, **13**, 831–832.

Prader, J. (1949) Diagnose und Therapie infizierten Wurzelkaniles. Basel: Benno Schwabe. Quoted by Guthrie *et al*, cited above.

Prader, J. (1962) Die Auswirkungen im Hämopulpogramm bei der konservativen Pulpitisbenhandlung mit einem Glukokortikoid – Antibioticum – Komkinations – praparat. *Schw. Mschr. Zahnheilk.*, **72**, 743. Quoted by Baume (1966) cited above.

Reynolds, R. L. (1966) The determination of pulp vitality by means of thermal and electrical stimuli. *Oral Surg.*, **22**, 231–240.

Sorenson, F. M., Phatek, N. M. and Everett, F. G. (1962) Thermal pulp tester; a new instrument. *J. dent. Res.*, **41**, 961–965.

Weast, R. C. (1972) (ed.) *Handbook of Chemistry and Physics*, 53rd ed. p F98. Cleveland: The Chemical Rubber Co.

# 7

# External stimuli provoking pain in teeth

The external stimuli causing pain in teeth may occur naturally or be applied for diagnostic reasons as described in Chapter 6. The most common natural stimuli are hot and cold foods, cold air, foods with a high concentration of sugar, e.g. chocolate and toffee, and application of pressure as in biting. Mechanical stimuli, such as the application of a finger nail to the neck of a tooth, also cause pain. Patients may observe these occurrences quite accurately and give a helpful account which is valuable in diagnosing. However, when pain occurs it does not follow that disease is necessarily present and the purpose of this chapter is to describe the physical conduction of the stimuli and to show how this influences pain production and cessation independently of any disease. Physiological factors are not considered, so nerves and the precise situation of nerve endings hardly enter the discussion, although of course they must eventually be involved.

## THERMAL STIMULI

Thermal change passes through teeth as expanding isotherms, and this has been demonstrated by the iridescent display produced by heating or cooling liquid crystals (Newton and Mumford, 1970). Extracted human teeth were cut by means of a diamond disc along various planes, and the cut surfaces coated with a black paint which was allowed to dry. Liquid crystals were then applied and also allowed to dry. Thermal stimuli were applied to various external surfaces of the teeth and as thermal change was conducted through them this was revealed as progressive rainbow colours produced by the liquid crystals, each colour representing an isotherm (Figs. 7.1, 7.2, 7.3). Thermal change spreads throughout the entire crown and is thus gradually dissipated, being in this respect quite different from an electrical stimulus which is more confined and not dissipated.

Whether or not pain occurs from thermal stimuli depends upon the temperature of the stimulating material and its mass, the area of contact it makes with the tooth, the mass of the tooth, the width of the tooth (or remaining tooth substance) between the point of application of the stimulus and the place where neural excitation occurs, and the thermal conductivity of the tooth.

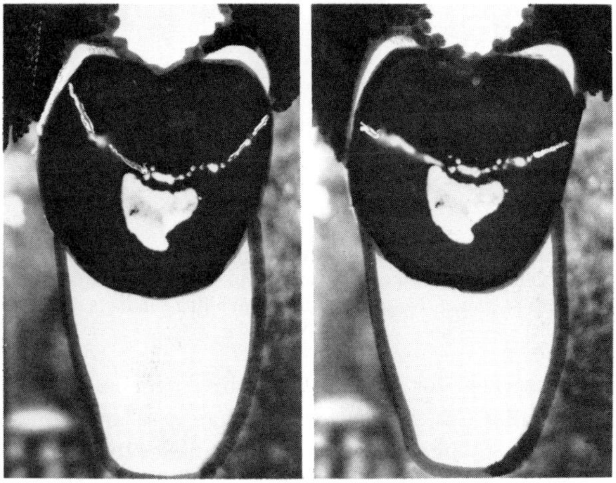

**Fig. 7.1.** A lower molar, divided facio-lingually, with the cut surface of the crown coated with black paint followed by a clear layer of liquid crystals. When a pledget of cotton wool soaked in ethyl chloride was applied to the occlusal surface a cold isotherm spread from the pledget in an expanding manner as illustrated.

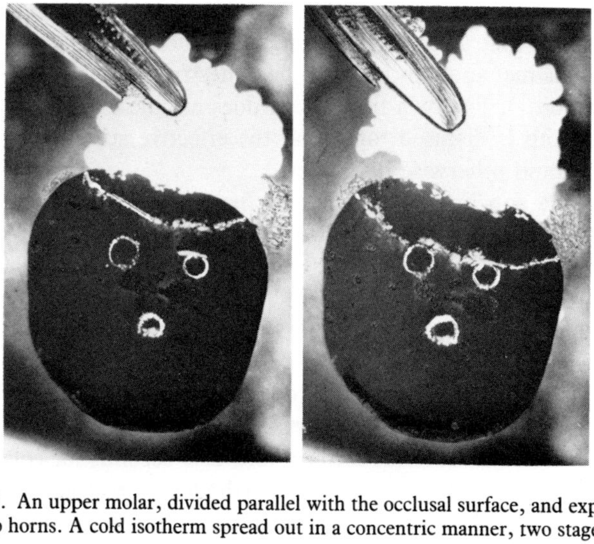

**Fig. 7.2.** An upper molar, divided parallel with the occlusal surface, and exposing the pulp horns. A cold isotherm spread out in a concentric manner, two stages being shown.

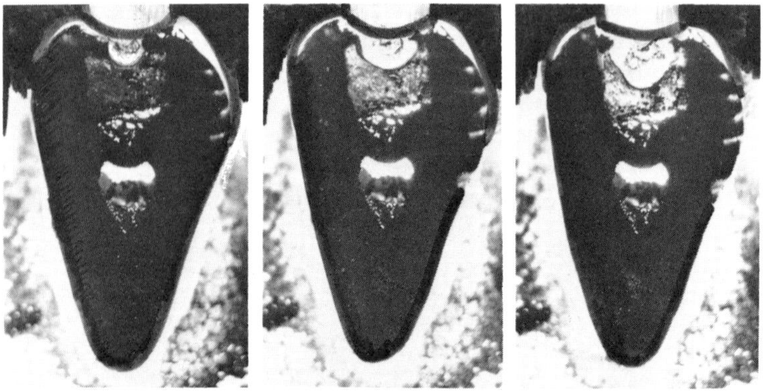

**Fig. 7.3.** A lower molar with an occlusal amalgam filling was sectioned facio-lingually. On applying heated gutta percha to the occlusal surface heat passed through the tooth as shown. Notice how the metal filling conducts the heat.

This means that, for a given stimulus, pain is more likely to occur in a smaller (less massive) tooth than in a larger one because the temperature change is greater in the smaller tooth.

Pain is more likely to occur where only a thin layer of tooth tissue is present at the point of application of the stimulus because a given stimulus gives a greater thermal gradient:

$$\frac{\text{Temperature of stimulus} - \text{Temperature where excitation occurs}}{\text{Distance between the two places}}$$

This means that stimuli which might not normally cause pain can do so if enamel and dentine have been destroyed by caries or cavity preparation, or lost by a fracture. It does not mean that the pulp of such a tooth is diseased; only that the effective stimulus is greater than it would otherwise have been.

It might appear that the patient first perceives pain when the temperature of the pulpo-dentinal junction is raised to approximately 47°C (Hensel and Mann, 1956), or lowered to 29°C (Naylor, 1964) and, in dogs, it has been shown that there are many nerve impulses from the pulp when the temperature of the pulpo-dentinal junction is raised to 45°C (Funakoshi and Zotterman, 1963). However, Trowbridge et al (1980) found that when hot and cold stimuli were applied to teeth the patient responded in 1.28 seconds for heat and 1.49 seconds for cold. After the teeth had been extracted (for orthodontic reasons) the same stimuli were applied but the pulpodentinal junction temperature did not change for 3.68 seconds. The explanation they gave is that the thermal change produced fluid movements in the dentinal tubules and hence pain before thermal change could reach the pulpodentinal junction.

The speed at which the temperature changes at the pulpodentinal junction depends partly on the stimulus. A greater amount of heat applied to the surface produces not only a greater increase of temperature at the pulpo-dentinal junction but also starts to produce the increase more quickly (Fig. 7.4). Once the pulp is affected by the heat it is subject to thermal expansion so the pulpal pressure rises, but the vasomotor state is also a factor to be considered (see below).

It should be understood that removing the source of heat does not terminate the stimulus immediately because the effective stimulus is the change in temperature of the tooth at the place where excitation occurs. Pain can therefore continue after the external stimulus is removed, this being frequently experienced both clinically and in everyday life. For extracted teeth a 5 second application of heated gutta percha to the surface allowed the temperature at the pulpodentinal junction to continue to increase for nearly 20 seconds longer (Trowbridge et al, 1980).

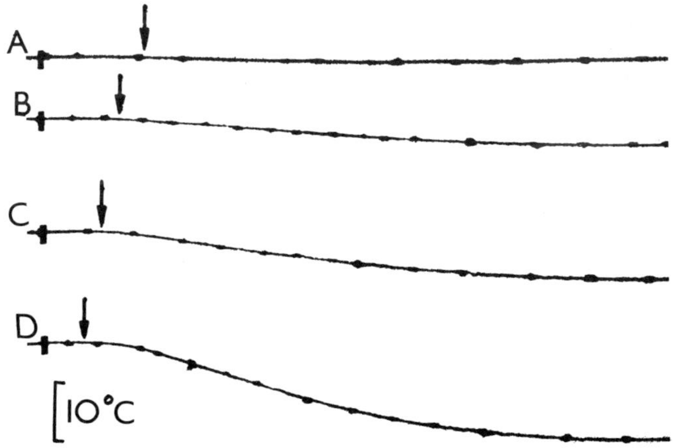


**Fig. 7.4.** A stick of gutta percha was heated in a flame and then applied to the labial enamel of a freshly extracted upper canine, the temperature of the pulpo-dentinal junction being recorded by a thermocouple. A downward deflection indicates a rise in temperature. The rectangular marker indicates the time when the gutta percha was applied.. The arrow indicates the time when the temperature started to change as shown on the original traces. Lines A, B, C, D show the temperature changes when the gutta percha was initially heated for 2·5, 5, 7·5 and 10 seconds respectively.

It has been suggested that under conditions of transient thermal change the thermal diffusivity is important, this being the thermal conductivity divided by the product of the specific heat and the density (Braden, 1964). He gave the following figures. The thermal conductivity of enamel is $2{\cdot}2 \times 10^{-3}$ cal/cm/sec/°C, and that of dentine is $1{\cdot}5 \times 10^{-3}$ cal/cm/sec/°C; i.e. 0·93 W/mK and 0·63 W/mK. The thermal diffusivity of enamel is $4{\cdot}2 \times 10^{-3}$ $cm^2$/sec, and that of dentine is $2{\cdot}6 \times 10^{-3}$ $cm^2$/sec; i.e. $4{\cdot}2 \times 10^{-7}$ $m^2$/s and $2{\cdot}6 \times 10^{-7}$ $m^2$/s.

**Pressure changes from thermal stimuli**

Application of thermal stimuli does not simply give rise to a temperature change since pressure changes also occur. Thus, application of water at 50°C to the intact crown for 10 seconds raised the pulpal pressure by 10–15 mm of mercury, and a blast of air for 10 seconds lowered the pressure by 4 mm of mercury (Brännström, Lindén and Åström, 1967). Clinical procedures also caused these fluid movements as when heated impression compound was applied to the tooth, or the tooth was subjected to drilling (Brännström, Lindén and Johnson, 1968).

Working on the canine teeth of dogs, Van Hassel and Brown (1969) found that the pulpal pressure rose linearly from the normal 36 mm of mercury by 2·5 mm of mercury for each degree rise in temperature. On cooling the tooth, the pressure fell more slowly at 1·6 mm mercury per °C.

## OSMOTIC STIMULI

Substances which cause pain in teeth by osmotic action include concentrated sugars such as occur in confectionery. When such sweets adhere to the margins of a 'leaking' filling, or when osmotic agents are applied to dentine for testing purposes, fluid is drawn through the dentinal tubules. Fluid flow has been observed microscopically when suction was applied to fractured dentine (Stevenson, 1965) and is associated with pain which lasts for the duration of the stimulus (Brännström, 1960a).

The rate of fluid flow through the tubules under osmotic pressures can be as high as 4·8 nanolitres per second (Anderson, Matthews and Goretta, 1967). This flow rate declines with repeated application of osmotic stimuli (Fig. 7.5) and may be related to a decline in the incidence of pain reported by human subjects whose teeth were subjected to repeated osmotic stimulation (Anderson and Ronning, 1962; Anderson, Matthews and Shelton, 1967; Lin-

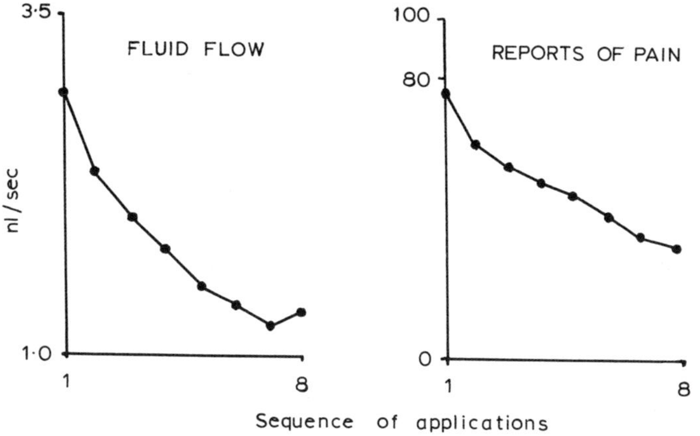


**Fig.** 7.5. Fluid flow and reports of pain on applying osmotic solutions. (Simplified and placed together, from Anderson, Matthews and Goretta, 1967.) On the left is the mean flow of dentinal fluid on application of saturated calcium chloride solution at 37°C. On the right are the subjects' reports of pain as a percentage of the applications of calcium chloride solutions (200–2800 atmospheres).

dén and Brännström, 1967). This is compatible with the view that pain could be caused by stimulation of pulpal receptors following disturbance transmitted through dentine by non-nervous means (Anderson, Curwen and Howard, 1958; Anderson and Naylor, 1962; Anderson, 1963). Occasionally pain can be sufficiently severe to be described as throbbing, and an osmotic pressure of 25 atmospheres appears to be the lowest which will elicit pain (Anderson and Ronning, 1962; Anderson and Matthews, 1967). Recent investigations of Horiuchi and Matthews (1973) have tended to support the above results but with reservations. After solutions of sodium chloride or dextrose had been alternately applied to dentine for 5 days there was a significant increase in the number of nerve impulses recorded — in cats (Northeast, 1980).

## MECHANICAL STIMULI

A stream of air over the dentine causes evaporation from the dentinal tubules and results in pain (Brännström, 1960a, b. c). Movement of fluid, and pain, can also be produced by applying dry absorbent paper; in this case pain is not simply due to touching the dentine because it is not elicited if the paper is wetted before being applied (Brännström and Åström, 1964). Also, water covering the dentine has to evaporate before there can be evaporation from the exposed dentinal tubules (Brännström and Johnson, 1978).

The way in which fluid movement acts as a stimulus has also been demonstrated in another way by Brännström (1961). When he applied an instrument to cut dentine with a force of 1 kilogram, equivalent to 100 $kg/cm^2$ (9·81 $MN/m^2$) there was no pain, and he presumed that this was because the instrument pressure was taken up by the hard tissue of dentine so that it was not transmitted to the fluid in the dentinal tubules. On the other hand, pressure applied by air or water to specially prepared cavities caused pain at pressures as low as 2 $kg/cm^2$ (0·196 $MN/m^2$), presumably because it was transmitted to fluid in the dentinal tubules. Brännström and Åström (1972) concluded that an outward flow of fluid in the tubules was more likely to cause pain than an inward movement, but it depends upon the rate of flow of dentinal fluid and this in turn depends upon whether the outer surface of the dentine is kept moist or not (Brännström, 1979); if movement is sufficiently rapid even a small amplitude might be sufficient to cause pain, as when using a probe.

When dentine is exposed the condition of the tubule apertures is an important influence on sensitivity. Surfaces exposed by fracture are more sensitive than are surfaces exposed by grinding which leaves the tubule apertures blocked by debris. The debris can be removed by application of 50 per cent citric acid, and this increases sensitivity to stimuli such as scraping with a probe, dry absorbent paper and a short blast of air (Johnson, 1974; Johnson and Brännström, 1974). This observation is clinically significant because people imbibe acid drinks, and this habit could easily contribute to the important and difficult problem of cervical sensitivity. Any attempt by the dentist to promote blockage of the tubules could be frustrated if the patient continues to drink acid fruit juices thereby removing any blocking material.

Johnson also sheds light on the role in pain production of gutta percha temporary restorations. Photographs taken with the scanning electron microscope revealed that some tubule apertures, initially blocked by grinding debris, were patent in cavities which had been filled with gutta percha for a few days, and this would make the cavities more sensitive.

Another mechanical stimulus shown to produce pain in teeth is leverage pushing apart the walls of a cavity. Forces as low as 1·5 kg produced pain in a few cases, and forces of 5·5 kg caused pain in half the cases tested (Robinson, 1964).

How does this evidence relate to the pain produced by dental instruments on the dentinal surface? Clinically it appears that the instrument must be moving to produce maximum pain — a rotating bur or a sliding probe — so it seems reasonable to suppose that they are exerting an intermittent pressure on the fluid in the dentinal tubules thereby causing pain. If a probe is pushed into the dentine at the dentino-enamel junction it has a plunger effect, producing fluid movement in the underlying tubules. If drawn across the surface of dentine a probe makes a groove which affects numerous dentinal tubules and even deforms them (Brännström, 1979). However, Anderson, Hannam and Matthews (1970) have remarked that it is difficult to imagine how lightly stimulating dentine with a sharp probe could cause a significant mechanical disturbance at a receptor in the pulp, surrounded as it is by vascular tissue in which the pressure is continually changing by up to 10 mm Hg with each heart beat. The heart beat itself can occasionally give rise to nerve impulses in the teeth of dogs — and this 'spontaneous' nerve activity (Fig. 7.6) becomes continuous if a pressure stimulus is applied (Narhi, 1978). This author also showed the relationship between hydrostatic pressure and neural impulses (Fig. 7.7). In such experimental work there is a risk that impulses could be artifactual rather than real nerve impulses (Horiuchi and Matthews, 1974),

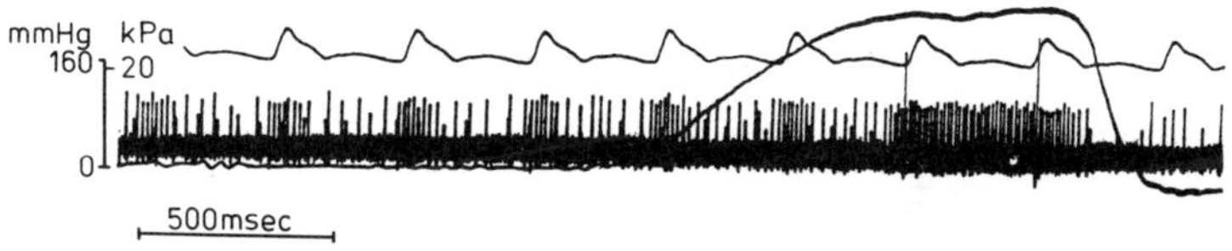


**Fig. 7.6.** Spontaneous activity in pulpal nerve fibre (in the dog). Neural impulses appear in bursts synchronously with the heart beat (upper trace). Impulses become continuous when a pressure stimulus is applied (Narhi, 1978).

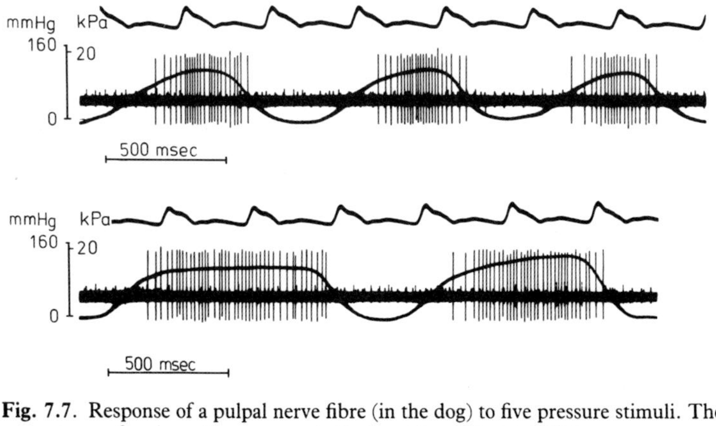


**Fig. 7.7.** Response of a pulpal nerve fibre (in the dog) to five pressure stimuli. The upper trace of each portion represents the heart beat (Narhi, 1978).

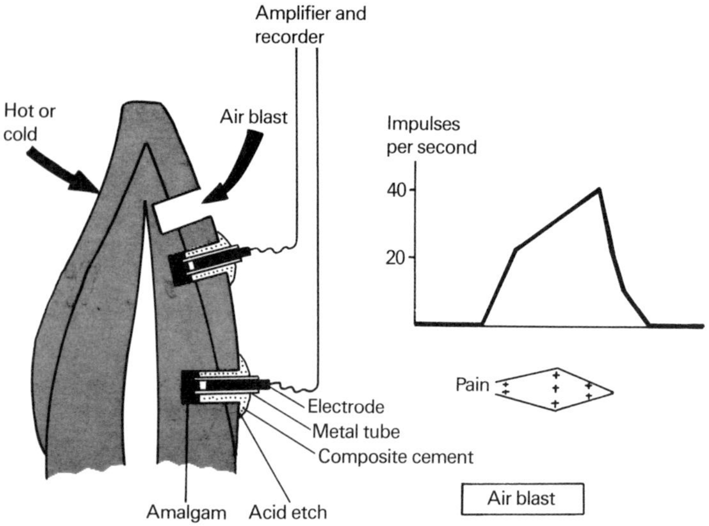


**Fig. 7.8.** *Left.* Experimental arrangement.
*Right.* Effect of an air blast stimulus on pulpal nerve activity, showing increase in nerve impulses per second, associated with pain which increases and then decreases. The air blast duration is shown. Similar results were obtained using hot and cold stimuli (Edwall and Olgart, 1977).

but Edwall and Olgart (1977) have overcome these objections, using fixed electrodes with large contact areas in human teeth (Fig. 7.8). They have also been able to correlate the stimulus with both nerve activity and the sensation.

## ELECTRICAL STIMULI

Electrical stimuli are at once the most natural and the most artificial of the stimuli applied to teeth. They are natural in that conduction through the tissues is electrolytic, depending on ionic movement, and ionic movement is fundamental to nerve excitation (Chapter 2). They are artificial in that electrical stimuli are not applied to teeth in the natural way that thermal stimuli are when eating and drinking. However, electrical stimuli have the great advantage over other stimuli that they can be precisely defined by electronic methods.

### Path of electric current

The stimulating electrode placed on the tooth is usually the cathode, whilst the anode or indifferent electrode is placed elsewhere, usually in the patient's hand. The electric current (as conventionally described) passes through the hand, arm, neck and head to leave the body via the tooth and the dental electrode. In passing through the body the current is distributed throughout the tissues in inverse proportion to the electrical resistance encountered. In the soft tissues the resistance is negligible compared with that of the hard dental tissues, and is about several thousand ohms. The resistance of dentine may be as much as 500 thousand ohms and that of the enamel 10 million ohms depending amongst other factors on the size of the electrode used (Mumford, 1956, 1967).

Within the tooth, current passes through the pulp, along the dentinal tubules and through the enamel as illustrated by the specimens in Fig. 7.9, and diagrammatically in Fig. 7.10. The above specimens were obtained by passing the coloured cation of methylene blue through extracted teeth under the influence of an electric field, and then grinding the teeth to reveal the blue colouration (Mumford, 1959a). Notice how the path taken by the electric current differs from that of thermal change which spreads throughout the crown. The above view of the electric current path is supported by subsequent investigations of Newton and Mumford (1969). They determined the path taken by water flowing through analogues of human teeth, illustrated in Fig. 7.11).

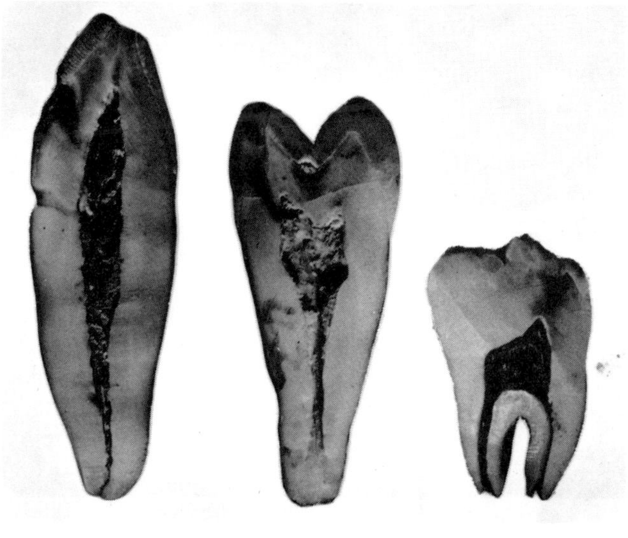

**Fig. 7.9.** Path of electric current as indicated by the passage of the coloured cation of methylene blue. The canine tooth is represented in Fig. 7.10.

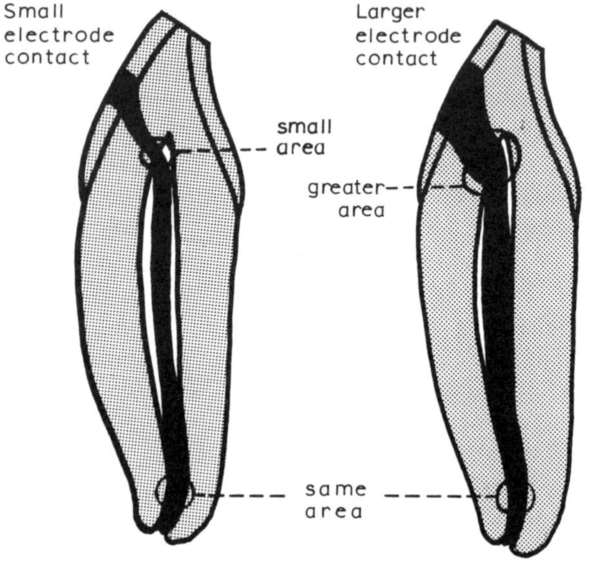


**Fig. 7.10**. Diagrams of the paths taken by an electric current passing through a tooth, showing the influence of electrode contact area. With a larger contact area the affected area of the pulpo-dentinal junction is greater. (Mumford and Newton, 1969a.)

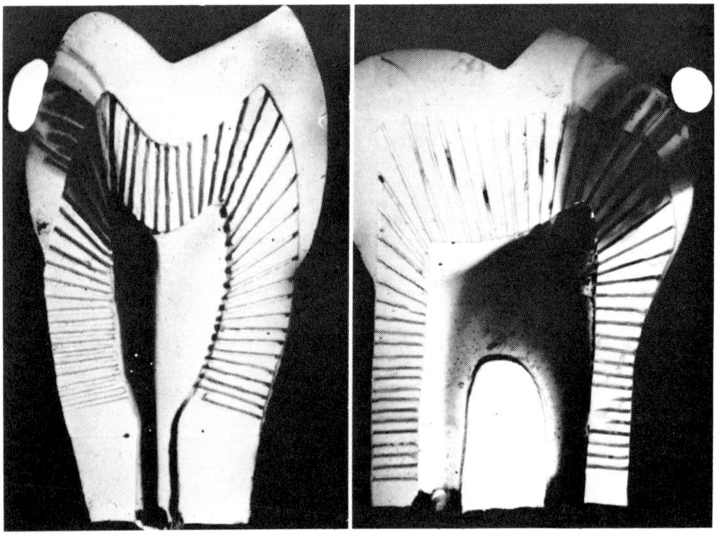

**Fig. 7.11**. These are analogues (made of plaster of Paris) of the premolar and molar in Fig. 7.9. The dark zones indicate the path taken by water flowing past potassium permanganate crystals. Notice the similarity of water flow to the electrical flow in Fig. 7.9.

**Zone of excitation**

Because of the electrical characteristics of teeth, increasing the electrode area on the enamel surface increases the area through which current flows in enamel and dentine but does not increase the area in the pulp canal (Fig. 7.10). This means that if excitation of nerves occurred primarily in the pulp canal the current needed in the two cases illustrated would remain the same. In fact it has been shown that increasing the electrode area necessitates an increase in current to produce excitation, so it follows that excitation occurs at or near the pulpo-dentinal junction, the increased current being needed to maintain the current density (current per unit area).

Naturally, the coronal pulp cannot be stimulated when it is dead and, if the radicular pulp is still vital, a response from the patient could be misleading. To avoid such a situation it is possible to use twin coronal electrodes, one being placed on the labial and the other on the lingual surface of the crown, the hand electrode being dispensed with (Mumford, 1959b). In this case the current takes the path shown in the specimen (Fig. 7.12), the analogous situation with fluid flow being shown in Fig. 7.13 (Newton and Mumford, 1969).

As a factor in the sensitivity of dentine it seems worth drawing attention to an observation of Rushton (1927). He found that the

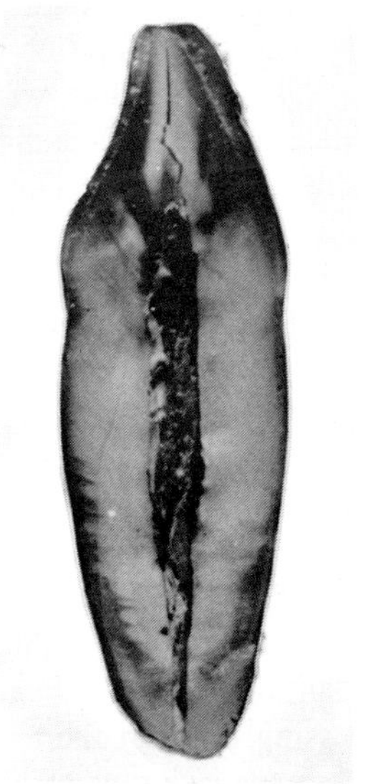

**Fig. 7.12.** Path of electric current between one electrode placed labially and another placed lingually.

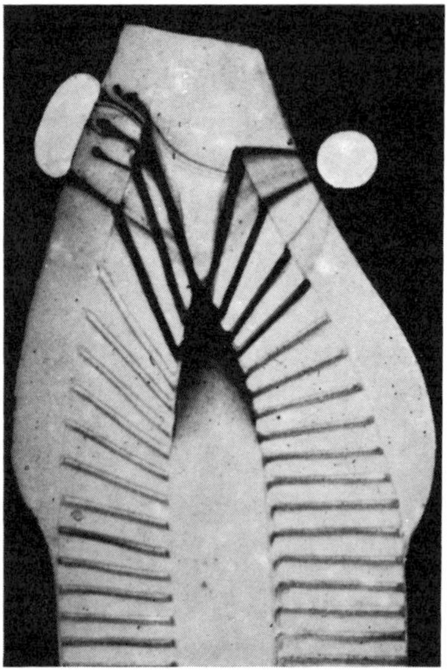

**Fig. 7.13.** Water flowing through a plaster analogue from an inlet on the labial surface to an outlet on the lingual surface. Notice similar path to that of the electric current in Fig. 7.12.

angle formed between a nerve and the direction of electric current applied to it was a factor in nervous excitation. He stated that the threshold varies inversely as the cosine of the angle between the current and the nerves. This means that, with nerve fibres lying in the dentinal tubules, the stimulating current would lie in the most favourable line, and this would result in low pain perception thresholds.

A further factor in sensitivity is the way in which current is conducted along the dentinal tubules rather than through the more solid intertubular part of the dentine, so the current density is really greater again than might be expected. The number of dentinal tubules per unit area of dentine may be taken as 45 000 $mm^{-2}$ and the diameter of the tubules as 2 $\mu m$ (Fromme and Riedel, 1970; Forsell-Ahlberg *et al.*, 1975; Garberoglio and Brännström, 1976; Whittaker and Kneale, 1979). The total area of tubules to overall area is therefore one to seven. Looked at simplistically, for an electrical stimulus, this is an amplification factor of seven to one — ignoring any current passing through the more highly resistant intertubular dentine, and any capacitative effects which are not properly understood in teeth (Mumford, 1980).

**Time to stimulate**

Electrical stimuli reach nerve fibres in the pulp almost instantaneously, whereas time is needed for thermal change at the tooth surface to spread through to the pulp (Fig. 7.4). A similar delay occurs when chemicals are applied to dentine because chemicals require a few seconds to diffuse to the pulp (Yamada and Sakada, 1961).

## STREAMING POTENTIAL AS A POSSIBLE CAUSE OF PAIN

It is obvious that fluid movements in dentine are produced by various physical agencies and that these agencies also cause pain. It is therefore reasonable to suppose that the actual fluid movement could be directly responsible for exciting nerve endings, perhaps by altering the ionic environment of the nerve endings, but another possibility is that the direct cause of excitation might be an electrical potential that is generated by the fluid movement. This is called a streaming potential and develops as described below. If the hypothesis could be substantiated it would have the merit of relating all the different stimuli described in this chapter.

Within the dentine there is a solid-liquid interface in each dentinal tubule where the wall of the dentinal tubule meets the fluid within it. At this interface there exists an electrical double layer and because the tubule wall preferentially adsorbs ions from the liquid, an imbalance arises between the charge on the wall and the charge in the liquid, with the result that an electrical potential difference exists, and this is called the zeta potential. Movement of fluid through dentine disturbs this potential difference by moving the liquid phase with its ionic layer, so that the electrical potential difference then exists along the tubules and is called the streaming potential. This streaming potential has been measured by Mumford and Newton (1969b) who applied fluid under pressure to extracted

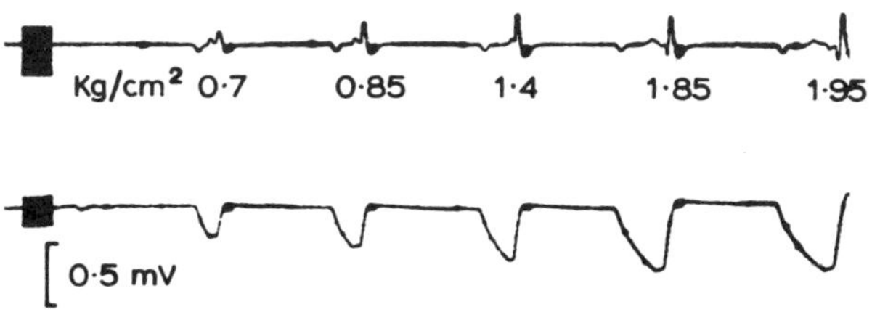


**Fig. 7.14.** Fluid pressure applied to dentine (upper trace) produced electrical potentials (lower trace).

human teeth and found that pressures of 2 kg/cm$^2$ produced potential differences across the dentine of 0·15–1·0 mV, the mean being 0·5 mV (Fig. 7.14). Horiuchi and Matthews (1973) also found a streaming potential of approximately 0·5 mV. The pressure of 2 kg/cm$^2$ was used because this pressure was found to be the lowest pressure which was just sufficient to cause pain when applied to human teeth *in vivo* (Brännström, 1961); in effect 2 kg/cm$^2$ is a pain perception threshold stimulus.

There is a theoretical relationship between the above factors given by the Helmholtz-Schmoluchowski equation:

$$E = \frac{P \varepsilon \zeta}{4\pi\eta\lambda}$$

where E is the streaming potential, P the applied pressure, ε the dielectric constant, ζ the zeta potential, η the viscosity and λ the conductivity of the fluid within the capillary system, in this case the dentine. Mumford and Newton (1969b) found appropriate values for the above factors from various sources and substituted them in the above equation to obtain

$$E = \frac{150 \times 30}{1{\cdot}06 \times 10^5 \times 12 \times 10^{-3}} = \pm\ 3{\cdot}5\ \text{mV}.$$

It will be seen that this value for the streaming potential was seven times that which they actually measured, and whether or not such potentials could cause excitation of nerve endings in the area of the pulpo-dentinal junction is not yet known. Whatever the final explanation may be it is to be expected that the rate of fluid flow will be an important factor.

## REFERENCES

Anderson, D. J. (1963) Chemical and osmotic excitants of pain in human dentine. In *Sensory Mechanisms in Dentine*, ed. Anderson, D. J., pp. 88–93. Oxford: Pergamon.
Anderson, D. J., Curwen, M. P. and Howard, L. V. (1958) The sensitivity of human dentine. *J. dent.* Res., **37**, 669–677.
Anderson, D. J., Hannam, A. G. and Matthews, B. (1970) Sensory mechanisms in mammalian teeth. *Physiological Reviews*, **50**, 171–195.
Anderson, D. J. and Matthews, B. (1967) Osmotic stimulation of human dentine and the distribution of dental pain thresholds. *Archs. oral Biol.*, **12**, 417–426.
Anderson, D. J., Matthews, B. and Goretta, C, (1967) Fluid flow through human dentine. *Archs. oral Biol.*, **12**, 209–216.
Anderson, D. J., Matthews, B. and Shelton, L. E. (1967) Variations in the sensitivity to osmotic stimulation of human dentine. *Archs. oral Biol.*, **12**, 43–47.
Anderson, D. J. and Naylor, M. N. (1962) Chemical excitants of pain in human dentine and dental pulp. *Archs. oral Biol.*, **7**, 413–415.

Anderson, D. J. and Ronning, G. A. (1962) Osmotic excitants of pain in human dentine. *Archs. oral Biol.*, **7**, 513–523.

Braden, M. (1964) Heat conduction in teeth and the effect of lining materials. *J. dent. Res.*, **43**, 315–322.

Brännström, M. (1960a) Dentinal and pulpal response. I. Application of reduced pressure to exposed dentine. *Acta odont. Scand.*, **18**, 1–15.

Brännström, M. (1960b) Dentinal and pulpal response. II. Application of an air stream to exposed dentine. Short observation period. *Acta odont. Scand.*, **18**, 17–28.

Brännström, M. (1960c) Dentinal and pulpal response. III. Application of an air stream to exposed dentine. Long observation periods. *Acta odont. Scand.*, **18**, 235–252.

Brännström, M. (1961) Dentinal and pulpal response. V. Application of pressure to exposed dentine. *J. dent. Res.*, **40**, 960–970.

Brannström, M. (1979) The transmission and control of dentinal pain. In *Mechanism and Control of Pain*, ed. Grossman, L. I., pp. 15–35. New York: Masson.

Brännström, M. and Åstrom, A. (1964) A study of the mechanism of pain elicited from the dentine. *J. dent. Res.*, **43**, 619–625.

Brännström, M. and Åstrom, A. (1972) The hydrodynamics of the dentine; its possible relationship to dentinal pain. *Int. dent. J. (Lond.)*, **22**, 219–227.

Brännström, M. and Johnson, G. (1978) The sensory mechanisms in human dentin as revealed by evaporation and mechanical removal of dentin. *J. dent. Res.*, **57**, 49–53.

Brännström, M., Lindén,-A. and Åström, A. (1967) The hydrodynamics of the dental tubule and of pulp fluid. A discussion of its significance in relation to dental sensitivity. *Caries Res.*, **1**, 310–317.

Brännström, M., Lindén, L.-Å. and Johnson, G. (1968) Movement of dentinal and pulpal fluid caused by clinical procedures. *J. dent. Res.*, **47**, 679–682.

Edwall, L. and Olgart, L. (1977) A new technique for recording of intradental sensory nerve activity in man. *Pain*, **3**, 121–125.

Forsell-Ahlberg, K., Brännström, M. and Edwall, L. (1975) The diameter and number of dentinal tubules in rat, cat, dog and monkey. *Acta Odont. Scand.*, **33**, 243–250.

Fromm, H. G. and Riedel, H. (1970) Messungen über die Weite der Dentinkanälchen an nichtenmineralisierten bleibenden Zähnen und Milchzähnen. *Deutsche zahnärztlichen Zeitschrift*, **25**, 401. Quoted by Forsell-Ahlberg et al (see above).

Funakoshi, M. and Zotterman, Y. (1963) A study in the excitation of dental pulp nerve fibres. *In Sensory Mechanisms in Dentine*, ed. Anderson, D. J., pp. 60–72. London: Pergamon.

Garberoglio, R. and Brännström, M. (1976) Scanning electron microscopic investigation of human dentinal tubules. *Archs. oral Biol.*, **21**, 355–362.

Hassel, H. J. Van and Brown, A. C. (1969) Effect of temperature changes on intrapulpal pressure and hydraulic permeability in dogs. *Archs. oral. Biol.*, **14**, 301–315.

Hensel, H. and Mann, G. (1956) Temperaturschmerz und Wärmleitung in menslichen Zahn. *Stoma*, **9**, 76–85.

Horiuchi, H. and Matthews, B. (1973) *In-vitro* observations on fluid flow through human dentine caused by pain-producing stimuli. *Archs. oral Biol.*, **18**, 275–294.

Horiuchi, H. and Matthews, B. (1974) Evidence on the origin of impulses recorded from dentine in the cat. *J. Physiol. (Lond.)*, **243**, 797–829.

Johnson, G. (1974) The hydrodynamics of the dentin and its clinical applications. Stockholm: Tryckeri Balder AB.

Johnson, G. And Brännström, M. (1974) The sensitivity of dentin. Changes in relation to conditions at exposed tubule apertures. *Acta. Odont. Scand.*, **32**, 29–38.

Lindén, L.-Å. and Brännström, M. (1967) Fluid movements in dentine and pulp. An *in vitro* study of flow produced by clinical solutions on exposed dentine. *Odont. Revy*, **18**, 227–236.
Mumford, J. M. (1956) Direct current electrodes for pulp testing. *Dent. Practit. dent. Rec.*, **6**, 235–238.
Mumford, J. M. (1959a) Path of direct current in electric pulp testing using one coronal electrode. *Brit. dent. J.*, **106**, 23–26.
Mumford, J. M. (1959b) Path of direct current in electric pulp testing using two coronal electrodes. *Brit. dent. J.*, **6**, 243–245.
Mumford, J. M. (1967) Resistivity of human enamel and dentine. *Archs. oral Biol.*, **12**, 925–927.
Mumford, J. M. (1980) Transmission mechanisms in dental pain. *Brit. J. oral Surg.*, **17**, 198–217.
Mumford, J. M. and Newton, A. V. (1969a) Zone of excitation when electrically stimulating human teeth. *Archs. oral Biol.*, **14**, 1383–1388.
Mumford, J. M. and Newton, A. V. (1969b) Transduction of hydrostatic pressure to electric potential in human dentin. *J. dent. Res.*, **48**, 226–229.
Narhi, M. (1978) Activation of dental pulp nerves of the cat and the dog with hydrostatic pressure. *Proc. Finn. Dent. Soc.*, **74**, Suppl. 5.
Naylor, M. N. (1964) Studies on sensation to cold stimulation in human teeth. *Brit. dent. J.*, **117**, 482–486.
Newton, A. V. and Mumford, J. M. (1969) Current paths through analogues of human teeth. *Archs. oral Biol.*, **14**, 699–705.
Newton, A. V. and Mumford, J. M. (1970) Thermal flow through human teeth. *Dent. Practit. dent. Rec.*, **21**, 84–86.
Northeast, S. E. (1980) The effects of silicate cement fillings on the response of intradental nerves to chemical and osmotic stimulation of dentine in the cat. *Int. Ass. Dent. Res. (Brit. Div.) Abstr.* 224.
Robinson, A. D. (1964) A preliminary investigation of the pain response to mechanical deformation of the teeth. *Archs. oral Biol.*, **9**, 281–286.
Rushton, W. A. H. (1927) The effect upon the threshold for nervous excitation of the length of nerve exposed, and the angle between current and nerve. *J. Physiol* (Lond.), **63**, 357–377.
Stevenson, T. S. (1965) Odontoblast aspiration and fluid movement in human dentine. *Archs. oral Biol.*, **12**, 1149–1157.
Trowbridge, H. O., Franks, M., Korostoff, E. and Emling, R. (1980) Sensory response to thermal stimulation in human teeth. *J. Endo.*, **6**, 405–412.
Whittaker, D. K. and Kneale, M. J. (1979) The dentine-predentine interface in human teeth. A scanning electron microscope study. *Brit. dent. J.*, **146**, 43–46.
Yamada, M. and Sakada, S. (1961) The effects of some chemicals on cervix dentis. *J. dent Res.*, **40**, 975–987.

# 8

# Pain due to enamel factors

The title of this chapter may provoke surprise because it is not usual to think of enamel as being involved in the production of pain. Loss of enamel by attrition, abrasion and erosion does not cause pain, and even considerable loss of dentine from these causes is not associated with much pain. However, a physical factor to be considered is the fluid present in enamel. Apart from any defects, there is about 2 per cent of water in enamel and this is at least partly mobile, so it might possibly have some bearing on pain. A fluid outflow of 4000 nanolitres per $cm^2$ in 24 hours (about 0·05 nl/$cm^2$/sec) has been recorded *in vitro* by Bergman and Siljestrand (1963), and *in vivo* by Bergman and Lindèn (1965).

The movement of water from enamel is illustrated by drying of enamel which occurs when teeth are isolated under rubber dam and which is associated with a rise in its electrical resistance (Mumford, 1966). When dry, the enamel looks whiter than the undried enamel, whether this is on adjacent teeth or part of the same tooth. The whiteness can be observed within half an hour of isolating teeth from the mouth, and lasts for about the same length of time after the rubber dam has been removed so that the enamel is again exposed to saliva. It follows that it requires this time for water to be taken up once more. The enamel is obviously more changeable in this respect than was once supposed, which means that there is a chance of pain from this source possibly by osmotic activity. The presence of enamel lamellae and cracks will increase this possibility.

A neurological factor to be considered is that nerve fibres might pass along the entire length of the dentinal tubules to reach the dentino-enamel junction and it has even been suggested that nerve fibres end in enamel spindles (Römer, 1899). These were sometimes regarded as sensory receptors, but this is not nowadays accepted.

**Damaged enamel**

When the enamel has been damaged the possibility of pain occuring is increased. Thus, in some teeth with superficial caries limited to enamel Brännström and Lind (1965) have found histological changes in the pulp, and these changes could conceivably lead to pain.

Numerous otherwise normal teeth are seen with many minute enamel cracks or crazing which can be seen only when light strikes the teeth at certain angles. In some cases patients complain of sensitivity in such teeth, and this is often the case after a blow, although sensitivity of this kind is seldom great and quickly diminishes. The underlying pulp sometimes becomes mineralised and this process is usually ascribed to the effect of trauma on the pulp, but the indirect effect on the pulp of these minute cracks in enamel and the accompanying sensitivity might be quite important.

A more severe crack in the enamel than the minute ones described above may cause severe pain and it is by no means easy to diagnose the cause in such cases. Pain occurs on eating citrus fruits and also when eating foods that exert a plunger action, such as fruit pastilles. A diagnostic point is that sharp pain is said to occur on releasing the pressure (Stanley, 1969). This condition is usually referred to as the cracked tooth syndrome (see Chapter 9).

A somewhat mysterious case of pain from enamel is considered of interest, although no explanation is offered. A science graduate, working with dentists on dental problems, presented with pain which occurred on touching the enamel on the labial aspect of the left upper central incisor. On examination it was found that a sharp pain occurred whenever a tiny area at the middle of the labial enamel was touched with a probe. The patient was prevented from seeing what the dentist was doing while several teeth were probed to try to confuse her, without resting the dentist's hand on her face which might have afforded her a clue to the probe position. Pain occurred only from the one tiny area of labial enamel. To avoid any possibility of galvanic activity causing the pain a sharpened orange-wood stick was used as a probe but sensitivity was still noted. Incredibly, radiographic examination revealed a satisfactory root filling! It has been shown (in cats and monkeys) that even lightly touching the tooth surface can produce impulses in periodontal nerve fibres (Kerr and Lysak, 1964) but such a response would have been well within the normal physiological range.

**Shock from the dental unit**

A patient complained of a sharp pain when the dentist's finger touched a tooth which was one of the group isolated by rubber dam. The patient was holding the compressed air syringe, and pain occurred when the dentist touched the tooth provided he was also manipulating the foot control. There was thus a complete electrical circuit through the dentist, the dental unit and the patient. The rubber dam effectively confined the current path thus allowing a high current density within the pulp. Under these conditions similar pain occurred in several patients, with several different units. Of course, this was not due to any fault in the tooth but it is mentioned here because pain occurred when the enamel was touched.

REFERENCES

Bergman, G. and Lindén, L.-Å. (1965) Techniques for microscopic study of the enamel fluid *in vivo*. *J. dent. Res.*, **44**, 1409.

Bergman, G. and Siljestrand, B. (1963) Water evaporation *in vitro* from human dental enamel. *Archs. oral Biol.*, **8**, 37–38.

Brännström, M. (1967) Fluid movements in dentine and pulp. *Odont. Revy*, **18**, 227–236.

Brännström, M. and Lind, P. O. (1965) Pulpal response to early dental caries. *J.dent. Res.*, **44**, 1045–1050.

Kerr, F. W. L. and Lysak, W. R. (1964) Somatotopic organization of trigeminal ganglion neurones. *Arch. Neurol.*, **11**, 593–602.

Mumford, J. M. (1966) Drying of enamel under rubber dam. *Brit. dent. J.*, **121**, 178–179.

Römer, O. (1899) Zahnhistologische Studie. Freiburg: Felsenfeld.

Stanley, H. R. (1969) The cracked tooth syndrome. *J. Amer. Acad. Gold Foil Operators*, **11**, 364–367.

# 9

## Pain due to factors affecting dentine

It is probably true to say that there is no such condition as dentine pain divorced from pulpal pain since pulp tissues must always be involved to some extend, the minimum pulpal involvement being that pain is mediated eventually by nerve fibres within the pulp. It might even be said that the part of dentine that matters in the origin of pain is really pulpal tissue since the odontoblastic processes are extensions of pulpal cells, and cutting normal dentine effectively involves producing many thousands of minute pulp exposures. Nevertheless it seems reasonable to consider one broad division of toothache cases as being due primarily to factors affecting dentine. This division includes cases where the teeth are otherwise normal in every way, as well as those with various degrees of dentine damage. Such damage may be associated with changes in the pulp of slight or greater severity, but there need be no pulp disease for pain to occur.

### PAIN IN NORMAL TEETH

Occasionally patients are referred for consultation because they sometimes suffer dental pain although the dentist can find no fault in the teeth concerned. One source of such pain is when the patient eats ice cream, and pain occurs in the lower anterior teeth. The crowns of these teeth are relatively small, which means that contact with any cold food or drink produces a greater fall in temperature than would occur in larger teeth. Moreover, the distance from the outer surface to the pulp is less than in other teeth so, for a given cold stimulus, the thermal gradient is greater in lower anterior teeth and the temperature of the pulpo-dentinal junction falls faster (Fig. 9.1). Pain occurs shortly after the ice cream is bitten and continues for a brief time afterwards, outlasting the stimulus for a few seconds because the dentine has been cooled and requires this short time to return to its normal temperature. What matters in causing pain is not the temperature at the tooth surface but that at the

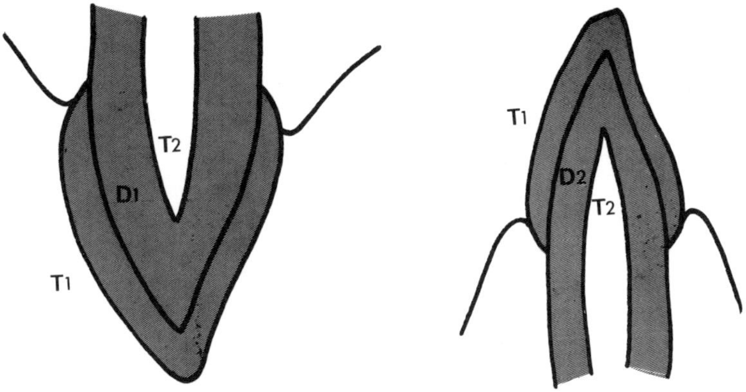


**Fig. 9.1**. The thermal gradient is the difference between the outside temperature (T1) and the inside temperature (T2) divided by the distance between (D). In the more slender lower incisor D2 is less than D1 in the canine so the thermal gradient is greater for the incisor which is more likely to hurt.

sensory receptors near the pulpo-dentinal junction. At least, that is true if the receptors are excited directly by thermal change, but it is possible that the initial excitation is indirectly caused by fluid movement in the dentinal tubules produced by the thermal change. This view is based on the work of Trowbridge et al (1980) who found that patients reported pain after application of thermal stimuli to teeth in less time than it took for thermal change to occur at the pulpo-dentinal junction. (See also Chapter 7 under Thermal change). As the person continues to eat ice cream pain becomes less likely because the temperature of the tooth gradually approaches that of the ice cream, so the thermal gradient decreases.

In a similar way, pain may occur from drinking hot liquids. This is even more likely if a person drinks hot coffee soon after taking a cold dessert. This is because the dentine has become colder than normal; application of heat to the outer surface therefore produces a large temperature gradient so that heat is conducted quickly through the tooth, and there is a rapid swing in temperature at the pulpo-dentinal junction (and more fluid movement) so that pain occurs. Such pain can, of course, occur in diseased teeth so a careful examination is needed, but if the teeth are normal the patient can be reassured. The solution of the problem is to avoid such severe temperature changes, but the increase in number of home refrigerator units seems likely to produce more such cases for the dentist to handle.

Following periodontal surgery, after the gingival packs have been removed, the teeth involved are more exposed to cold air and hot and cold foods, so pain is more likely to be experienced.

During the winter, some people complain of pain which occurs in their teeth when they leave a warm building to go into the cold outdoors. This is because of the cold air, and sometimes it can be reproduced in the surgery by a cold blast of air or a quick intake of breath.

Pain may also arise on moving in the opposite direction, from the cold outdoors to a warm room. The cause in this case is probably the vasodilation that occurs, but this is really a pulpal factor.

*Treatment*

Having listened to the complaint and examined the teeth the dentist is able to give reassurance that all is well. Extremes of heat and cold can be avoided.

**Sensitive dentine**

This occurs at the neck of a tooth and is also known as sensitive cementum. The affected area is sensitive to physical contacts and some patients complain that touching the area with a fingernail causes a brief pain lasting for only about a second. Such a stimulus can be avoided but if cavity preparation is needed just touching the zone with a bur is sufficient to make the patient jerk, and occasionally to jump convulsively with his arms and legs moving too. Toothbrushing is also a problem, partly because of the physical stimulus, partly because of the thermal stimulus if cold water is used and partly because of the toothpaste which can have both a thermal and chemical effect.

*Aetiology*

At the neck of the tooth dentine is not covered by enamel and may not be covered by gingiva, so that it is exposed. This may be made worse by restorative procedures which cause gingival recession, such as cervical fillings, crowns, badly placed denture clasps and 'gum stripper' partial dentures. The dentinal tubules thus exposed may be closed off by secondary dentine formation at the pulpal end, by mineralisation along the tubules producing a sclerosed zone, or by plugs forming at the external end. Unfortunately, some zones are sensitive, presumably by failure of the above mechanisms to occur or, perhaps, because any plugs peripherally have been inadvertently removed. This can happen if acid is applied. For example, before a glass ionomer cement filling is used the cavity is treated by citric acid to clean it and this procedure has been shown to remove any plugs from the dentinal tubules as well as widening the tubule orifice by removal of peritubular mineralised tissue (Johnson and Brännström, 1974; Brännström, 1979).

It should come as no surprise if citric acid present in citrus fruits also does the same thing, and many patients complaining of sensitive cervical dentine are found to take citrus fruits and drinks regularly. Davis and Winter (1977) exposed dentine to fresh orange juice and found, by using a scanning electron microscope, that the peritubular dentine was preferentially dissolved, the effect being almost as bad as from 1 per cent citric acid. A carbonated drink was less bad, and apple juice half as bad as the orange juice. Eventually repetitive stimulation seems to leave the teeth sensitive so that some patients with this condition are hardly able to eat and their lives become miserable, a state that affects their families too.

People who do not consume citrus fruits and drinks may nevertheless drink other soft drinks and these may be almost as harmful, as suggested above. It is also thought that the condition occurs in some cases because of the acid present in dental plaque. Once the condition develops pain interferes with proper oral hygiene and plaque becomes worse (thus providing a vicious circle).

*Treatment*

Scaling and polishing are carried out, as are any necessary restorative procedures together with elimination of any ledges on existing restorations. Oral hygiene is important because plaque is thought to be partly responsible in some cases, so careful instruction is given on correct tooth cleaning methods and one or more suitable toothbrushes must be obtained. For those who use a rotating method of toothbrushing it is desirable to spend some time brushing along the dental arches to be sure of thorough cervical cleaning, and this also stimulates the exposed cervical dentine, hopefully to provoke closure of the affected tubules. Toothbrushing in itself can be painful but it is helpful if warm water is used rather than cold water. Even if painful it must be done!

Having obtained a clean area the dentist (or dental hygienist) applies a desensitising paste to the sensitive zones using a soft rubber polishing cup. Such a paste may be Lukomsky's paste which is a mixture of one third kaolin, one third glycerin and one third of 2 per cent sodium fluoride. Stannous fluoride may also be used, as may pastes containing 1 per cent formaldehyde or 10 per cent strontium chloride. Traces of these materials may be left at the gingival margins at the close of treatment so that their effect is prolonged. Also the patient is advised to use a toothpaste which contains one of these agents. Once again traces of material may be left at the gingival margins at the end of toothbrushing.

Unfortunately, in the author's experience, these materials have not always helped, possibly because of failure to understand the importance of citrus fruits and acid soft drinks. These must be stopped even though the suggestion upsets some people because they partly drink soft drinks because they are trying to cut down on caffeine by drinking less tea and coffee. They can always try drinking water.

It is worth considering a calcium hydroxide paste. When this was applied to the dried sensitive zones it gave good reduction of sensitivity both immediately and almost as good in the longer term (Levin, Yearwood and Carpenter, 1973). Unfortunately this was not verified by Brännström, Isacsson and Johnson (1976), and Brännström (1979) concluded that almost any application which blocked the tubules for a couple of weeks was advisable; this gave time for any inflammation to subside and for some mineralisation to occur.

It is also possible to apply a varnish to the necks of the teeth affected and these should be preferably dry. It is desirable to avoid eating for some hours, preferably overnight, so the varnish is applied late in the day. The varnish contains sodium fluoride.

When using fluoride it is necessary to have sufficient concentration for a sufficiently long time to obtain adequate penetration of the dentinal tubules. To improve penetration the paste may be applied with an 'ionizing toothbrush'. This has a small 1·5V dry battery within the handle, an electrode at the base of the tufts and another electrode on the back of the brush head. The electric current generated is supposed to carry the fluoride ions into the tubules by electrophoresis. Perhaps it does but only a small part of the current can pass through the tooth because the electrical resistance of the tooth is so much greater than that of the saliva. Nevertheless, there could be a novelty value encouraging oral hygiene practice.

Another method is to apply an acid etch composite filling material or a glass ionomer cement. These have the advantage that little or no cavity preparation may be needed, but the acid etching must extend far enough onto the enamel to obtain adequate retention.

Finally, it may be necessary to drill away the sensitive zone from each tooth and place a suitable filling. This method, at least, works but care must be taken to avoid any new damage to the gingiva since gingival recession is an important factor in causing sensitive cervical dentine.

A word of warning is called for in giving advice to people who eat or drink citrus foods. The dentist may be tempted to advise tooth brushing immediately afterwards; unfortunately, it has been shown that at this time the tooth is much more vulnerable to abrasion, even if a toothbrush is used only with water (Davis and Winter, 1980).

### Sensitivity of dentino-enamel junction

Many clinicians believe that the dentino-enamel junction is more sensitive than other zones but there appears to be no scientific evidence to show this. Nerve fibres do not seem to reach as far as the junction, so activity would presumably be mediated by the odontoblasts and/or fluid flow. In connection with this it should be noted that a stimulus applied to the junction would have access to far more dentinal tubules than in deeper parts of dentine because of the considerable branching that occurs (Anderson, 1963). Moreover, at the cervix of the tooth the dentine is sometimes excruciatingly sensitive and this is the part that would have been the dentino-enamel junction had the enamel been covering it.

It is possible that with the old laborious cutting methods the dentino-enamel junction seemed specially sensitive after having been drilling in enamel or the carious part of the tooth, but this is less significant nowadays with modern local anaesthetics and water-cooled, high speed cutting instruments.

## PAIN IN TEETH WITH DISEASED OR LOST TISSUE

### Dental caries

In view of the existence of an enormous number of carious lesions it is surprising that there are not even more cases of toothache than there are already, and it can only be concluded that caries of itself seldom directly causes pain. Of course it is indirectly responsible for a great deal of pain because it progressively destroys tooth tissue thereby leaving the underlying pulp and dentine less well protected from external stimuli and, eventually, it reaches the pulp allowing ingress of micro-organisms and onset of pulpitis.

A carious cavity is subjected to mechanical stimulation of various kinds. Hard objects in food may strike directly on to dentine, or soft food such as bread can press into a cavity exerting a plunger action and forcing fluid through the dentinal tubules to cause pain.

A similar effect occurs and is useful when investigating early caries in pits and fissures. If a probe is pressed into a defect and causes a brief sharp pain this is due to it excerting a plunger effect and forcing fluid along the dentinal tubules. It follows that the defect extends to dentine, and indicates caries which must be treated. If there is no pain this may be because the defect is limited to enamel and treatment might not be necessary.

Foods containing high concentrations of sugar exert an osmotic effect, and strong alcoholic drinks may also withdraw fluid from the dentinal tubules, both of these stimuli causing pain.

Hot and cold foods including liquids enter the carious cavity and thus come closer to the pulpo-dentinal junction. As described earlier, the temperature gradient across the remaining dentine is inversely proportional to the thickness of the remaining dentine, so the temperature of the pulpo-dentinal junction rises more rapidly than in the normal tooth (Fig. 9.2). Moreover, there is less remaining tooth substance to be heated so the available heat can produce a relatively higher rise in temperature, with resulting pain.

Fortunately defence reactions of the dentine and pulp tend to prevent pain from these sources by closing the tubules. This occurs either by mineralisation within the tubules forming a sclerotic zone (translucent zone) or by formation of a calcified layer along the pulpal aspect of the dentine leading to death of the contents of the dentinal tubules in a dead tract. At the periphery of such zones the dentinal tubules may be quite normal so that during cavity preparation it is possible to encounter dentine of varying sensitivity.

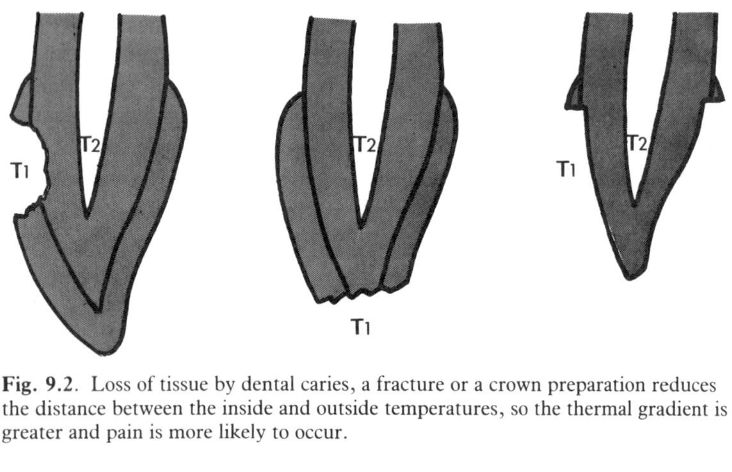


**Fig. 9.2.** Loss of tissue by dental caries, a fracture or a crown preparation reduces the distance between the inside and outside temperatures, so the thermal gradient is greater and pain is more likely to occur.

*Treatment*

Caries is excavated, taking care not to expose the pulp, and a dressing is placed. (See later in this chapter under Temporary restorations.)

**Trauma and operative procedures**

Trauma and operations on teeth produce a rapid loss of tissue and there is no time for defence reactions to occur in the dentine and pulp. If the injured area is not suitably protected, pain arises from mechanical, thermal and chemical stimuli, as described above (Fig. 9.2). There is, however, a difference between the two factors. Fracture leaves the dentinal tubules open whereas cutting appears to leave them blocked, at least superficially (Anderson and Ronning, 1962). This explains why, in experimental work, dentine surfaces exposed by fracture are more sensitive than dentine which has been ground (Johnson and Brännström, 1974). The same is not necessarily true with accidental fractures because the pulp may be concussed or even dead. These results are supported by the observation of Stevenson (1967) that fluid movement from the tubules occurred following fracture but not after wet cutting and grinding.

*Effect of repeated stimulation*

It used to be a common practice to treat prepared cavities by applying absolute alcohol with the object of drying them and perhaps sterilising them too. This was accompanied by considerable pain because of removal of heat to vaporise the alcohol, and also by withdrawal of fluid from the dentinal tubules, and is not usually practised nowadays. The procedure was too painful to be repeated but, in experimental conditions, when exposed dentine is subjected to repeated stimulation by liquids of high osmotic pressure there is a progressive decrease in the pain produced. This is regarded as being due to dentinal changes (Anderson, Matthews and Shelton, 1967), possibly plugging of the pulpal end of the dentinal tubules by the odontoblastic process (Lindén and Brännström, 1967). An important factor is the amount of fluid flow, Anderson, Matthews and Goretta (1967) having shown that this diminishes with repeated applications as do the percentage of pain reports (Fig. 7.5). However, this reduction in the number of responses is only true for liquids of high osmotic pressure. For lower osmotic pressure there is not a fall of sensitivity, which suggests that the sensory mechanism is being inactivated at the higher concentrations (Anderson and Matthews, 1967). Pain on applying zinc phosphate cement is probably due to its osmotic effect, but acidity and temperature are also factors.

*Effect of time from preparation*

Clinical observation seems to show that if a cavity is not finished at the first appointment, completion at a later visit is more than usually painful. This is in accordance with investigations of Anderson, Matthews and Shelton (1967) who found more reports of pain a week after cavity preparation, and of Brännström, Lindén and Johnson (1969) — one week after preparation cavities were more sensitive to probing or a short air blast but less sensitive to application of pressure by compressed air.

Hypersensitivity after a lapse of time is specially noticeable when removing temporary restorations of gutta percha or zinc oxide-eugenol. After leaving gutta percha in a cavity for a week it was more sensitive than immediately after cutting (Anderson and Ronning, 1962) and this may be associated with hyperaemia of the underlying pulp (Massler, 1956). However, it seems more likely that it is due to the gutta percha removing debris that was originally blocking the tubules. This has been shown by use of the scanning electron microscope (Johnson, 1974).

*Effect of cavity depth*

A hot or cold stimulus is more painful when applied to deep cavities because the reduced amount of dentine between the cavity and the pulp allows a higher thermal gradient than in shallow cavities (see earlier). The temperature also rises (or falls) more because there is less tooth substance.

Pain from applied pressure also occurs more readily in deep than in shallow cavities, because the former have dentinal tubules which are both shorter and wider (Brännström, Lindén and Johnson, 1969). This is assuming that there has been no time for defence reactions to occur in the dentine and pulp underlying the cavities.

It has also been shown that materials such as calcium hydroxide paste placed in deeper cavities of dogs teeth produce a greater number of nerve impulses than with shallow cavities (Yamada and Sakada, 1962). In other words, the stimulus would be more effective in deeper cavities.

*Effect of age*

The results of electrical stimulation show that there is no fundamental difference in sensitivity of dental nerves in older people (Mumford, 1965; Harkins and Chapman, 1976). However, when operating on teeth in older people, they do seem to be less sensitive than in young adults, and this is presumably because of age changes in the dentine and pulp. The dentinal tubules have become narrower and possibly closed by mineralisation and secondary dentine formation, while the pulps horns and pulp have receded.

These changes mean that mechanical, thermal and chemical stimuli are less effective whereas the electrical stimulus has the same effect since it passes right through the tooth (Chapter 7). The two apparently contradictory findings are therefore entirely compatible.

*Effect of secondary dentine*

Secondary dentine formation affects the incidence of pain in two ways. Firstly, by adding to the thickness of dentine the effectiveness of external stimuli — mechanical, thermal and chemical — is reduced. Secondly, the absence of dentinal tubules or their reduced number diminishes the fluid flow that can occur and also prevents or reduces ingress of nerve terminals.

The time needed for secondary dentine to form is no doubt variable but Brännström (1960) suggests that a month may be sufficient.

**Attrition, abrasion and erosion**

Loss of tooth tissue from these factors is usually sufficiently slow to allow defensive changes to occur in dentine and pulp, and as a rule pain is not a feature, but this depends both on the rate at which change occurs and the extent. However, great loss of tissue may not be associated with pain (Fig. 9.3), whereas relatively small loss of tissue (Fig. 9.4) can allow pain from hot, cold and sweet foods, and from gentle stroking with a probe. Sometimes sensitive occlusal areas occur which are only 1–2 mm in diameter. It should be expected that these would be more sensitive after acid food or drinks (Johnson and Brännström, 1974).

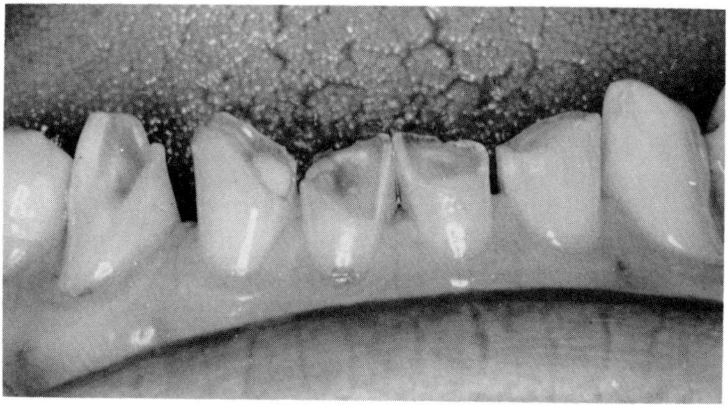

**Fig. 9.3.** Considerable attrition may not be associated with pain.

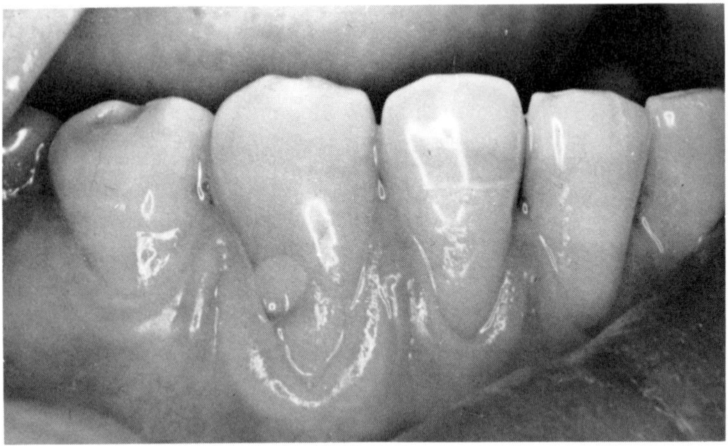

**Fig. 9.4.** A small amount of attrition was associated with pain in this patient. It occurred in the lower premolar on touching the worn area of the occlusal surface.

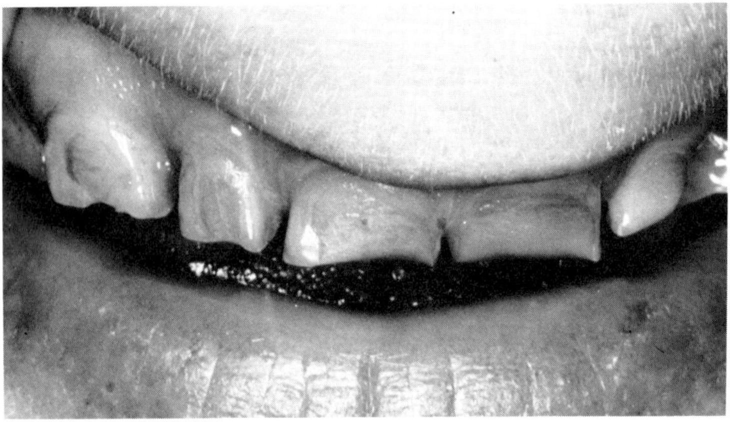

**Fig. 9.5.** Considerable erosion was not associated with pain in this patient.

The lady whose eroded teeth are shown in Fig. 9.5 had eaten fresh grapefruit and drunk lemon juice for 20 years but noticed only mild sensitivity which occurred on imbibing these foods. She presented for treatment only because the teeth looked unsightly. The apparent incompatibility of this kind of case with the greater sensitivity suggested by the work of Johnson and Brännström is presumed to be due to the much longer time involved.

## PAIN IN RESTORED TEETH

### Inadequately lined restoration

When a metal restoration has been inserted the underlying dentine is protected from mechanical stimuli, but pain may still occur from application of hot and cold stimuli. This is first noticed following the operative procedure once the local anaesthetic has worn off. Closely related is the condition of hyperalgesia produced by injudicious polishing of the restoration.

*Treatment*

Although pain occurs on eating or drinking hot or cold foods and lasts for the period of application or a little longer no treatment is needed, other than reassurance. Meanwhile, such foods should be avoided for a few days, and pain usually ceases to occur. If pain continues the case history should indicate whether a lining has been placed or not, or if it might be inadequate but this might be revealed only by removing the restoration (Fig. 9.6). A suitable temporary restoration is placed and this usually stops the pain.

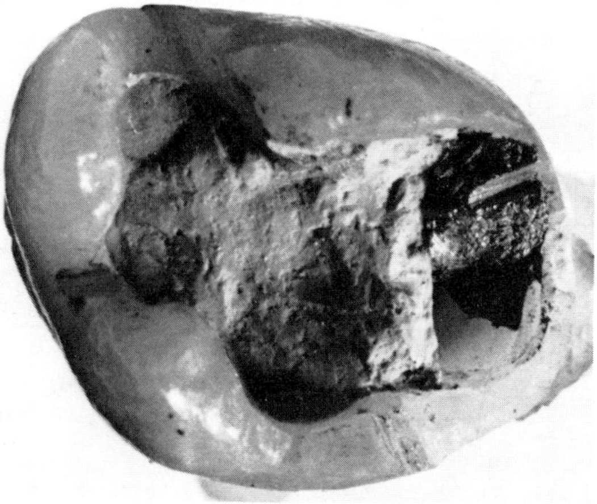

**Fig. 9.6.** There was a thick zinc phosphate lining on the pulpal wall of the cavity but none on the palatal axial wall, so the amalgam (dark) almost reached the pulp.

### Secondary expansion of amalgam

Contamination by water of silver amalgam which contains zinc can produce a great secondary expansion of the set amalgam. This expansion can theoretically cause pain by exerting pressure on the walls of the restored tooth, but it is doubtful whether this actually occurs. Many thousands of amalgam restorations must be contaminated by saliva, but the author has not knowingly seen a case where secondary expansion of the amalgam filling was the cause of pain.

**Leaking restoration**

There are millions of amalgam restorations which have deficient margins and any of these could be leaking but, fortunately, the small gap between metal and tooth seems to be filled by growth of metallic crystals and corrosion products. Nevertheless, some margins leak and pain occurs from fluid movement reaching dentine. This may be produced by food with high sugar concentrations withdrawing fluid, or by food which exerts a plunger action on the deficient zone (Fig. 9.7). The same effect can occur from loss of the cement used to place gold inlays. In association with bridges, pain from this source is specially important because the deficient seal might not otherwise be noticed. The loose retainer is held in place by the rest of the bridge, caries starts and rapidly destroys tissue although the disease is hidden by the retainer, sometimes even on close examination. Compared with this, a leaking amalgam filling does not readily allow recurrent caries.

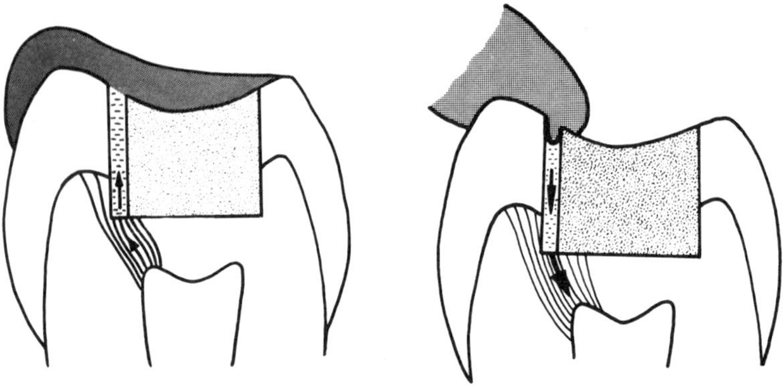

**Fig. 9.7**. Deficient amalgam restoration with fluid in the defect.
*Left*. Confectionary produces a high concentration of sugar solution in the defect so that fluid is withdrawn from the dentinal tubules causing pain.
*Right*. Chewing a carrot or other tough food has a plunger effect which forces fluid along the dentinal tubules causing pain.

When a gold pinlay (Fig. 9.8 upper) has a cement bond which has broken down pain can occur when the patient bites on it, and this may be misleading because pain on biting is usually regarded as indicating periodontitis. Moreover, percussing such a pinlay also

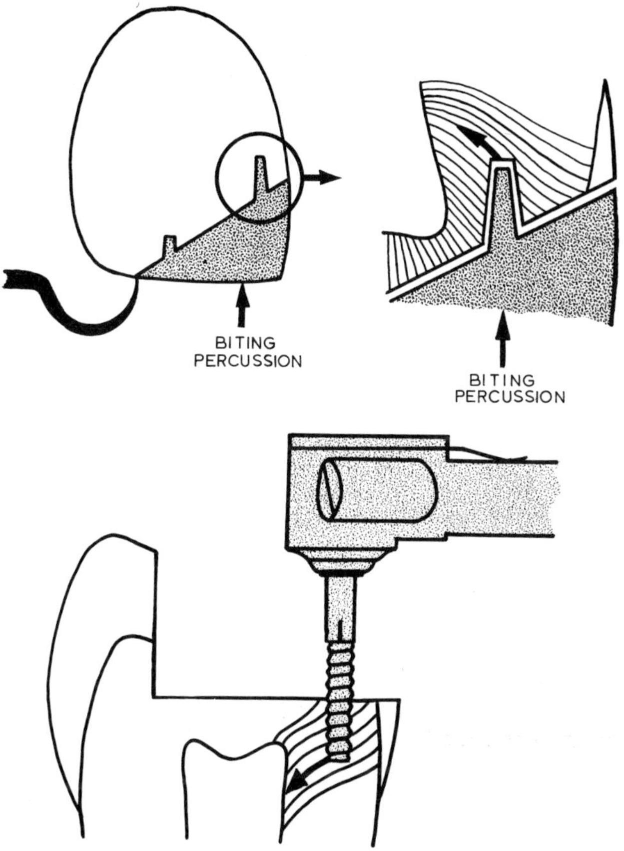


**Fig. 9.8**. *Upper*. Probing the margin of this loose pinlay caused pain. Pain also occurred on biting and percussion because fluid was forced through the dentinal tubules.

*Lower*. When the threaded pin is driven into the pinhole fluid in the pinhole forces fluid through the dentinal tubules causing pain.

causes pain, again usually taken as indicating periodontitis. The explanation is that a force applied to the pinlay is transmitted to fluid which has percolated between it and the tooth. Since pressure is force divided by area, at the pulpal end of pinholes where the area is small the pressure is considerable and is sufficient to force fluid through dentinal tubules thereby causing pain.

Pain can also occur in this way when a threaded dentine pin is inserted using a handpiece that allows rapid placement. Such pain can be so sharp that the operator may fear that it has penetrated the pulp. Pain is less likely to occur if the pin hole is first dried, and also if a geared-down handpiece is used (Fig. 9.8, lower).

There is a further source of confusion because it is often thought that pain on percussion is always present when there is pain on biting, but this is not so. When biting into tough food, such as a raw carrot or an apple, it acts as a plunger in a defect such as those just described, causing fluid to be forced through dentine causing pain. On the other hand, percussing the tooth does not affect the defective zone, so the patient's response is normal. In the case of the pinlay (Fig. 9.8) percussion was applied to the gold since it was the most accessible place, so pain occurred as described.

Thermal expansion and contraction play a part in causing pain. All restorative materials have coefficients of thermal expansion which are different from those of enamel and dentine, so temperature changes lead to differential dimensional changes which, if the cement seal breaks, allow fluid movement and possibly pain.

*Treatment*

When there is an easily accessible, non-carious, defective margin, it is possible to clean it with a probe, dry it with a jet of air, and fill it with amalgam or cement (possibly as a temporary measure). A localised carious lesion can have a small cavity cut and the caries removed before placing a small filling alongside the original restoration. A loose or defective restoration is removed and a suitable temporary restoration placed. In each case cessation of pain confirms the diagnosis.

**Fractured restoration**

In effect a fractured restoration is similar to one which has a leaking margin. It is not always easy to detect but the narrow and weak parts of amalgam restorations must be examined with this in mind. An apparently insignificant crack could open when the teeth move during masticatory movements (Fig. 9.9). When a restoration

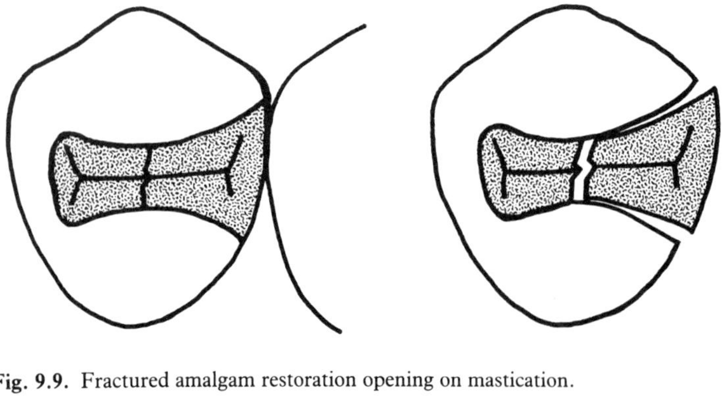

**Fig. 9.9.** Fractured amalgam restoration opening on mastication.

breaks, it would be better for the patient if it fell out altogether rather than be held loosely in place by contact point pressure causing pain and allowing recurrent caries to develop.

*Treatment*

The entire restoration is removed and replaced, using a suitable lining. If only part of a large restoration has fractured off it may be possible to replace just the one part.

**Cracked tooth**

The cracked tooth syndrome seems to be occurring more frequently, presumably because more patients are keeping their teeth until later life, although the condition also occurs in younger people. As a rule such a tooth will already have been weakened by caries and possibly weakened further by the surgical preparation e.g. when a keyway is cut to retain an incisal tip gold inlay. Perhaps after many years of normal function the tooth might be momentarily painful on biting a hard object, and this pain may be dull or sharp. Such pain recurs a number of times but after a while the incisal part of the tooth, complete with inlay, breaks off (Fig. 9.10). This is less likely to happen now that dentists tend to restore teeth with crowns, but a more frequent site for the cracked cusp to occur is the cheek teeth, especially if cavity preparation has been overzealous (Fig. 9.11).

Before the cusp finally fractures the usual diagnostic tests may not help but in addition to pain on biting on the tooth, there may be a pain on releasing the biting pressure. Also, pain seems to occur in one particular occlusal position and, after biting, there may remain a mild sense of 'tension' in the tooth for one or two seconds. As might be expected, sweet or acid food may also produce pain, and vague discomfort might have been present for a long time, becoming gradually painful. Eventually pain occurs more frequently and at greater intensity because the crack gradually deepens. This is associated with penetration of fluid and growth in the crack of microorganisms, the toxins of which produce increased pulpal sensitivity (Brännström, 1979). Pain may be so severe as to confuse even experienced clinicians as the following case indicates.

A consultant dentist suffered severe pain in an upper premolar, which both he and the author ascribed to acute pulpitis. He refused endodontic treatment (partly for experimental reasons) and eventually pain ceased. It was supposed that the pulp had died but a few weeks later the entire lingual cusp fractured off, leaving den-

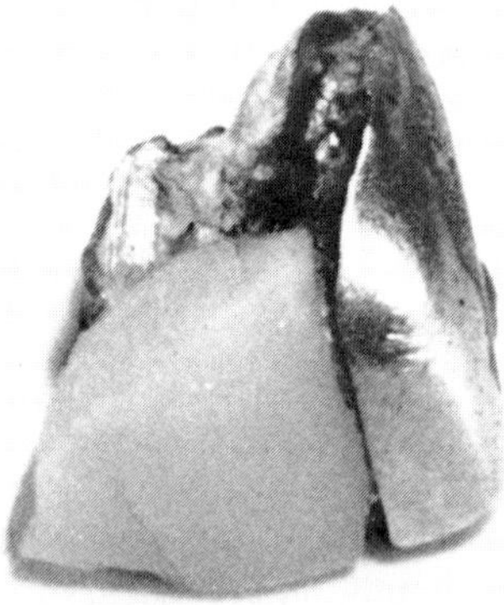

**Fig. 9.10.** Fractured crown of an upper lateral incisor with a class IV gold inlay. There was a dull pain of about 1 second duration on biting incisally, during 3 days before this tooth fractured. The pulp was vital and there was no further pain.

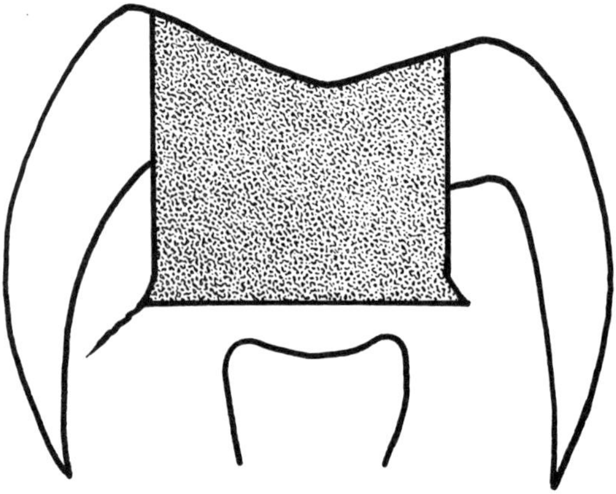

**Fig. 9.11.** Another place where a cusp starts to crack.

tine of normal appearance and sensitivity. The pulp was clearly not dead and the final diagnosis was of a cracked tooth.

Stanley (1969) has suggested testing for such a crack by getting the patient to bite on a rubber wheel or applicator stick placed over the suspected site. Brännström (1979) suggests use of ice, application to the cracked cusp being painful whereas application to the normal cusp is not. Perhaps a dye such as methylene blue could be used to detect the crack (Hill, 1957). A probe is often useful, and if it can be pressed into the crack, movement of a cusp, together with pain, may establish the diagnosis.

*Treatment*

It is usual to wait until the cusp fractures off but if pain is severe the associated restoration is removed, at which stage the defect may become obvious. The tooth is restored or dressed according to circumstances.

**Pain due to galvanism**

When dissimilar metals are placed in an electrolyte an electromotive force develops, the value of which depends on the electrode potentials of the metals concerned (Table 9.1). Since saliva and the tissue fluids of tooth, bone and soft tissues are electrolytes, if gold and amalgam restorations are placed in the same mouth, an electromotive force arises of approximately 0·5 volts (Schoonover and Souder, 1941; Schriever and Diamond, 1952; Mumford, 1957; Farrell, 1958).

**Table 9.1.** Electrode potentials of some metals used in the mouth (Kortüm, 1965)

| | | | |
|---|---|---|---|
| Aluminium | −1.66 | Mercury | +0.789 |
| Zinc | −0.763 | Silver | +0.799 |
| Tin | −0.136 | Platinum | +0.85 |
| Copper | +0.337 | Gold $Au^+$ | +1.5 |

It is usually stated that saliva is the cell electrolyte (Lain and Caughron, 1936; Reinhard, Solomon and Goltz, 1939; Schoonover and Souder, 1941; Skinner, 1954; Farrell, 1958), but this explanation is unacceptable. If this were the case, whenever the metals came into contact then (apart from local corrosion currents) the electric cell would cease to exist and any electric current that passed at the moment would be confined to the metal and saliva, so it would not reach pulpal nerves to be able to stimulate them (Mumford, 1957).

On the contrary, it is considered that pain occurs in the following way. Although an electric cell does arise from the metals contacting saliva, it is essential for pain production that the electric cell includes the electrolytes with the dentine, pulp, bone and soft tissues. When the metals make contact, as when they are in opposing teeth which occlude, there is a short circuit which allows the current to rapidly reach a peak value (Fig. 9.12) and it is at this moment that a brief pain occurs if it is going to. If the teeth are kept occluded so that the restorations remain in contact the electric cell polarises and the current intensity falls (Fig. 9.12). Separation of the teeth allows the cell to recover so that further contact of the

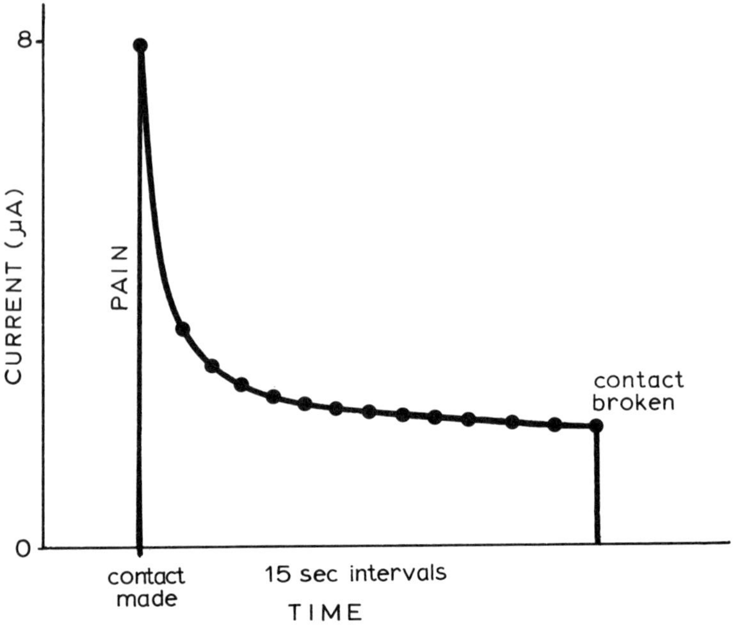


**Fig. 9.12.** The rapid rise of current is associated with pain provided the current density is sufficient. The current then diminishes as the cell polarises.

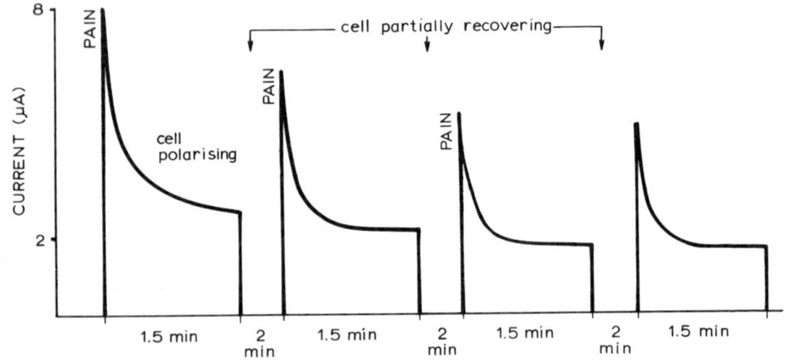


**Fig. 9.13.** As contact was made the current reached its peak value and then decreased as polarisation occurred. After 1·5 minutes contact was broken and the cell was allowed to recover for 2 minutes. In the mouth, pain occurs with the abrupt onset of current as indicated, and may be repeated. Since the cell does not recover completely pain eventually ceases to occur.

restorations may allow a current to pass of sufficient intensity to cause a further brief pain (Fig. 9.13). However, recovery is incomplete (Fig. 9.13) so pain eventually ceases to occur. In addition to polarisation the electric cell also deteriorates by surface changes on the metals.

Whether the current is strong enough to cause pain depends on various factors. Firstly, the electromotive force which arises depends upon the metals involved (Table 9.1). Comparisons of combinations actually used in conservative dentistry showed that between 22 carat gold and silver amalgam it averaged 470 millivolts; with 17 carat gold and silver amalgam it averaged 575 millivolts, and with 22 carat and 17 carat gold, 119 millivolts (Mumford, 1957). The electromotive force is independent of the electrode area so it is not affected by the size of a restoration or the presence of a cement lining as long as the metal contacts some part of dentine.

Secondly, the electrical resistance of the dentine and soft tissues is important. This varies from approximately several kilohms to 500 kilohms, depending mainly on the thickness of the remaining dentine (Mumford, 1956). From these two factors, the possible steady currents can be calculated by Ohm's law, though for brief currents capacitative effects would have to be considered.

Thirdly, the current density is important, i.e. the current passing through a unit area, In the gingiva and bone, current can spread out, but in the tooth its path is restricted (Mumford, 1959) so, for a given current, the current density is greater in the tooth than in the soft tissues. Since nerve stimulation depends on current density pain is felt, if at all, in the tooth. In addition, the tooth is richly innervated so the electrical stimulus is highly efficient, stimulating many nerve fibres and generating many neural impulses which summate in the brain to give rise to painful sensation.

If there is no pain it is because the current density is not sufficient to stimulate the nerves, and this accounts for the fact that pain is not necessarily obtained with higher electromotive forces.

A further factor could be whether or not the pulp is in a state of hyperalgesia (see Chapter 10).

*Clinical manifestations of galvanism.*

Pain due to galvanism occurs in several ways. The most common is that of a patient who complains of a brief pain lasting approximately a second whenever he closes his mouth. Examination reveals opposing teeth restored with dissimilar metals, one of which has been recently placed. Pain occurs even though no occlusal force is applied, mere contact of the teeth being sufficient, and it does not matter whether the patient keeps his teeth in contact or separates them, the pain still stops because it occurs only when the circuit is made and the current rapidly reaches its peak value (Fig. 9.12). In fact, the patient involuntarily separates his teeth; if contact is made once more the brief pain recurs and this can be repeated a number of times until the current falls below the level necessary to cause pain, i.e. below the pain perception threshold value. The clinical situation is represented in Fig. 9.14, left. This explanation is considered more likely than that in Fig. 9.14, right, because in the latter case the circuit would offer approximately twice the electrical resistance due to the additional thickness of dentine. For a given electromotive force the current would therefore be approximately half that for Fig. 9.14, left. (NOTE. The above explanation is simplified. The true flow of current is expected to be through all the tissues in inverse proportion to the electrical resistances encountered).

Pain due to galvanism may occur when a person touches a metal filling with another metal object such as a fork, spoon or paper clip

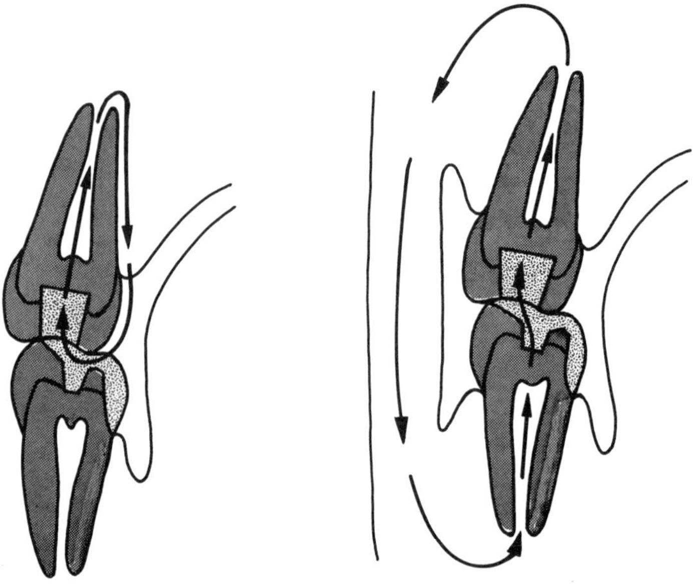

**Fig. 9.14.** When the upper tooth, restored by amalgam, occludes with the lower tooth, restored by gold, there is a current as shown, and this may be sufficient to cause pain. The circuit on the left is considered to be the one responsible, but that on the right is possible.

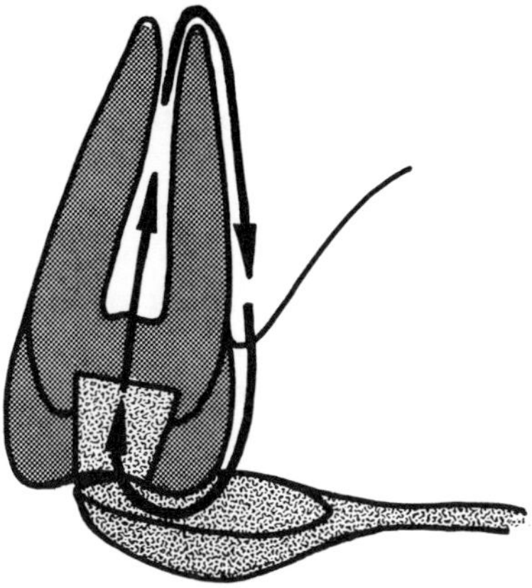

**Fig. 9.15**. A domestic spoon or other metallic object can make contact with a restoration and may cause pain.

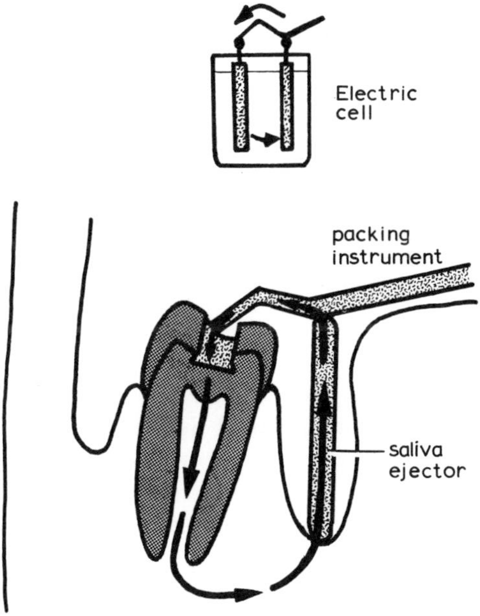


**Fig. 9.16**. When packing an amalgam restoration there may be pain because of the electric circuit illustrated.

(Fig. 9.15). This metal object is thus equivalent to the gold inlay in Fig. 9.14, left. This is also the explanation of the peculiar sensation experienced when 'silver paper' is accidently chewed with chocolate; it is really a mild pain.

From the foregoing explanation it will be appreciated that dissimilar metal restorations which never come into contact do not cause pain unless the two are momentarily connected by a fork, spoon or dental instrument.

Pain due to galvanism sometimes occurs during operative procedures when it can be disconcerting to both the patient and the operator. For example, the metal back of a mouth mirror may make contact with a metal filling so that the patient 'jumps' without apparent cause, the explanation being as in Fig. 9.15. Similarly, pain unexpectedly occurs occasionally when a saliva ejector makes indirect contact with silver amalgam as the material is being packed into a cavity (Fig. 9.16).

*Treatment*

The intensity of pain due to electrolytic activity is seldom severe, and rapidly diminishes. Indeed, some patients find it somewhat fascinating and repeatedly produce it by making intermittent contact. Since it ceases to occur usually within hours, but maybe in days, treatment is seldom needed. The patient may ask for an explanation so this can be given, with reassurance that all is well. However, in a few cases pain may be sufficiently severe to justify removal of the restoration, especially if an adequate insulator lining has not been placed. The tooth is dressed or restored according to circumstances.

Galvanism is also mentioned in Chapter 15.

**Temporary restorations**

Temporary restorations have several functions, chief of which is protection of the remaining dental tissues. The latter will already have suffered considerable damage so the temporary restoration should be non-irritant. It should also make a good seal with the dental tissues, for failure to achieve this allows ingress of oral fluids which take part in producing pain. Perhaps the worst material in this respect is gutta percha which is used because it can be so easily removed when the permanent restoration is ready — a useful property but one which must be weighed against pain due to seepage. Moreover, once the gutta percha has been removed from the cavity, the underlying dentine is usually exquisitely sensitive, a feature which may be at least partly due to hyperaemia of the underlying pulp (Massler, 1956), but it may also be because the gutta percha removes debris that had previously blocked the dentinal tubules (Johnson, 1974). This may not be the only factor as shown by similar sensitivity on removing zinc oxide-eugenol cement which is regarded as providing a good seal.

A temporary restoration should be strong enough to withstand occlusal stress without wearing or crumbling away, and without fracturing. If either should happen, external stimuli will more easily reach dentine and cause pain. For this reason a fortified zinc oxide-eugenol cement may be used or a little cotton wool incorporated. The author prefers a two part temporary restoration, calcium hydroxide being placed on the pulpal and axial dentine, followed by zinc phosphate cement; this is mixed to a thick creamy consistency, intermediate between the cementing consistency and the lining consistency. It is contoured to be free of the gingiva and also to occlude properly. For anterior teeth a temporary crown may be necessary and can be aesthetically satisfying, but care must be taken to protect the underlying dentine with a protective layer such as zinc oxide-eugenol cement.

For posterior teeth a contoured aluminium shell crown is recommended. Occasionally this can cause pain in an unusual way if it is used as a temporary restoration in the presence of a newly placed amalgam filling. Aluminium is a highly reactive metal but it is normally covered by a thin invisible layer of aluminium oxide which is very tenacius and impermeable, and protects the underlying metal (Kortüm, 1965). Even when the metal is abraded the oxide rapidly re-forms, probably within a second, but mercury attacks and destroys the abraded metal in the presence of water (Fig. 9.17, right), producing an amalgam and hydrogen with considerable heat which may cause pain (Mumford, 1968). The patient complains that the aluminium feels hot and the saliva around it is 'fizzy'.

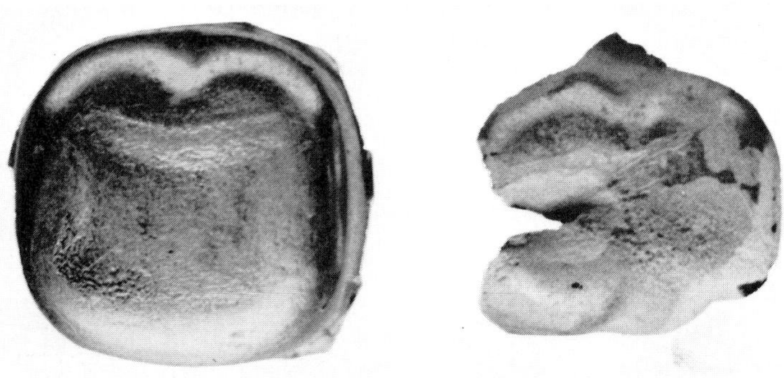

**Fig. 9.17.** A temporary aluminium shell crown (left) is quickly destroyed (right) if abraded in the presence of mercury and moisture. The reaction produces an amalgam, hydrogen, and also heat which may cause pain.

## SOME FEATURES OF PAIN DUE TO DENTINAL FACTORS

### Localisation

Localisation of pain to a tooth is difficult and, according to Anderson, Matthews and Shelton (1967), localisation to a part of a tooth is impossible. However, this refers to localisation only by the neural impulses arriving at the brain from the tooth, whereas a clinical situation is much more complex than this and involves visual and other sensory modalities. Thus, a patient who deliberately touches sensitive cervical dentine knows which tooth he has stimulated. He experiences pain and knows which tooth is involved, but it is the stimulus that is localised rather than the sensation. However, the clinician still has his answer. When the patient complains that pain occurs from a more widely distributed stimulus, e.g. a hot drink, the case can be investigated by using a stimulus which is localised to one tooth at a time, e.g. a stick of heated gutta percha. Similarly it is possible to localise the source of pain to a very tiny area of, say, the neck of a tooth by using a probe to stimulate it.

### Onset

It is probably correct to say that pain associated with dentinal factors never occurs spontaneously; it is always provoked by an external stimulus. This is one of the chief differences between it and pain arising from disease of the pulp and periodontal tissues which does occur spontaneously, i.e. without any recognisable external stimulus. Pain from these diseases does, of course, become worse as a result of external stimuli, as will be shown in later chapters.

### Quality

The vocabulary available for describing pain is not really good enough to do so and, no doubt, this is partly related to the complex neurophysiological states involved. Patients are naturally influenced by their previous experience and describe the pain accordingly, 'like the drill', 'like eating ice cream', etc. However, a direct request to describe the quality of pain without the patient being given any guidance usually meets with a bewildered response. Given a choice of words, about half of the patients suffering pain due to dentinal factors choose the word 'ache' whereas the other half choose 'pain'. Similarly there is an even division between the words 'dull' and 'sharp'. This is not what might be expected because dentine pain is usually regarded as being sharp and bright.

### Quantity

It is not yet possible to quantitate pain, and in algesimetric investigations it is usual to measure either the stimuli which produce it or the drugs which control it. However, although no numerical values can be stated human subjects can give some indication of the intensity of pain, and can grade it on an ordinal scale. For this purpose humans submitting to experimentally induced pain have recorded its level on a revolving smoked drum (Armstrong *et al.*, 1953; Smith, 1962; Keele and Armstrong, 1964), by push buttons which control the rate of a counting mechanism (Rogers and Lim, 1966), or by drawing graphs (Melzack and Eisenberg, 1968). More modern methods may include push buttons and automatic time recording (Nayman, 1979).

Patients suffering pain in and about the teeth have been asked to draw graphs to indicate the intensity and duration of pain (Mumford, 1969) and the accompanying figures illustrate the results obtained in cases of toothache due to dentinal factors. These illustrations have been drawn with the intensities mild, moderate and severe equally spaced, but this should not be taken to mean that the change in intensity between mild and moderate equals that between moderate and severe.

These graphs make it quite obvious that there are two stages of pain in many cases. The first is provoked by the stimulus and lasts a short time at high intensity. It may cease altogether (Fig. 9.18) or fade to a lower intensity which lasts for a longer time (Fig. 9.19). This lower intensity pain is probably the same as that illustrated in Figs. 9.20 and 9.21.

Fig. 9.21 illustrates an important point in understanding dentine pain, including sensitive cervical dentine. At first, stimulation caused pain which subsided completely, but repetitive stimulation presumably produced a mild inflammation in the underlying pulp

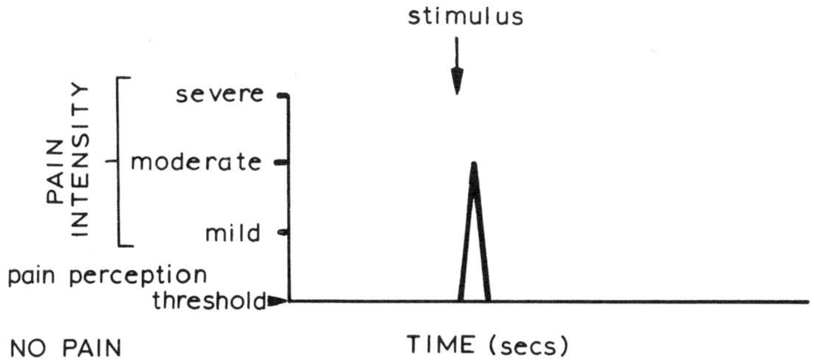


**Fig. 9.18**. In this case pain lasted for seconds after the exposed dentine was touched by a probe or the patient's finger nail. On cleaning her teeth pain lasted for minutes.

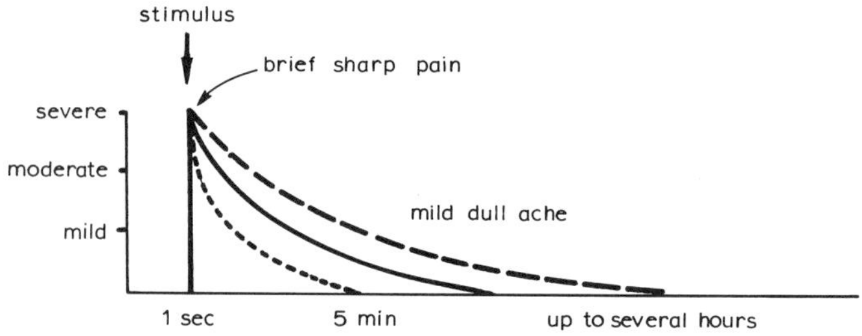


**Fig. 9.19**. Brief sharp pain followed by a dull ache. The patient who drew these curves suggested a median (continuous line). She said that she 'let her drinks cool, and her ice cream go soggy'.

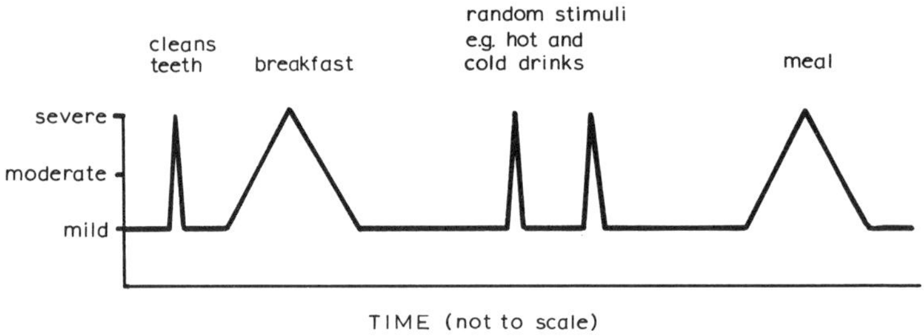


**Fig. 9.20**. Basic low intensity pain with exacerbations due to various stimuli. In this case an amalgam restoration had broken away leaving the dentine unprotected.

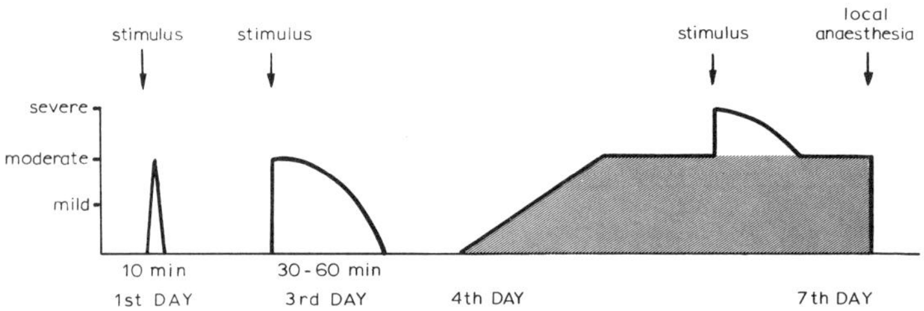


**Fig. 9.21**. This patient had exposed cervical dentine. At first, stimulation caused pain which subsided completely. Later, a constant pain developed and remained at a steady level unless stimulation caused a more severe pain to be superimposed. All pain ceased on anaesthetising the tooth, and no further pain occurred after a cervical cavity was prepared, lined and filled with amalgam. If the pain (shaded) had been due to pulp disease it would presumably have returned when local anaesthesia ended (see text).

leading to increased sensitivity of the nerve endings in the area. Thus, stimuli which would normally not have caused pain were able to do so and, with assistance from the mild inflammation, the basic pain was maintained. Once a dressing was placed further stimuli were no longer able to get through, so sensitisation of underlying nerves was of no consequence, and pain ceased abruptly. Since any inflammation could not instantly cease its intensity must have been very mild so that any neural impulses produced were below the level of perception.

**Two phases of pain**

Following peripheral injury, it is sometimes possible to detect two pains because of the different conducting rates of the nerve fibres involved, the first pain occurring when neural impulses arrive in the brain by fast conducting A delta fibres; the second by slowly conducting unmyelinated small fibres (C fibres). For these first and second pains to be separately recognisable needs time and distance for the volleys of neural impulses in the two nerve types to separate, so the phenomenon is best experienced when one stubs one's toe. Whilst this may be the factor concerned in producing the two phases of dentine pain, the effect might also depend on adaptation, some nerve fibres taking longer than others to adapt, and it could be that these are responsible for the longer lasting second phase of pain. Change in the stimulus intensity with time is also a factor. Recently, Brännström and Åström (1972) have speculated that the longer lasting pain might be due to heat whereas the shorter pains might be due to cold and drilling.

There is also the possibility of chemical changes occurring in the dentine and pulp, and these might be responsible for the second stage pain, the longer duration of which might be due to these chemicals requiring some time to diffuse away or become inactivated (Chapter 10).

Finally, the central nervous system might be partly responsible in some cases by maintaining a short term memory of the pain, a form of sensory afterglow. Not much is known about this as yet although it is common knowledge that visual images persist (usually in a reversal form) for some time after removing the light stimulus, such as by closing the eyes.

**Apparent volume of pain**

In addition to the intensity and duration of pain the apparent volume of tissue involved is a factor which should be noted. This is not appropriate for individual teeth but it is when sensitive cervical dentine involves a number of teeth. The patient can give some indication of the volume, but only a somewhat vague approximation for it is so subjective. Perhaps for this reason the clinician usually settles for an estimate of the area involved, and this can be noted on a drawing of the face. (Examples of such drawings occur in later chapters.)

## REFERENCES


Anderson, D. J. (1963) General discussion. In *Sensory Mechanisms in Dentine*, p. 96. Oxford: Pergamon.

Anderson, D. J. and Matthews, B. (1967) Osmotic stimulation of human dentine and the distribution of dental pain thresholds. *Archs. oral Biol.*, **12**, 417–426.

Anderson, D. J., Matthews, B. and Goretta, C. (1967) Fluid flow through human dentine. *Archs. oral Biol.*, **12**, 209–216.

Anderson, D. J., Matthews, B. and Shelton, L. E. (1967) Variations in the sensitivity to osmotic stimulation of human teeth. *Archs. oral Biol.*, **12**, 43–47.

Anderson, D. J. and Ronning, G. A. (1962) Osmotic excitants of pain in human dentine. *Archs. oral Biol.*, **7**, 513–523.

Armstrong, D., Dry, R. M. L., Keele, C. A. and Markham, J. W. (1953) Observations on chemical excitants of cutaneous pain in main. *J. Physiol. (Lond.)*, **120**, 326–351.

Brännström, M. (1960) Dentinal and pulpal response. III. Application of an air stream to exposed dentine. Long observation periods. *Acta odont. Scand.*, **18**, 235–252.

Brännström, M. (1961) Dentinal and pulpal response. V. Application of pressure to exposed dentine. *J. dent. Res.*, **40**, 960–970.

Brännström, M. (1979) The transmission and control of dentinal pain. In *Mechanisms and Control of Pain*. ed. Grossman, L. I., pp. 15–35. New York: Masson.

Brännström, M. and Aström. A. (1972) The hydrodynamics of the dentine; its possible relationship to dentinal pain. *Int. dent. J. (Lond.)*, **22**, 219–227.

Brännström, M., Isacsson, G. and Johnson, G. (1976) The effect of calcium hydroxide and fluorides on human dentine. *Acta odont Scand.*, **34**, 59–67.

Brännström, M., Lindén, L.-Å. and Johnson, G. (1969) Fluid flow and pain response in the dentine produced by hydrostatic pressure. *Odont. Revy*, **20**, 1–16.

Davis, W. B. and Winter, P. J. (1977) Dietary erosion of adult dentine and enamel. Protection with a fluoride toothpaste. *Brit. dent. J.*, **143**, 116–119.

Davis, W. B. and Winter, P. J. (1980) The effect of abrasion on enamel and dentine after exposure to dietary acid. *Brit. dent. J.*, **148**, 253–256.

Farrell, T. H. (1958) A preliminary investigation into the electrical properties of human teeth. *Brit. dent. J.*, **104**, 353–359.

Harkins, S. W. and Chapman, C. R. (1976) Detection and decision factors in pain perception in young and elderly men. *Pain*, **2**, 253–264.

Johnson, G. (1974) *The hydrodynamics of the Dentine and its Clinical Applications*. Stockholm: Tryckeri Balder A. B.

Johnson, G. and Brännström, M. (1974) The sensitivity of dentin. Changes in relation to conditions to exposed tubule apertures. *Acta odont. Scand.*, **32**, 29–38.

Keele, C. A. and Armstrong, D. (1964) *Substances producing Pain and Itch*. London: Arnold.

Kortüm, G. (1965) *Treatise on Electrochemistry*, 2nd edition. Amsterdam: Elsevier.

Lain, E. S. and Caughron, G. S. (1936) Electrogalvanic phenomena of oral cavity caused by dissimilar metallic restorations. *J. Amer. dent. Ass.*, **23**, 1641–1652.

Levin, M. P., Yearwood, L. L. and Carpenter, W. N. (1973) The desensitizing effect of calcium hydroxide and magnesium hydroxide on hypersensitive dentin. *Oral Surg.*, **35**, 741–746.

Lindén, L.-Å. and Brännström, M. (1967) Fluid movements in dentine and pulp. *Odont. Revy*, **18**, 227–236.

Massler, M. (1956) Effects of filling materials on the pulp. *N. Y. J. dent.*, **26**, 183–198.

Melzack, R. and Eisenberg, H. (1968) Skin sensory afterglows. *Science*, **159**, 445–447.

Mumford, J. M. (1956) Relationship between the electrical resistance of human teeth and the presence and extent of dental caries. *Brit. dent. J.*, **100**, 239–244.

Mumford, J. M. (1957) Electrolytic action in the mouth and its relationship to pain. *J. dent. Res.*, **36**, 632–640.

Mumford, J. M. (1959) Path of direct current in electric pulp testing using one coronal electrode. *Brit. dent. J.*, **106**, 23–26.

Mumford, J. M. (1960) Pain due to galvanism. *Brit. dent. J.*, **108**, 299–301.

Mumford, J. M. (1965) Pain perception threshold and adaptation of normal human teeth. *Archs. oral Biol.*, **10**, 957–968.

Mumford, J. M. (1968) Corrosion of aluminium shell crowns. *Brit. dent. J.*, **124**, 423–424.

Mumford, J. M. (1969) Measurement of toothache. *J. Brit. Endo. Soc.*, **3**, 48–51.

Nayman, J. (1979) Measurement and control of postoperative pain. *Ann. Roy. Coll. Surg. (Eng.)*, **61**, 419–426.

Reinhard, M. C., Solomon, H. A. and Goltz, H. L. (1939) Further experiments in oral galvanism. *J. Amer. dent. Ass.*, **26**, 1846–1848.

Rogers, R. W. and Lim, R. K. S. (1966) Measurement of subjective pain in man. *Pharmacologist*, **8**, 206, Abstr.

Schoonover, I. C. and Souder, W. (1941) Corrosion of dental alloys. *J. dent Res.*, **28**, 1278–1291.

Schriever, W. and Diamond, L. E. (1952) Electromotive forces and electric currents caused by metallic dental fillings. *J. dent Res.*, **31**, 205–209.

Skinner, E. W. (1954) *The Science of Dental Materials*, 4th edition. Philadelphia: Saunders.

Smith, R. (1962) The vocabulary of pain. In *The Assessment of Pain in Man and Animals*, ed. Keele, C. A. and Smith, R., pp. 32–40. Edinburgh: Livingstone.

Stanley, H. R. (1969) The cracked tooth syndrome. *J. Amer. Acad. Gold Foil Operators*, **11**, 364–367.

Stevenson, T. S. (1967) Odontoblast aspiration and fluid movement in human dentine. *Archs. oral Biol.*, **12**, 1149–1157.

Trowbridge, H. O., Franks, M., Korostoff, E. and Emling, R. (1980) Sensory response to thermal stimulation in human teeth. *J. Endo.*, **6**, 405–412.

Yamada, M. and Sakada, S. (1962) Electrophysiologic observations on the effects of capping materials on the pulp nerve fibres. *J. dent. Res.*, **41**, 1359–1366.

# 10

# Endogenous algogenic substances

In the last chapter stress was laid on external stimuli causing pain in teeth even in the absence of pulp disease. These stimuli also cause pain when the pulp is diseased or they make existing pain become worse, but external stimulation is not always essential because pain can occur spontaneously due to inflammation being associated with factors which are in themselves pain producing (algogenic). Notice that the word spontaneously is being used in the clinical sense that there is no obvious stimulus causing the pain.

## HYPERALGESIA

When damage causes acute inflammation there is dilatation of the arterioles, the capillary bed opens up, the vessel walls become more permeable and there is an outflow of fluid into the tissues. In some parts of the body, such as the skin, this fluid can be accommodated by an increase in volume, but the dental pulp is largely confined by dentine so its volume cannot increase, which means that pressure must rise, and this increase in pressure is associated with severe pain. For the same reason pain is made momentarily worse in some cases due to the increase in pressure produced by the arrival of each arterial pulse, the result being throbbing pain. The above explanation of pain is true as far as it goes, and is sufficient and satisfying for most patients, but it is not the whole story.

Most inflammatory pain occurs in association with hyperalgesia in which there is an increase in sensitivity, shown by a reduced pain perception threshold, and an increase in sensibility shown by the exaggerated response to stimuli (Hardy, Wolff and Goodell, 1950). The latter effect can be seen in some cases of acute pulpitis when application of too much heat in diagnostic tests causes such severe pain that it 'sends the patient through the roof'; naturally this unfortunate result is usually avoided by controlling the amount of heat applied. The former effect, however, a diminished pain perception threshold, has not been demonstrated for teeth (Mumford, 1967).

On a speculative note, this state of affairs in teeth may be similar to that of secondary hyperalgesia as described by Hardy, Wolff and Goodell (1950), in which the pain perception threshold is normal but response to noxious stimuli is exaggerated.

## CHEMICAL MEDIATORS OF PAIN

Keele and Armstrong (1964) considered it unlikely that hyperalgesia was due to increased tension of tissue fluid since it can develop before swelling occurs. They suggested that the most important factor in causing inflammatory pain is the greatly increased sensitivity of pain nerve endings to all kinds of stimuli so that stimuli not normally causing pain do so, and stimuli normally causing slight pain cause pain which is agonising. Lewis (1942) had already pointed out that the painful state could not be due simply to damage of nerve endings at the time of injury, but must result from something arising as a result of the injury after a variable delay, and that such substances acted on the pain nerve endings rendering them hyperexcitable. He showed the importance of chemical mediators, and drew particular attention to the release of H-substance (histamine).

Keele and Armstrong (1964, 1968) considered the role of endogenous algogenic agents — substances naturally present in the body which are released in certain circumstances in amounts sufficient to cause pain. These chemicals can cause pain in two ways, either by exciting sensory nerve terminals directly, or by making them more susceptible to mechanical, thermal or other stimuli. The latter state of increased susceptibility is hyperalgesia, and both effects may result from the one algogenic agent. Algogenic agents may be considered in two main groups, intracellular and extracellular.

### Intracellular algogenic substances

To be effective these must be released from the cells into the extracellular tissue fluid in which pain receptors lie. Probably the most important is 5-hydroxytryptamine (also known as serotonin) which is released from blood platelets as they disintegrate during the inflammatory process. This chemical produces a prolonged hyperalgesia, or lowering of the threshold of excitation, and is liberated especially in thrombosis and embolism (Sicuteri, 1968).

According to Sicuteri 5-hydroxytryptamine does not in itself cause pain, but it does leave the receptors more susceptible to potassium ions which are another intracellular algogenic substance and are released when erythrocytes break up (Keele and Armstrong, 1968). It may also have a part to play in causing headaches (Sicuteri, 1972). Benjamin (1959) considered the possibility that the essential action of acetylcholine, 5-hydroxytryptamine and bradykinin (see below) might be their ability to release potassium ions. However, potassium ions are only active in concentrations of 500 micrograms per ml compared with effective concentrations of less than 1 microgram per ml for 5-hydroxytryptamine and bradykinin (Keele and Armstrong, 1968).

Histamine is another intracellular algogenic agent and is present in nearly all tissues of the body, concentrated in the granules of mast cells (Keele and Armstrong, 1968; Busse, 1979). It is released in an explosive manner so acts rapidly on sensory nerves as well as on the smooth muscle of blood vessels producing dilatation of arterioles, capillaries and venules (Busse, 1979).

Acetylcholine acts on nerve endings rather than on the nerve fibres directly and affects both myelinated and unmyelinated fibres, being active in concentrations as little as 0·5 micrograms per ml. It is potentiated to a limited extent by 5-hydroxytryptamine. Since acetylcholine is a potent algogenic agent Keele and Armstrong (1964) considered the possibility that the other mediators of the autonomic nervous system (adrenaline and noradrenaline) might act similarly, but found them a good deal less potent.

Substance P (so-called because it was a 'P'owder) is now known to be a peptide. It is present in about a fifth of the cell bodies in the trigeminal ganglion, all of them associated with unmyelinated fibres (Hökfelt et al, 1975). Their central processes go to the trigeminal spinal nucleus where they end in the marginal layer and the substantia gelatinosa. These are the small primary afferent fibres which carry the impulses mediating painful sensations, and it has been shown by Jessell and Iversen (1977) that they release the substance P as a transmitter, the mechanism being calcium dependent (Schenker, Mroz and Leeman, 1976; Jessell, 1977; Iversen, 1979).

### Extracellular algogenic substances

The most important of the extracellular algogens is a group of polypeptides which can be formed in plasma by various modes of activation; these are the plasma kinins, chief of which is bradykinin. Bradykinin is rapidly destroyed by kininase, present in plasma and lymph, so needs to act on receptors which are close by. There are several forms of bradykinin and they are effective algogenic agents in small doses that do not cause any sign of injury, these amounts being comparable with those of hormones and chemical mediators (Lim, 1967b). Lim appeared to regard bradykinin as the main pain producing agent because it was effective in smaller doses than 5-hydroxytryptamine which required a dose 35 times greater, histamine (44 times) or acetylcholine (340 times). However, Keele and Armstrong (1968) gave equal figures for the pain producing dose of 5-hydroxytryptamine and bradykinin, namely in concentrations of less than one microgram per ml. The kinins contribute to the classical signs of inflammation — vasodilatation, redness, increased vascular permeability associated with exudation, swelling and pain, but full confirmation of their role is still required (Movat, 1979).

The effect of the plasma kinins is enhanced by the previous activity of 5-hydroxytryptamine released from blood platelets (Sicuteri, 1968).

Keele and Armstrong (1968) suggested that the significance of histamine might be that it increased the permeability of capillaries thus allowing escape into the interstitial spaces of the various components of the plasma kinin-forming system.

Human serum caused pain when applied to the base of a skin blister previously caused by application of cantharadin (Armstrong, Dry, Keele and Markham, 1953). These investigators showed that, compared with acetylcholine, the onset of pain was delayed (for 10–45 seconds) and more prolonged. The active component of serum may be 5-hydroxytryptamine (Keele and Armstrong, 1964).

Various other substances have been considered as algogenic including acids derived from inflammatory exudates, such as lactic acid.

Since so many chemical agents can excite pain receptors it seems reasonable to regard them as chemoreceptors (Lim, 1967a, b, 1968), although excitation does not depend on specific chemical configuration and may depend ultimately on the electrical charge on the receptors and the charge of the algogenic agents. It may also be that heat acts by chemical mediation (Hardy, 1962; Keele and Armstrong, 1968).

**The prostaglandins**

Another group of substances which have been considered algogenic are the prostaglandins which are widely distributed in the tissues and influence many physiological processes. Evidence is accumulating to suggest that they are involved with defence reactions such as inflammation, pyrexia and pain (Piper 1973) and they have been recovered from exudates. They are thought to sensitise receptors rather than causing pain directly (Ferrieira, Moncada and Vane, 1973) and act synergistically with other inflammatory mediators to produce oedema and overt pain (Ferrieira, 1979). They may act by release of amines from mast cells (Crunkhorn and Willis, 1971).

## APPLICATION TO TEETH

Anderson and Naylor (1962) prepared standard cavities in the premolars of human subjects and applied acetylcholine, histamine, 5-hydroxytryptamine and potassium chloride as solutions made isotonic with sodium chloride at a pH of 7·0–7·5, but they did not cause pain. The pulps were carefully exposed and the solutions were again applied, the experimental method being thus analogous to the blister base preparation of Armstrong *et al.* (1953), and all of the solutions caused pain. Brännström (1962) also found that an isotonic solution of potassium chloride caused pain when applied to the pulp but not when applied to dentine. Presumably these materials affect nerve endings which are accessible in the pulp but not in dentine.

Aspiration of odontoblasts almost certainly results in damage to the cells and would cause liberation of injury products which could stimulate nociceptor endings in the pulp or even in the dentinal tubules (Brännström and Åström, 1964; Anderson, Matthews and Goretta, 1967). However, aspiration of odontoblasts does not always cause pain (Kramer, 1954).

Experiments on unanaesthetised human pulps as described by Anderson and Naylor (1962) are obviously difficult and potentially very painful even without the application of chemicals. For this reason they were unable to pursue their investigations, so were not able to explain why some substances did not cause pulpal pain even though they were effective algogens when applied to a skin blister base (Anderson, 1963).

Substance P has now been demonstrated in human teeth where it may play a part in the development of inflammation (Olgart et al, 1977; Olgart, 1979). However, when applied to the exposed pulp, substance P did not excite nerve fibres, so its role in the dental pulp is still obscure (Gazelius et al, 1977).

A polypeptide similar to bradykinin was reported in the pulp (Kroeger, 1968) and has been found in the exudate collected from the exposed pulp (in dogs); mechanical, thermal or electrical stimulation applied to the exposed pulp triggered the release of this substance (Inoka, Toyoda, and Yamamoto, 1973; Kudo et al, 1975; Inoki et al, 1979). Although evidence is incomplete it must be supposed that pain-producing agents are active in the dental pulp just as they are in other parts of the body. Naturally, the anatomical configuration of the dental tissues will have an influence on the inflammatory process, as will be described in the next chapter.

Evidence is not yet available about the role of prostaglandins in pulpitis (Haegerstam and Edwall, 1977).

## REFERENCES


Anderson, D. J. (1963) Chemical and osmotic excitants of pain in human dentine. In *Sensory Mechanisms in Dentine*, ed. Anderson, D. J., pp. 88–93. Oxford: Pergamon.

Anderson, D J., Matthews, B. and Goretta, C. (1967) Fluid flow through human dentine. *Archs. oral Biol.*, **12**, 209–216.

Anderson, D J. and Naylor, M. N. (1962) Chemical excitants of pain in human dentine and dental pulp. *Archs. oral Biol.*, **7**, 413–415.

Armstrong, D., Dry, R. M. L., Keele, C. A. and Markham, J. W. (1953) Observations on chemical excitants of cutaneous pain in man. *J. Physiol.* (*Lond.*), **120**, 326–351.

Benjamin, F. B. (1959) Release of intracellular potassium as the physiological stimulus for pain. *J. appl. Physiol.*, **14**, 643–646.

Brännström, M. (1962) The elicitation of pain in human dentine and pulp by chemical stimuli. *Archs. oral. Biol.*, **7**, 59–62.

Brännström, M. and Åström, A. (1964) A study on the mechanism of pain elicited from the dentine. *J. dent. Res.*, **43**, 619–625.

Busse, W. W. (1979) Histamine: mediator and modulator in inflammation. In *Handbook of Inflammation, Vol. 1. Chemical Messengers of the Inflammatory Process*, ed. Houck, J. C., pp. 1–45. Amsterdam: Elsevier/North Holland.

Crunkhorn, P. and Willis, A. L. (1971) Cutaneous reactions to intradermal prostaglandins. *Brit. J. Pharmacol.*, **41**, 49–56.

Ferrieira, S. H. (1979) Prostaglandins. In *Handbook of Inflammation, Vol. 1, Chemical Messengers of the Inflammatory Process*, ed. Houck, J. C., pp. 113–151. Amsterdam: Elsevier/North Holland.

Ferrieira, S. H., Moncada, S. and Vane, J. R. (1973) Prostaglandins and the mechanisms of analgesia produced by aspirin-like drugs. *Brit. J. Pharmacol.*, **49**, 86–97.

Gazelius, B., Olgart, L., Edwall, L. and Trowbridge, H. O. (1977) Effects of substance P on sensory nerves and blood flow in the feline dental pulp. In *Pain in the Trigeminal Region*, ed. Anderson, D. J. and Matthews, B., pp. 95–101. Amsterdam: Elsevier/North Holland.

Haegerstam, G. and Edwall, L. (1977) Sodium acetylsalicylate and the role of prostaglandins in the mechanisms of intradental pain. *Acta odont. Scand.*, **35**, 63–67.

Hardy, J. D. (1962) The pain threshold and the nature of pain sensation. In *The Assessment of Pain in Man and Animals*, ed. Keele, C. A. and Smith, R., pp. 170–201. Edinburgh: Livingstone.

Hardy, J. D., Wolff, H. G. and Goodell, H. (1950) Experimental evidence of the nature of cutaneous hyperalgesia. *J. clin. Invest.*, **92**, 115–140.

Hökfelt, T., Kellerth, J. O., Nilsson, G. and Pernow, B. (1975) Substance P: localisation in the central nervous system and in some primary sensory neurons. *Science, N.Y.*, **190**, 889–890.

Inoki, R., Toyoda, T. and Yamamoto, I. (1973) Elaboration of a bradykinin-like substance in dogs' canine pulp during electrical stimulation and its inhibitation by narcotic and non-narcotic analgesics. *Naumyn-Schmeiderberg's Arch. Pharmacol.*, **279**, 387–398.

Inoki, R., Matsunoto, K., Kudo, T., Kotani, Y. and Oka, M. (1979) Bradykinin as an algesic (pain producing) substance in the pulp. *Naumyn-Schmiederberg's Arch. exp. Path. Pharmak.*, **306**, 29–36.

Iversen, L. L. (1979) The chemistry of the brain. *Scient. Amer.*, **241**, 118–128.

Jessell, T. M. (1977) Opiate inhibition of substance P release from the rat trigeminal nucleus, *in vitro*. *J. Physiol.* (*Lond.*), **270**, 56p.

Jessell, T. M. and Iversen, L. L. (1977) Opiate analgesics inhibit substance P release from rat trigeminal nucleus. *Nature* (*Lond.*), **268**, 549–551.

Keele, C. A. and Armstrong, D. (1964) *Substances producing Pain and Itch*. Baltimore: Williams and Wilkins.

Keele, C. A. and Armstrong, D. (1968) Mediators of pain. In *Pharmacology of Pain*, ed. Lim, R. K. S., Armstrong, D. and Pardo, E. G., pp. 3–24. Oxford: Pergamon.

Kramer, I. R. H. (1954) The relationship between pain and changes in the dental pulp following the insertion of fillings. *Brit. dent. J.*, **96**, 9–13.

Kroeger, D. C. (1968) Possible role of neurohumoral substances in the pulp. In *Biology of the Dental Pulp Organ: a Symposium*, ed. Finn, S. B., pp. 333–346. Alabama: Univ. Alabama Press.

Kudo, T., Kawagoe, M., Hayashi, T., Takezawa, J. and Inoki, R. (1975) Inhibitory effect of apernyl on production of bradykininlike substance in pulp. *J. dent. Res.*, **54**, 1082–1086.

Lewis, T. (1942) *Pain*. New York: Macmillan.

Lim, R. K. S. (1967a) Pain mechanisms. *Anesthesiol.*, **28**, 106–110.

Lim, R. K. S. (1967b) Pharmacologic viewpoint of pain and analgesia. In *New Concepts in Pain and its Clinical Management*, ed. Way, E. L., pp. 33–47. Philadelphia: Davis.

Lim, R. K. S. (1968) Neuropharmacology of pain and analgesia. In *Pharmacology of Pain*, ed. Lim, R. K. S., Armstrong, D. and Pardo, E. G., pp. 169–217. Oxford: Pergamon.

Movat, H. Z. (1979) Kinins and the kinin system as inflammatory mediators. In *Handbook of Inflammation, Vol. 1. Chemical Messengers of the Inflammatory Process*, ed. Houck, J. C., pp. 47–112. Amsterdam: Elsevier/North Holland.

Mumford, J. M. (1967) Pain perception threshold on stimulating human teeth and the histological condition of the pulp. *Brit. dent. J.*, **123**, 427–433.

Olgart, L. (1979) Influence of pharmacologic agents on blood flow and sensory nerves in the pulp. In *Mechanism and Control of Pain*, ed. Grossman, L. I., pp. 69–85. New York: Masson.

Olgart, L., Hökfelt, T., Nilsson, G. and Pernow, B. (1977) Localisation of substance P-like immunoreactivity in nerves in the tooth pulp. *Pain*, **4**, 153–159.

Piper, P. J. (1973) Distribution and metabolism. In *The Prostaglandins: Pharmacological and Therapeutic Advances*, ed. Cuthbert, M. F., pp. 125–150. London: Heinemann.

Schenker, C., Mroz, E. A. and Leeman, S. E. (1976) Release of substance P from isolated nerve endings. *Nature* (*Lond.*), **264**, 790–792.

Sicuteri, F. (1968) Sensitization of nociceptors by 5-hydroxytryptamine in man. In *Pharmacology of Pain*, ed. Lim, R. K. S., Armstrong, D. and Pardo, E. G. pp. 57–86. Oxford: Pergamon.

Sicuteri, F. (1972) Headache as possible expression of deficiency of brain 5-hydroxytryptamine (central denervation supersensitivity). *Headache*, **12**, 69–72.

# 11

# Pain due to pulp disease

The most important cause of pulpal pain is dental caries although caries in itself does not directly cause pain — if it did millions of people with numerous untreated lesions would need dental attention right away — but caries is indirectly responsible for pain in two ways. Firstly, it causes loss of tooth tissue which allows external stimuli to have a greater effect as described in earlier chapters. Secondly, it affects the pulp, perhaps even when caries is confined to enamel (Brännström and Lind, 1965), and when caries is still in dentine bacterial products from it gain access to the pulp and may be responsible for pain. Eventually caries invades the pulp which is not well placed to withstand the attack. This is partly because it has a blood supply which reaches it by only one route, the apical foramen; except for accessory canals in some cases, no alternative blood supply is available since the pulp is confined in dentine. The fact that this surrounding calcified tissue is unyielding is a further disadvantage because the pulp is unable to increase in volume, so cannot accommodate inflammatory exudates to any great extent. In such circumstances the pressure rises, and even in the normal pulp the pressure of tissue fluid (about 25 mm Hg) is already high compared with that in other tissues (Pohto, 1972). Moreover, the already narrow apical foramen becomes progressively narrower with age and, with these disadvantages, it is remarkable that the pulp ever survives invasion by caries which, bearing in mind the pulp's small size, is quite a massive onslaught.

Pulp disease is also caused by trauma, both accidental and operative. In accidental trauma fractures through the tooth may involve the pulp either in the clinical crown (Fig. 11.1) or less obviously in the root (Fig. 11.2). If a pulp, exposed in this way, is probed it is painful (assuming it is still alive) but many such teeth are only slightly painful, and some patients do not attend for treatment until the lapse of considerable time, sometimes many weeks. The explanation probably lies partly in the fact that there

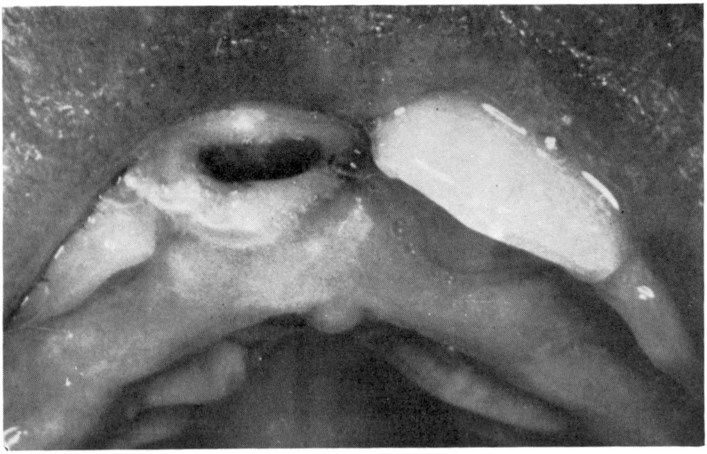

**Fig. 11.1.** The patient suffered a blow which fractured the crown of an upper central incisor, leaving the pulp exposed and bleeding.

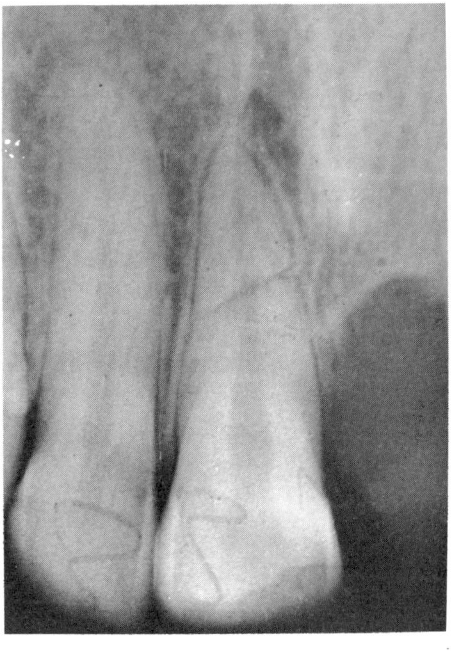

**Fig. 11.2.** A blow caused a fracture through the root but the pulp remained vital and the tooth has been retained for several years.

is drainage through the exposed area so that pressure is unable to build up. On the other hand, an exposure produced during operating procedures may be covered with a restoration, either because it is unnoticed or in a reasonable attempt to secure healing, but in either case the damaged pulp is sealed so that inflammatory products cannot escape.

Other factors causing pulp damage are heat that might be produced in drilling teeth without adequate cooling control, and chemicals applied to the cavity or placed as restorative materials.

It has also been suggested that pulp disease can be caused by electrolytic activity due to dissimilar metal restorations, but this is not accepted by the author. (The subject was discussed in Chapter 9.)

## PAIN AND HISTOLOGICAL APPEARANCE OF PULP

After many investigations it must be concluded that there is no overall correlation between a patient's experience of pain, the clinical condition and the histological appearance of the pulp (Stephan, 1937; Herbert, 1945; Björn, 1946; Vargas and Vivaldi, 1959; Seltzer, Bender and Ziontz, 1963; Baume, 1966, 1970a, b; Harndt, 1969; Lundy and Stanley, 1969; Tyldesley and Mumford, 1970; Matthews, Searle and Adams, 1974). There is, of course, considerable difficulty in obtaining first class histological preparations of the pulp and dentine combined, not least being the process of extracting the tooth which can distort the true pulpal appearance. However, there is no doubt that the appearance of pulpal sections can vary considerably from one area to another, and more than one recognisable pathological process may be seen; this adds to the difficulty so it is not surprising that Baume (1970b) and others have concluded that it is not possible to make a differential diagnosis of the pulp state by clinical means.

The problem is well illustrated by Table 11.1 (prepared by Dr W. R. Tyldesley). Examination of the first line of this table illustrates one aspect of the difficulty for it shows that 12 of the 142 painful teeth had histologically normal pulps. Moreover, the last column shows that throbbing pain occurred in 24–50 per cent of cases for each of the different histological conditions listed, including 33 per cent for teeth with histologically normal pulps. It might be thought that in such cases some diseased part had been missed by taking too few histological sections, but multiple sections were examined (Tyldesley and Mumford, 1970).

It can reasonably be argued that, in diagnosing pain cases, the histological condition of the dental pulp is not known anyway, and microscopic examination can at best give confirmatory evidence. Indeed, Seltzer, Bender and Nazimov (1965) have argued in favour of classifying pulp disease in clinical terms rather than on a histological basis and the author finds some sympathy with this view. However, a ceaseless effort must be maintained to improve the diagnosis of pulpal conditions and to define both those conditions that we do understand and those we do not understand. This is not just an academic view because, in the author's opinion, it is necessary to prepare for a major advance in dentistry in which teeth, at present being extracted, will be conserved by simple endodontic procedures not involving tedious and time-consuming methods of root canal treatment. Already, pulp capping can be effective, e.g. a long-term follow-up of 130 cases has shown that 87·3 per cent of pulps were still vital after an average post-operative time of 11·7 years (Haskell et al, 1978).

## PULP EXPOSURES

Pain is frequently experienced by patients when there is an exposed pulp but, as might be expected, the histological condition of the pulp in such cases is very variable. There may be acute pulpitis, chronic pulpitis, or degenerative changes, the pulp might appear normal or it might be dead, pain in the latter case arising from periapical disease. It follows that the exposure itself is not the essential feature with which pain (or lack of pain) can be correlated. However, pain is not the only feature enabling a diagnosis to be made, the history of the case being very important, especially the time factor (Mumford, 1968). For example, there may have been a recent operation on the tooth, perhaps several days to several weeks before pain started; this is quite a common time lapse in which pain develops after pulp exposures. The case history provides valuable help with information recorded at previous visits such as cavity depth, etc.

Once the restoration has been removed from such a tooth the exposed pulp may be visible on inspection, although it is often easier to detect it by means of a probe. Damage from this instrument should be avoided if the pulp is to be preserved, but if the pulp is to be removed or the tooth extracted, and if it is anaesthetised, probing does not matter. In the absence of anaesthesia, probing a vital pulp causes pain of variable intensity, being slight in chronic pulpitis but severe in other cases. The author has had a probe pushed into a vital non-anaesthetised pulp and was momen-

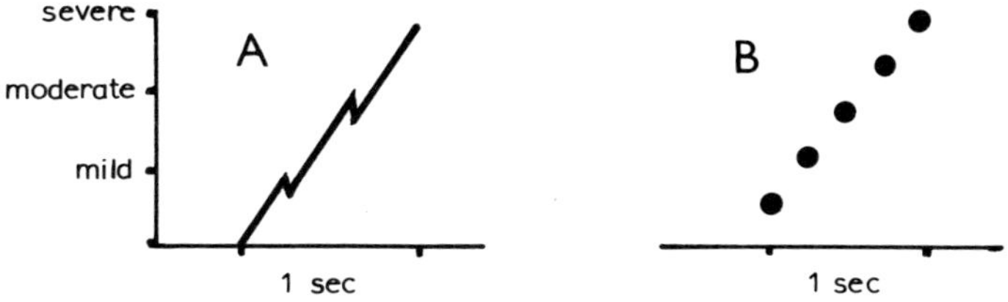


**Fig. 11.3A.** The author had a probe pushed into a non-anaesthetised vital pulp and 'saw' the lightning illustrated. He also 'heard' the 'de de de de de' with each stroke of the graph shown. (The incident was neither masochistic nor in the interests of science, but accidental.)
B. A middle-aged male suffered a brief pain of unbearable intensity when the right side of his lower lip was touched. He drew the dots illustrated, describing the pain as 'dot dot dot dot dot like Morse code'.

tarily incapacitated by the pain which would have been absolutely intolerable had it persisted for longer than it did. It lasted for about one second, while he not only felt the pain but 'saw lightning' and 'heard' it (Fig. 11.3, A). The explanation of this severe pain is that numerous nerve terminals were subjected to intense stimulation at the same moment, with the result that a veritable bombardment of neural impulses was transmitted to the central nervous system from this one tiny area of the body. Speculating, it is supposed that this pain is similar to that experienced by some patients suffering from pulpitis and perhaps related to that of trigeminal neuralgia. These conditions will both be considered later, but Fig. 11.3, B, shows how a patient with suspected trigeminal neuralgia illustrated his pain (having been given a card on which co-ordinates had been drawn by the author). These two cases are compared in Fig. 11.3 to show the resemblance; the time scale is the same, and both pains gave a sensation of thudding represented by the dots in one case and the zigzag in the other. Also, in both cases pain appeared to stop at its peak, unlike pain illustrated by graphs elsewhere in this chapter and in Chapter 9. It might be expected that there would be a contrasting period of calm after such an onslaught, any residual mild sensation remaining unnoticed. Also there would not have been time for algogenic chemicals to become active, but the physical disturbance of the pulp and the vascular reaction might have been expected to leave at least some after pain.

## HYPERAEMIA

This is an early state of disturbed pulpal circulation with increased vascularity, which is able to resolve, so that the pulp returns to normal. Pain is caused by stimuli which do not normally cause it, and is described as transient, lasting only for the duration of the stimulus and subsiding immediately the stimulus is removed. This view is misleading in several ways. Firstly, by this definition it would only be possible to diagnose hyperaemia retrospectively, i.e. when it had already resolved. Secondly, pain due to external stimuli depends on the nature of the stimulus, especially its intensity, and this, in turn, depends upon the physical state of the tooth as described in Chapter 7. If tooth substance has been lost by caries or trauma then hot and cold food and liquids, or cold air, will produce a greater than usual temperature change at the pulpo-dentinal junction, so of course there may be pain, but the pulp could be normal. If the cavity or fracture is suitably dressed this will provide insulation against heat and cold so the effective stimulus is diminished and pain is likely to cease, so it cannot reasonably be claimed that hyperaemia has resolved!

The suggestion has also been made that a 'hyperaemic' pulp responds to a lower than normal electrical stimulus, but there is no satisfactory evidence for this (Mumford, 1967).

However, there is one clinical situation in which a condition exists that might be called hyperaemia, and that is when a metal restoration has been polished too energetically. If there was no sensitivity to thermal change before polishing, and sensitivity developed after polishing, and this sensitivity soon ceased, the pulp state could be called hyperaemia. However, this would be an unwarranted assertion since the pulp condition is not known. The word hyperaemia should not be used to describe the clinical condition. Instead it would be more accurate to use the word hyperalgesia which is the term used for other parts of the body. This is a proper expression of the symptoms and does not require histological verification which, in the vast majority of cases, is not even sought.

Because of the above uncertainty over hyperaemia and the difficulties in classifying histological conditions of the pulp, it has been suggested that the term 'initial inflammation' be used (Pheulpin, Fiore-Donno and Baume, 1967); this might progress to an acute or a chronic condition. The idea is to get away from a too rigid histopathological classification of pulp conditions that might exert an undue constraint on treatment, and it accords with the views of Seltzer, Bender and Nazimov (1965) mentioned earlier, as well as those of Tyldesley and Mumford (1970).

## ACUTE PULPITIS

The first stage of acute pulpitis involves dilatation of the capillaries. (This *is* hyperaemia). Since the flow in a capillary is proportional to the fourth power of its radius (Poiseuille's Law) a small increase in the diameter of the pulpal capillaries would be expected to result in a large increase in blood flow. However, direct observation on the living pulp in rats' incisors has revealed diminished flow in some cases (Scheinin, 1963).

The first significant point for pain production is that the dilated vessels have an increased permeability so that fluid escapes into the surrounding pulpal tissues causing an increase in pressure. This also has an adverse effect on venous drainage because the relatively thin walled vessels are less able to withstand the pressure, and stasis occurs. According to Scheinin (1963) stasis may involve a rhythmic back and forth movement of the contents of a vessel as well as a standstill, but in either case stasis lasts for no more than 30 minutes before thrombosis occurs. As described in the previous chapter, thrombosis is associated with the liberation of 5-hydroxytryptamine from the blood platelets, and this affects the nerve terminals rendering them more sensitive to noxious stimuli. Potassium ions are liberated from the erythrocytes, and plasma kinins are freed, the total result being pain which can be very severe.

### Three forms of pain

Pain from acute pulpitis may be first noticed in three main ways. The first arises as a result of a recognisable external stimulus, usually heat or cold, but may be on biting or on contact with sweet foods, and tends to be localised. This kind of pain is described as sharp, lasts for a relatively short time, and patients represent it as in Fig. 9.18. At first it occurs with the stimulus and is brief, lasting only seconds or minutes, but gradually its duration increases and it outlasts the stimulus, continuing for many minutes, patients representing it as in Fig. 9.19. It is not surprising that patients drew graphs similar to those drawn for 'dentine pain' because both pains are evoked by external stimuli.

The second form of pain occurs spontaneously (without any recognisable external stimulus), because of chemical changes in the pulp (described in Chapter 10, but not yet strictly proven for the pulp). It is described as a dull ache which may last only minutes

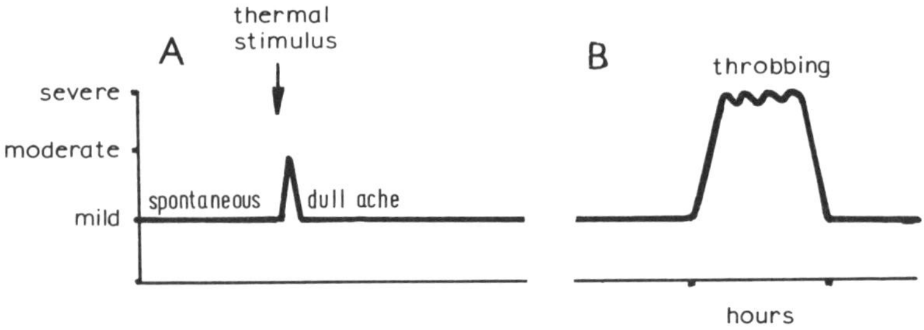


**Fig. 11.4A.** The patient who drew this graph had a continuous dull ache which arose spontaneously, plus brief exacerbations provoked by external stimuli.
B. A Similar case to A, but the exacerbations were more intense, lasted longer, were brought on by raising the blood pressure and consequently were described as throbbing.

but usually lasts for hours (unless analgesic drugs are taken). It is also more diffuse but exacerbations occur when external stimuli such as heat and cold are applied, and pain may then be more localised. If asked to do so the patient may draw a graph to represent it as shown in Fig. 11.4, A. The character of this pain may be modified by increased blood pressure due to activity such as climbing stairs, and this causes throbbing, but it is purely a pressure change — there is nothing fundamentally different about it. It might appear to be paradoxical but lying down may also bring on throbbing by allowing more blood to reach the head. In one patient, standing up stopped the throbbing whereas lying down started the throbbing again. A patient suffering from such pain drew a graph represented in Fig. 11.4, B. It is this type of pain which is usually described in the literature as constant, severe and throbbing, the tooth being sensitive to heat and sometimes cold. It is probably unavoidable in a general text but such a description is over-simplified, as may be seen from the accompanying tables. In 35 cases of pain caused by acute generalised pulpitis, 33 per cent described the pain as constant and severe, and 47 per cent as throbbing (Table 11.1). The tooth was said to be sensitive to heat in 60 per cent of cases, and sensitive to cold in 71 per cent of cases (Table 11.2).

As is usual in any dental practice, many of the painful teeth investigated by these authors were very carious or filled with metal, so pain on applying heat or cold was due at least partly to this physical condition. The point cannot be too strongly stressed that there are two chief variables, one physical as described earlier,

**Table 11.1** Patient's description of pain. The histological appearance was investigated without knowledge of the history or the clinical condition, i.e. blind-testing (Tyldesley and Mumford, 1970). Cases with intermittent or constant pain add up to 100 per cent, whereas throbbing is featured separately

| Histological finding in 142 cases | Intermittent mild pain, per cent of cases | Intermittent severe pain, per cent of cases | Constant mild pain, per cent of cases | Constant severe pain, per cent of cases | Throbbing pain, per cent of cases |
|---|---|---|---|---|---|
| Normal in 12 cases | 33 | 33 | 17 | 17 | 33 |
| Hyperaemia in 4 cases | 25 | 25 | 50 | 0 | 50 |
| Acute localised pulpitis in 25 cases | 4 | 56 | 28 | 12 | 24 |
| Acute generalised pulpitis in 35 cases | 21 | 40 | 6 | 33 | 47 |
| Acute and chronic pulpitis in 15 cases | 0 | 73 | 20 | 7 | 25 |
| Chronic pulpitis in 19 cases | 32 | 37 | 5 | 26 | 36 |
| Degeneration in 14 cases | 29 | 35 | 7 | 29 | 35 |
| Necrosis in 18 cases | 33 | 22 | 12 | 33 | 50 |

**Table 11.2.** Sensitivity to heat, cold and percussion. The histological condition was investigated without knowledge of the history or clinical condition, i.e. blind testing (Tyldesley and Mumford, 1970). H, sensitive to heat; C, sensitive to cold; P, sensitive to percussion

| Histological finding in 142 cases | H | C | P | HC | HP | CP | HCP | None |
|---|---|---|---|---|---|---|---|---|
| | | | | percentage of cases | | | | |
| Normal in 12 cases | 0 | 8 | 17 | 25 | 0 | 0 | 33 | 17 |
| Hyperaemia in 4 cases | 0 | 0 | 0 | 25 | 0 | 0 | 0 | 75 |
| Acute localised pulpitis in 25 cases | 4 | 16 | 4 | 8 | 8 | 4 | 36 | 20 |
| Acute generalised pulpitis in 35 cases | 6 | 11 | 9 | 11 | 3 | 9 | 40 | 11 |
| Acute and chronic pulpitis in 15 cases | 7 | 7 | 7 | 7 | 0 | 14 | 38 | 20 |
| Chronic pulpitis in 19 cases | 0 | 10 | 26 | 10 | 0 | 16 | 16 | 22 |
| Degeneration in 14 cases | 14 | 0 | 14 | 22 | 7 | 14 | 7 | 22 |
| Necrosis in 18 cases | 11 | 16 | 28 | 6 | 0 | 11 | 16 | 22 |

and the other pathological. Moreover, the physical stimulus itself varies considerably. Coffee or soup can be imbibed at various temperatures. In clinical tests a stick of gutta percha can be heated to different temperatures prior to being applied to the tooth, and this will clearly affect the percentage of teeth in which pain occurs on stimulation.

The third form of pain also occurs spontaneously. It is less common than the first two forms, and can be momentarily devastating. A male patient said, 'There was a series of short sharp jabs that halted me dead in my tracks'. A female patient described it as a violent shooting pain which left the area tender as though bruised — as though someone had hit her. This paroxysmal type of pain lasts for seconds and is repeated several times in a couple of days, by which time the patient is frightened and wants treatment immediately, together with some reassurance. However, by the time an appointment arrives the jabs of pain may have ceased to occur, perhaps because the pulp has died.

It is said that for teeth with acute pulpitis the pain perception threshold is lower than normal, and this would be expected from the basic principles described in the previous chapter, but it has never been satisfactorily demonstrated; indeed, using electrical stimulation, it has been clearly shown that many different histological states of the pulp, including acute pulpitis, are associated with pain perception thresholds similar to those for normal teeth (Mumford, 1967).

Occasionally the dentist is given a somewhat bizarre clue to the condition, and this manifests itself in several ways. Sometimes the patient opens his mouth and fans it vigorously with his hand or with papers. At other times cold water is held against the tooth, and on one occasion a patient even brought his own supply of cold water in a milk bottle. A patient familiar with the surgery may seize the compressed air syringe, insert the nozzle into his mouth and blow a cool draught on to the tooth. When questioned, the patient explains that coldness has a soothing effect. In a way this makes diagnosis more difficult since, as mentioned earlier, 71 per cent of patients with acute pulpitis said that the tooth was sensitive to cold. In one case both cold effects were noted, a young adult describing the pain as being caused by heat and cold, but also saying that a cold drink would counteract the pain from heat. Diagnosis is made even more difficult because many cases are sensitive to percussion, but this should not be surprising because inflammation tends to spread.

### Localisation of pain

It is generally considered that localisation of pulpal pain is poor, at least in comparison with pain of periodontal origin, although Sandberg (1963) did not think so. However it has been shown that, following electrical stimulation of teeth, human subjects did not localise the stimulated tooth very well (Friend and Glenwright, 1968; Mumford and Newton, 1971). The latter showed that only 22 out of 48 teeth stimulated were correctly localised, and even when the next tooth on either side was included there were still only 35 out of 48 correct localisations. This poor localisation might be because, on first exposure to a stimulus, the nervous system specifies it less precisely than after many exposures (Morrell, 1967), and since the dental pulp is not normally painful, this could account for why pain in it is not well localised. However, it is more likely to be because of anatomical convergence of pulpal nerves in the trigeminal nuclei and subsequent convergence at higher levels. In other words, it is supposed that each dental pulp does not have an individual representation anywhere in the brain.

In clinical cases localisation is improved because the patient usually knows which tooth has been stimulated, perhaps by seeing what the dentist is doing, but it is partly the stimulus which is localised rather than just the pain. It is partly for this reason that pain which arises spontaneously is more poorly localised.

Localisation of pain seems to be even poorer when pain becomes more intense. The explanation of this could be due to the fact that the terminal arborisations of neurones diverge (as well as converge). With mild pains neural impulses passing along the outermost arborisations may be too few to excite postsynaptic neurons because with such a system there is no synaptic security. With more intense pains, however, the increased number of neural impulses may secure transmission at synapses which are more peripheral, thus reducing localisation. In other words there is a breakdown of surround inhibition.

Localisation of pulpal versus periodontal pain will be considered in Chapter 12.

In some cases patients localise the pain in one jaw when the disease causing it is in the other jaw, and this is called referred pain (Chapter 17). Its character is the same as already described.

### Late stages

Although inflammation is a vital defence mechanism its effect in the enclosed pulp space is to increase damage. As pressure rises collapse of the thin walled veins causes drainage to decrease so that pressure rises further and pain also becomes worse, this being a classical case of the 'vicious circle'. Eventually the pulp dies, in which case pain from the pulp necessarily ceases, although pain from periapical disease may supervene, and may already have started before the pulp finally succumbs. The pulp is then in the condition illustrated in Fig. 11.5, and there is no response to electrical stimulation. However, three cases have been seen at preterminal stages when approximately four-fifths of the pulp were already dead (Fig. 11.6, left) but living nerve fibres were presumably still present in the apical fifth (Fig. 11.6, right) because the tooth still responded to electrical stimulation. At this stage the nerve bundles would be loosened, irregularly thickened and fragmented (Plačková, 1966). It seems likely that a delay of even a few hours would allow complete death of the pulp, including the nerves, and several cases have been seen where the change occurred between one examination and another done on the following day. When the condition of a patient changes in this manner it could be

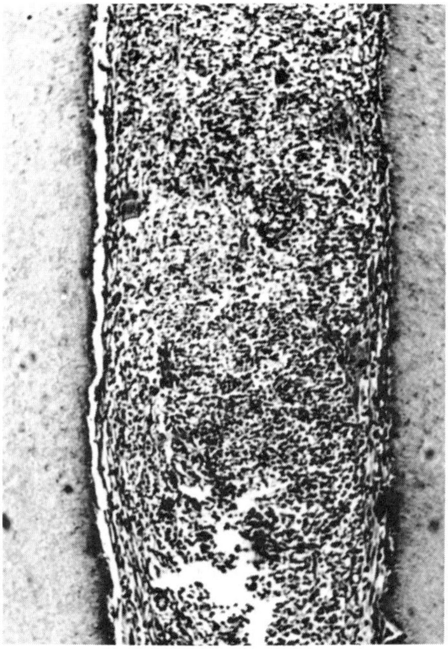

**Fig. 11.5.** Generalised acute pulpitis in its terminal state. Original magnification × 32.

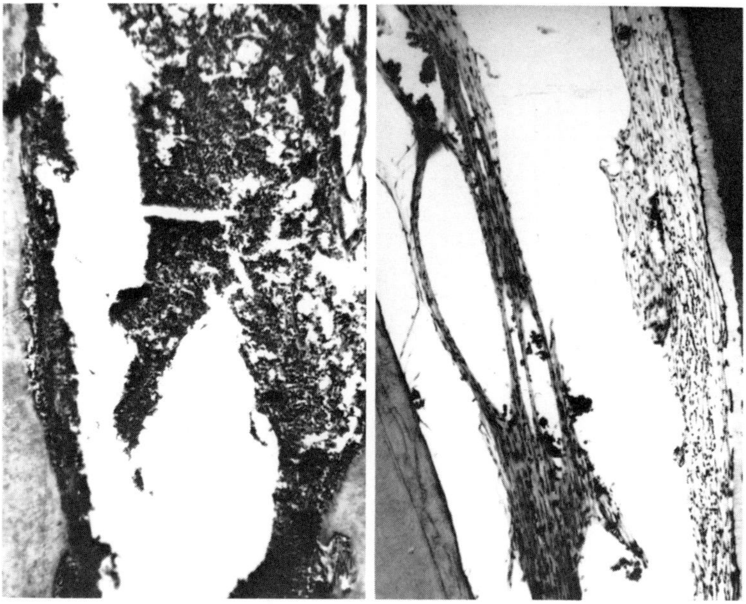

**Fig. 11.6.** Moribund pulp with about four-fifths dead (left) and only a small living remnant in the pulp canal (right). Original magnification × 32.

confusing but it should usually be helpful in providing additional clues to the condition.

### Localised acute pulpitis

Acute pulpitis may be localised rather than generalised, because of various factors already described. This could happen naturally by drainage occurring but most examples seen by the author are in association with cases where pulp capping has been practised. (This should not be taken as a criticism of pulp capping.) In such cases patients complain of pain in a tooth, the pulp of which has been exposed and capped some weeks earlier. Pain sometimes occurs as several short jabs but may also be continuous. The pulp of such a case is shown in Fig. 11.7. A similar localised acute abscess is seen in Fig. 11.8. When pain occurs in short sharp jabs this should be taken as indicating the need for pulpectomy or extraction.

It other cases of localised acute pulpitis pain is the same as in generalised acute pulpitis. It is worth remarking that there may be more than one fault, as in a patient who complained of pain, diffusely situated over the right zygomatic bone. It first started a week earlier, and pain occurred spontaneously three or four times during

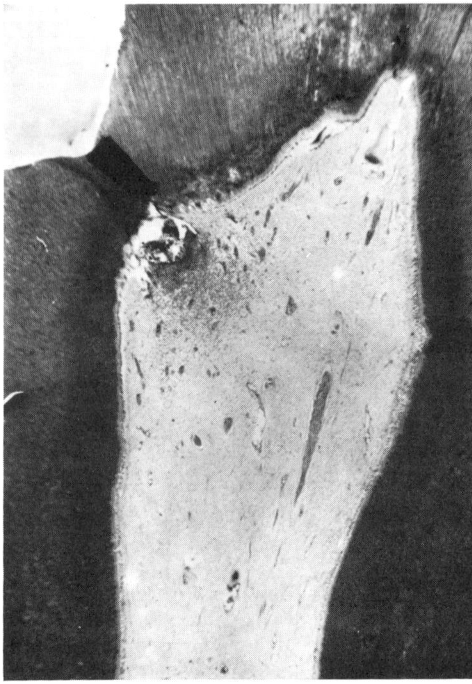

**Fig. 11.7.** Localised acute pulpitis. There is a circumscribed abscess surrounded by pulp with dilated blood vessels. Further afield the pulp looks normal. Original magnification × 25.

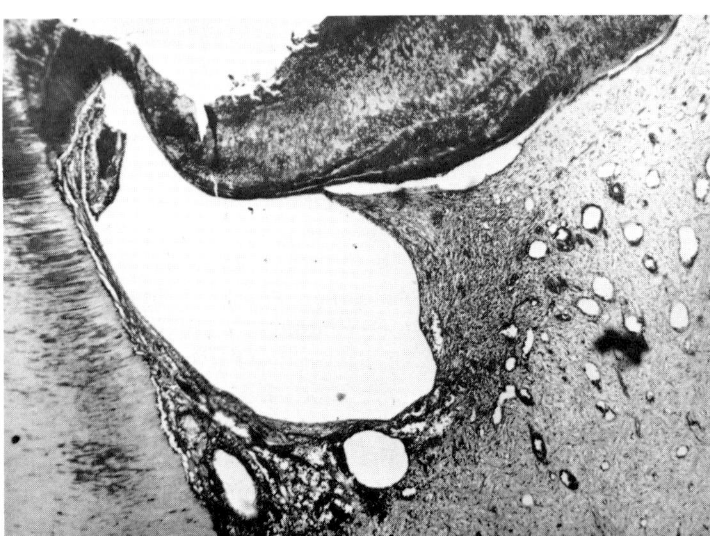

**Fig. 11.8.** Localised acute abscess. The pulp had been exposed and capped two months earlier. Pain occurred in short sharp jabs. Original magnification × 32.

that period, lasting for several hours. The right upper third molar was found to have a leaking amalgam filling which might have been wrongly regarded as causative, but closer examination revealed a pin point exposure.

## Treatment of acute pulpitis

The minimal form of acute pulpitis associated with a newly placed filling, and usually called hyperaemia, is associated with only mild pain which is stimulus-evoked and passes off quickly. This is left untreated, though a reassuring explanation is given to the patient. Hot and cold foods are avoided for a few days until the pulp recovers. If pain is more severe it is necessary to remove the filling, especially if a lining has not been used. A temporary restoration is placed using zinc oxide-eugenol cement, preferably of the quick-setting fortified variety. If the temporary restoration has to last a longer time it is better to apply a layer of calcium hydroxide paste followed by a layer of zinc phosphate cement. The latter two-part restoration is also better if there is any chance that the pulp has been exposed, or nearly so, because calcium hydroxide is less irritant to the pulp than is zinc oxide-eugenol cement. Also, the zinc phosphate layer offers better physical protection than does zinc oxide-eugenol cement which tends to crumble thus leaving the underlying tooth exposed to oral fluids, thermal stimuli and additional microorganisms. Instead of zinc phosphate a polycarboxylate cement may be used and this should ensure a better peripheral seal.

When there is a definite exposure it is reasonable to use a paste containing a corticosteroid with an antibiotic. The rationale of this treatment is that acute inflammation, though an important defense mechanism, is potentially destructive within the confined pulp space; inflammatory exudate cannot readily escape so there is pressure on the venules and this makes drainage even more difficult. The corticosteroid is anti-inflammatory so gives the pulp chance to recover, but it is then necessary to combat microorganisms with a broad-spectrum antibiotic so this is included in the paste (Ledermix brand). Schroeder (1979) finds this material valuable, but it is not universally favoured, partly because the first application has to be replaced. The author prefers to subject the pulp to as little manipulation as possible, with no probing of the pulp, removal of all or almost all caries, a layer of calcium hydroxide gently and widely applied, a zinc phosphate layer and then an amalgam restoration. This gives the best seal and maximum physical protection. If it succeeds no further manipulation is needed since the amalgam has already been placed. If it fails it is an easy matter to drill through the amalgam to perform a pulpectomy and the amalgam provides good walls to isolate the pulp.

As implied, it is quite likely that a pulpectomy will be needed and it may be better to do this at the earliest opportunity. It stops the acute pulpitis by removing the whole pulp, and has the advantage that spread of the inflammation to the periodontal tissues is less likely.

As a last resort it may even be necessary to extract the tooth. The treatment used will depend upon the severity of the pulpitis, the physical condition of the tooth, the nature of the dentition and the attitude of the patient.

**Measurement of pain**

Patients suffering from acute pulpitis have been given cards on which were drawn an ordinate with a pain intensity scale, and also an abscissa on which any time scale could be indicated (Mumford, 1969). Each patient was asked to draw a graph representing the intensity and duration of his pain, and results have been obtained such as those shown in Figs. 9.18–9.21, 11.3 and 11.4. Not only is there considerable variation between graphs drawn for similar conditions but graphs similar to these have been drawn by patients suffering from different conditions as far apart as sensitive cervical dentine and acute periapical periodontitis. Moreover, patients are often extraordinarily poor at making graphs, sometimes even at the university level of education, so this is not yet recommended as a useful approach to diagnosis except for those carrying out research on the subject.

The graphs are interesting in so far as they give a measurement of the pain suffered, although this is not an accurate measurement in the sense used in the physical sciences because the pain intensity scale is only in a subjectively determined order. However, the mild level is probably much the same for all patients, being only just noticeable. The severe level now includes what used to be called unbearable (Mumford, 1969) — pain which leaves the patient at least momentarily incapacitated; or when the patient is clearly sick with pain, feeling like knocking his head against a wall, and actually doing so in some cases; or when every meal is an ordeal and the patient has to get up from the table and walk about in desperation; or when the patient, normally very sensible, is in such pain that she is screaming, so that her husband is afraid that she is in a 'fit'. The word unbearable is slightly misleading since in a sense the pain has to be borne; what it means is that continuation of the pain would temporarily disrupt the patient's personality, i.e. cause him to 'break down'. In some cases this actually happens.

Although the pain intensity scale is only ordinal it is the best at present available (Smith, 1962; Rogers and Lim, 1966; Nayman, 1979). The abscissa, of course, is a real time scale though subject to the patient's estimate which is only approximate. Notice that the area between the curve and the abscissa is a crude measurement of the quantity of pain (time-intensity).

**Quality of pain**

The quality of pain described as sharp is apparently related to external stimuli though not always, whereas the quality called dull is more likely to be related to pain arising from endogenous factors. Thus, in one group of 25 teeth which all had exposed pulps there was some correlation between the quality of pain and the way in which it started (unpublished investigation). When pain occurred spontaneously the quality of pain was described by the patients as being dull in 5 cases and sharp in 2 cases. On the other hand, pain which occurred as a result of stimulation by heat, cold or biting was described as sharp in 14 cases and dull in only 2 cases. In this respect the quality of the pain is considered to be a factor worth watching, although it must be pointed out that Seltzer, Bender and Ziontz (1963) found no correlation between the character of the pain and the histological condition.

Throbbing pain is sometimes endowed with significance but all that can really be said is that the arterial pulse arrives in the inflamed area and causes a momentary increase in pressure which causes an increase in neural impulses which register as a brief increase in pain intensity. In fact, throbbing can be regarded as an intensity change rather than quality in itself. The bursts of neural impulses in rhythm with the arterial pulse have been demonstrated (in dogs) by Funakoshi and Zotterman (1963) and Narhi (1978).

In some cases there is toothache which is not throbbing while the patient is standing but only when he lies down. Throbbing ceases if he stands up again. This is because lying down produces an increase in pressure in the pulp which is just enough to allow the arterial pulse to produce the throbbing pain. Similarly, a dentist reported that he developed a slight toothache in an upper premolar only when he walked up several flights of stairs.

Table 11.1 includes a final column on throbbing pain which suggests that this feature does not help in making an exact diagnosis of the pulp's histological condition.

It has sometimes been suggested that a tingling sensation in the tooth caused by electrical stimulation indicates a degenerating pulp, but this is not accepted because it has been shown that more normal teeth give this sensation than any other sensation (Mumford, 1965). In fact, tingling probably only indicates the frequency of stimulation. Moreover, many different words are used to describe the sensation from a standard electrical stimulus so the quality of pain probably has no significance at the lower intensities. This is a feature of the state called metaesthesia by Keele (1962) to describe the lower levels of sensation produced by acetylcholine, potassium chloride, 5-hydroxytryptamine and bradykinin applied to an exposed blister base.

**Sequelae of acute pulpitis**

One sequel of acute pulpitis is periapical disease which will be described in the next chapter, but a number of cases have been seen in which further spread of disease seemed to stop once the pulp died even though no treatment was instituted. Naturally, such treatment (or lack of it) cannot be recommended because there could be an acute exacerbation at any time, most likely when the patient's resistance is low, e.g. while he has influenza and can least afford to have acute periapical inflammation. On the other hand, several molar teeth have been extracted because, although symptomless, the pulps were dead, yet examination of the apices failed to reveal patent apical foramina, cementum having apparently covered the areas. It seems likely that such teeth could have been left in place indefinitely if only more had been known about them, and there is clearly room for further research on this subject.

Chronic pulpitis may develop from an acute pulpitis, especially if the micro-organisms involved in the attack are of low virulence, or if the apical foramen has not fully formed, for this allows better drainage so that pressure does not build up as much as it would otherwise have done. Also the carious process or trauma might have left the pulp exposed so that fluid can escape through this opening. This partly explains why many patients with such pulp exposures have less pain than might have been expected, and often fail to seek treatment for months or even years. Naturally, after the lapse of some time there may be degenerative changes or chronic inflammation in the pulp.

## CHRONIC PULPITIS

From the foregoing discussion it is obvious that chronic pulpitis can be associated with a pulp exposure — open chronic pulpitis —

or it can be in a pulp which is entirely enclosed — closed chronic pulpitis. The former is likely to be less painful because drainage can occur, but in neither instance is much pain experienced, the condition not being sensitive to thermal change. In this respect a casual examination of Tables 11.1 and 11.2 could be confusing for it might wrongly suggest a high incidence of pain from chronic pulpitis, but these tables analyse only those cases where the patients complained of pain.

It is said that when teeth are tested by electrical stimulation a higher current than normal is required to elicit pain in cases of chronic pulpitis (a raised pain perception threshold) but this has not been satisfactorily demonstrated and values lie within the range for normal teeth which is approximately 2–20 microamps (Mumford, 1967).

When there is open chronic pulpitis there may be ulceration of the pulp at the exposed area, chronic ulcerative pulpitis, and this is sensitive to mechanical stimulation, e.g. by a probe, but much less than it would have been with a normal pulp.

Occasionally, especially in children, the pulp may proliferate through the exposure to form a pulp polyp (chronic hyperplastic pulpitis). The polyp lies in the carious cavity and is almost insensitive to probing (Fig. 11.9).

In other words, pain is not an important feature of chronic pulpitis unless acute exacerbations occur.

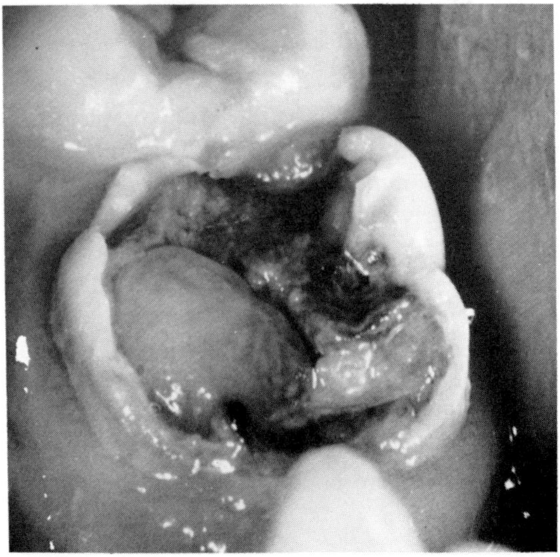

**Fig. 11.9.** Molar with a large carious cavity in which lies a pulp polyp (hypertrophic chronic pulpitis).

## ACUTE WITH CHRONIC PULPITIS

There may be an acute exacerbation of a chronic condition if the drainage becomes blocked, e.g. by the dentist placing a dressing in the cavity over an exposed pulp. Tyldesley and Mumford (1970) have called the corresponding histological condition 'acute with chronic pulpitis' because there are substantial numbers of polymorphonuclear leucocytes and chronic inflammatory cells together (Fig. 11.10). This term also applies, in the histological sense, to an acute condition which is subsiding to a chronic state, though the history of pain would be different. Some clinicians might prefer to describe such conditions as subacute pulpitis but this could imply a more stable state than exists.

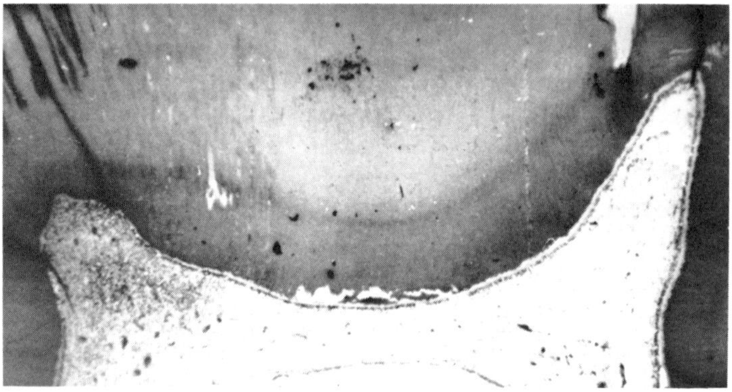

**Fig. 11.10.** Acute with chronic pulpitis localised to one part of the pulp underlying invading caries. Original magnification × 10·4.

Table 11.1 shows the nature of the pain complained of in acute with chronic pulpitis, the terms intermittent pain and constant pain being used in the commonly accepted manner, but it would be better to use properly estimated times. These were from several minutes up to 6 hours, pains of the shorter duration tending to be stimulus provoked whereas those of longer duration tend to arise spontaneously. It is noteworthy that percussion caused pain in about two-thirds of these cases. On electrical stimulation the pain perception threshold lies within the range for normal teeth.

After a while the chronic state may develop once more, only to be followed by acute exacerbations. This changing state of the pulp explains some cases where bouts of pain occur from time to time over a period of years.

*Treatment*

This follows the lines already suggested for acute pulpitis.

## PULP GANGRENE

When a pulp is badly damaged in association with gas producing micro-organisms pulp gangrene can develop. Pain occurs spontaneously or on biting or both, and heat sometimes provokes it. Pain is localised rather than diffuse, and described as a dull ache which lasts for hours or even days. In nearly all cases there is pain on percussion, and this can be expected because the disease spreads to involve the periodontal membrane.

Care should be taken when applying heat to such cases because the gas present is capable of great thermal expansion which causes pain and facilitates passage of micro-organisms through the apical foramen. Several cases have been seen where application of heat to such a tooth has left the patient in a state of agony which completely incapacitated him for several minutes. This can be better understood from the following values. The coefficient of thermal expansion of gas is 0·00367 per degree C, at constant pressure, being about ten times that of water which is 0·00036 per degree C, at 37° (Weast, 1972)

If the pulp space is opened there is an offensive smell of variable intensity. Even without local anaesthesia instruments can be passed into the pulp canal without pain, provided they are eased in; if they are pushed in too rapidly there may be a plunger effect causing fluid to be forced on to the periapical tissues thus causing pain.

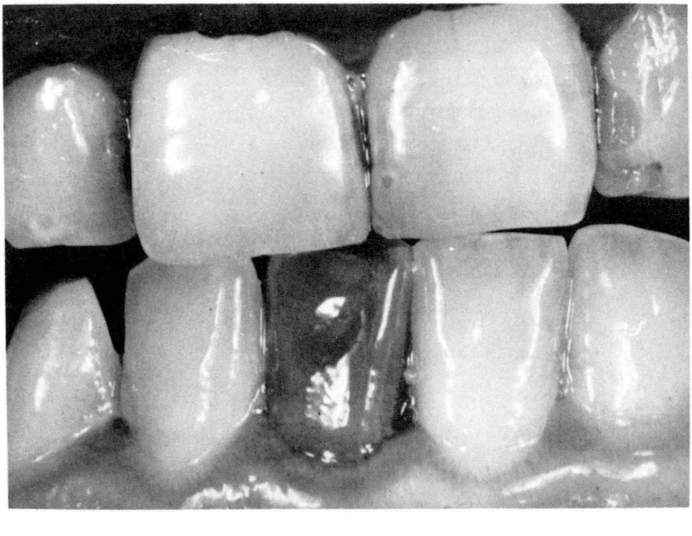

**Fig. 11.11.** Lower central incisor deeply discoloured as a result of pulp gangrene.

Applying a barbed broach fails to withdraw pulp tissue, but a greyish black jelly is found.

It will be obvious from the above description that the diagnosis should be pulp gangrene with acute periapical periodontitis. Eventually the tooth gradually discolours, becoming pale grey to dark purple (Fig. 11.11).

*Treatment*

Root canal treatment is indicated when there is a good dentition and this removes the source of pain. Bleaching is needed afterwards or even a jacket crown or post crown. For poor dentitions extraction is indicated.

## PULP NECROSIS

Occasionally it is said that there is no need to make a differential diagnosis between pulp necrosis and pulp gangrene since in both cases the pulp is dead, but the conditions are different. The term necrosis is used to indicate death of the pulp without microorganisms being necessarily present. The pulp dies slowly, losing fluid and becoming dry; in some cases the pulp disappears completely and when the pulp chamber is opened it is found to be empty. There is no unpleasant odour as there is with gangrene, and no pressure, so pain is not as likely to occur, and such cases are usually symptomless. Moreover the crown of the tooth can be completely intact and of normal colour so that the condition is only discovered by chance, such as in making comparative pulp tests when it is found that the affected tooth is insensitive. It may also be difficult to pass electric current through such a tooth because the drying out process leaves the tooth with a very high electrical resistance, whereas gangrenous fluid has a low electrical resistance which allows a high current to pass.

After pulp necrosis there is much less chance of acute periapical disease developing than is the case following pulp gangrene.

## PULP CONCUSSION

When a patient suffers a blow teeth may be fractured or dislocated and pulps may die. In addition it is said that they can be concussed, which implies that they remain vital but fail to respond to stimuli for a variable period after which normal sensitivity returns. This is comparable with the apparent diminution in sensitivity of soft tissues which have been subjected to accidental trauma. However, the author has not knowingly seen such a case of pulp concussion. It is possible that, immediately after an accident, haemorrhage from the gingival margin and swollen lacerated soft tissues may render accurate electrical pulp testing impossible by conducting electricity away from the pulp, so allowing no response when there might otherwise have been one.

## INTERNAL RESORPTION

Internal resorption of teeth (endodontoma) is not associated with pain, early cases being found radiographically (Fig. 11.12), and later ones by pulp showing through the crown — pink spot. However, the resorptive process gradually extends outwards to the periodontal membrane and, if the gingival margin is involved, infection supervenes and there may then be pain due to acute pulpitis (Figs. 11.13, 11.14).

### *Treatment*

At the stage when pain occurs it may be necessary to extract the tooth because pulpectomy and root canal treatment are seldom feasible. However, pain can cease of its own accord and the patient may prefer to suffer the pain a while rather than lose the tooth. In young people it is well worth while to retain the tooth for as long as possible so that eventually it is easier to provide a bridge, the abutment teeth being then more mature.

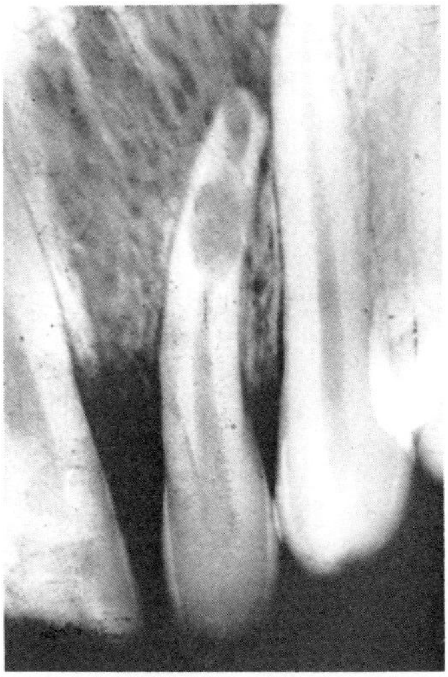

**Fig. 11.12.** Internal resorption of dentine (endodontoma).

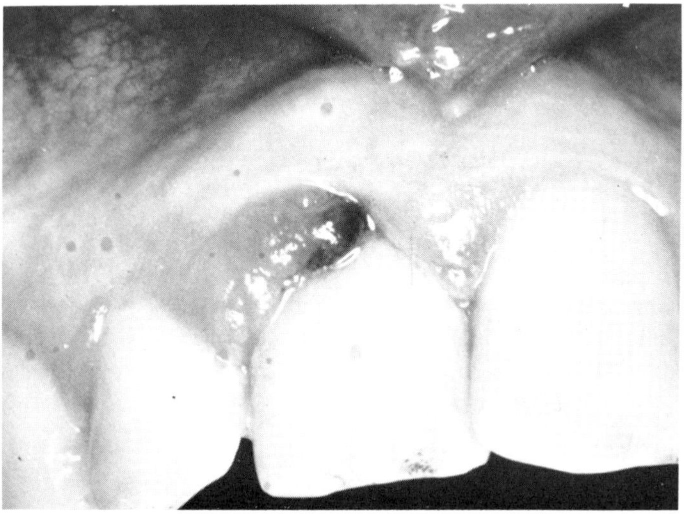

**Fig. 11.13.** Inflammation of the marginal gingiva due to the resorptive change shown in Fig. 11.14.

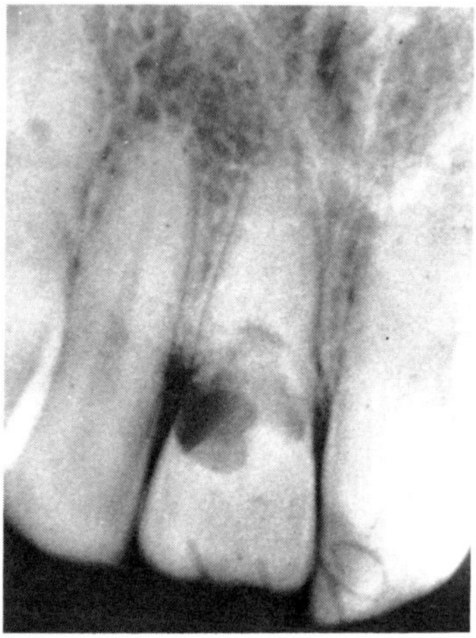

**Fig. 11.14.** Extensive internal resorption of dentine (endodontoma) perforating through to the periodontal membrane. Same case as Fig. 11.13.

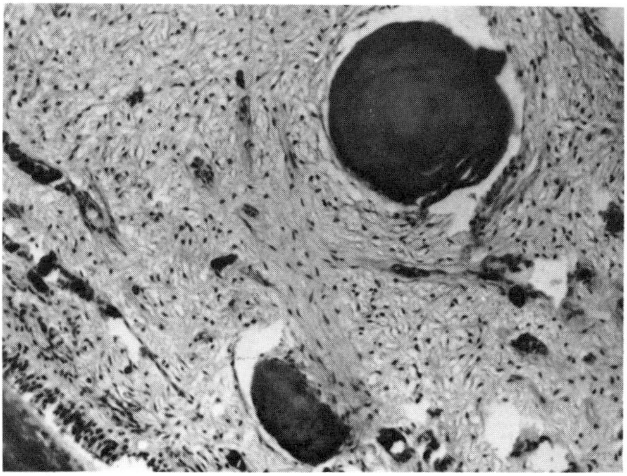

**Fig. 11.15.** A pulp stone (denticle) which did not cause pain. Original magnification × 32.

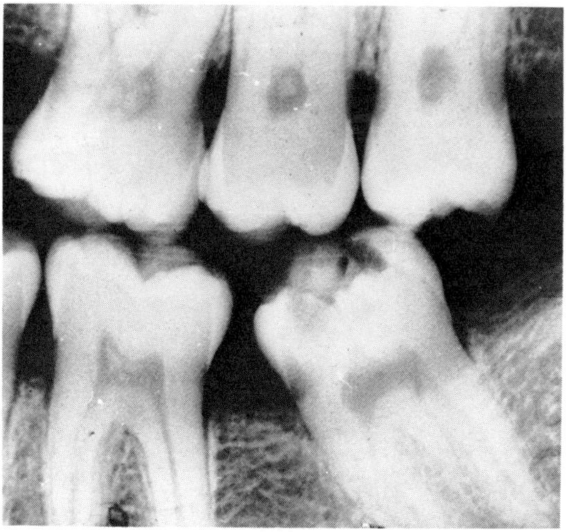

**Fig. 11.16.** Pulp stones are present in the coronal pulps of four of these molars. In the upper second molar what appears to be a pulp stone could be the sub-pulpal wall of dentine.

## CALCIFICATION

It is said that pain may occur as a result of pulp calcifications involving nerve fibres, affecting the neural connective tissue first (Bernick, 1967), but there is no real evidence for this. Moreover, pulp stones (Fig. 11.15) and other calcifications are frequently present without pain, and sometimes large 'pulp stones' pointed out on radiographs of molars are only the sub-pulpal wall of dentine (Fig. 11.16). However, encroachment of calcification on to nerve fibres could conceivably stimulate them in the way suggested by Fig. 11.17. Against this is the fact that a response to electrical stimulation within the normal range is sometimes obtained from pulps which are mainly calcified, such as that in Fig. 11.18.

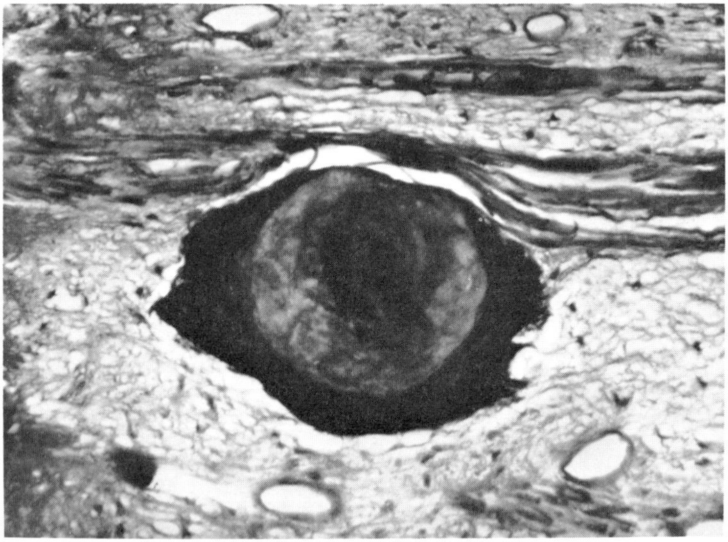

**Fig. 11.17.** Apparent compression of nerve fibres by calcification within the pulp. This might conceivably cause pain. Original magnification × 32.

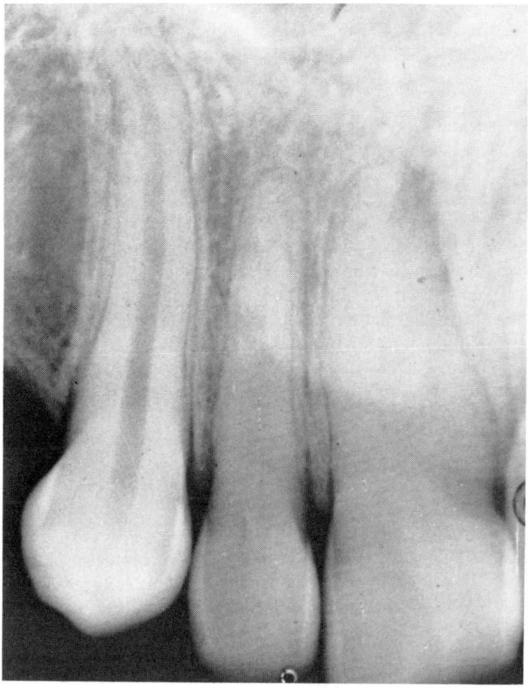

**Fig. 11.18** The pulps of the central and lateral incisors are calcified to a great extent. Compare with the pulp in the canine.

REFERENCES

Baume, L. J. (1966) Clinical and pathohistological aspects of current endodontic therapy. *Int. dent. J. (Lond.)*, **16**, 30–54.

Baume, L. J. (1970a) Dental pulp conditions in relation to carious lesions. *Int. dent. J. (Lond.)*, **20**, 309–337.

Baume, L. J. (1970b) Diagnosis of diseases of the pulp. *Oral Surg.*, **29**, 102–116.

Bernick, S. (1967) Effect of ageing on the nerve supply to human teeth. *J. dent. Res.*, **46**, 694–699.

Björn, H. (1946) Electrical excitation of teeth, and its application to dentistry. *Svensk tandl. Tidskr.*, **39**, Suppl.

Brännström, M. and Lind, P.O. (1965) Pulpal response to early dental caries. *J. dent. Res.*, **44**, 1045–1050.

Friend, L. A. and Glenwright, H. D. (1968) An experimental investigation into the localization of pain from the dental pulp. *Oral Surg.*, **25**, 765–774.

Funakoshi, M. and Zotterman, Y. (1963) A study in the excitation of dental pulpal nerve fibres. In *Sensory Mechanisms in Dentine*, ed. Anderson, D. J., pp. 60–70. Oxford: Pergamon.

Harndt, R. (1969) Die Erkrankungen der Pulpa und ihre Diagnose. *Deutsche zahnärztliche zeit.*, **24** (i), 389–400 (with English summary).

Haskell, E. W., Stanley, H. R., Chellemi, J. and Stringfellow, H. (1978) Direct pulp capping treatment: a long-term follow-up. *J. Amer. dent. Ass.*, **97**, 607–612.

Hassel, H. J. Van and Harrington, G. W. (1969) Localisation of pulpal sensation. *Oral Surg.*, **28**,753–760.

Herbert, W. E. (1945) A correlation of the clinical signs and symptoms and histological condition of the pulps of 52 teeth. *Brit. dent. J.*, **78**, 161–174.

Keele, C. A. (1962) Sensations aroused by chemical stimulation of the skin. In *The Assessment of Pain in Man and Animals*, ed. Keele, C. A. and Smith, R., pp. 28–31. Edinburgh: Livingstone.

Lundy, T. and Stanley, H. R. (1969) Correlation of pulpal histopathology and clinical symptoms in human teeth subjected to experimental irritation. *Oral Surg.*, **27**, 187–201.

Matthews, B., Searle, B. N., Adams, D. and Linden, R. (1974) Thresholds of vital and non-vital teeth to stimulation with electric pulp testers. *Brit. dent. J.*, **137**, 352–355.

Morrell, F. (1967) Electrical signs of sensory coding. In *The Neurosciences*, ed. Quarton, G. C., Melnechuk, T. and Schmitt, F. O., pp. 452–469. New York: Rockefeller Univ. Press.

Mumford, J. M. (1965) Pain perception threshold and adaptation of normal human teeth. *Archs. oral Biol.*, **10**, 957–968.

Mumford, J. M. (1967) Pain perception threshold on stimulating human teeth and the histological condition of the pulp. *Brit dent. J.*, **123**, 427–433.

Mumford, J. M. (1968) Time factor in toothache. *Brit. dent. J.*, **125**, 311–314.

Mumford, J. M. (1969) Measurement of toothache. *J. Brit. Endo. Soc.*, **3**, 48–51.

Mumford, J. M. and Newton, A. V. (1971) Convergence in the trigeminal system following stimulation of human teeth. *Archs. oral Biol.*, **16**, 1089–1097.

Närhi, M. (1978) Activation of dental pulp nerves of the cat and the dog with hydrostatic pressure. *Proc. Finn. Dent. Soc.*, **74**, Suppl. V.

Nayman, J. (1979) Measurement and control of postoperative pain. *Ann. Roy. Coll. Surg. (Eng.)*, **61**, 419–426.

Pheulpin, J. L., Fiore-Donno, G. and Baume, L. J. (1967) Les inflammations pulpaires: Leurs diagnostics cliniques et histopathologique. *Schweiz. Mschr. Zahnheilk.*, **77**, 701–728.

Plačková, A. (1966) Pathological changes in the innervation of the dental pulp during the carious process. *J. dent. Res.*, **45**, 62–65.

Pohto, P. (1972) Sympathetic adrenergic innervation of permanent teeth in the monkey (macaca irus). *Acta odont. Scandinav.*, **30**, 117–126.

Rogers, R. W. and Lim, R. K. S. (1966) Measurement of subjective pain in man. *Pharmacologist*, **8**, 206, Abstr.

Sandberg, L. O. (1963) Förmagen att okalisera en dental smärtretning; end experimentellklinisk undersokning. *Svensk tandl. Tidskr.*, **56**, 49. Quoted by Friend and Glenwright, cited above.

Scheinin, A. (1963) Flow characteristics of the pulpal vessels. *J. dent. Res.*, Suppl. 1, **42**, 438–441.

Schroeder, A. (1979) Control of pain in endodontic practice. In *Mechanism and Control of Pain*, ed. Grossman, L. I., pp. 121–137. New York: Masson.

Seltzer, S., Bender, I. B. and Nazimov, H. (1965) Differential diagnosis of pulp conditions. *Oral Surg.*, **19**, 383–391.

Seltzer, S., Bender, I. B. and Ziontz, M. (1963) The dynamics of pulp inflammation: correlations between diagnostic data and actual histologic findings in the pulp. *Oral Surg.*, **16**, 846–871 and 969–977.

Smith, R. (1962). The vocabulary of pain. In *The Assessment of Pain in Man and Animals*, ed. Keele, C. A. and Smith, R., pp. 32–40. Edinburgh: Livingstone.

Stephan, R. M. (1937) Correlation of clinical tests with microscopic pathology of the dental pulp. *J. dent. Res.*, **16**, 267–278.
Tyldesley, W. R. and Mumford, J. M. (1970) Dental pain and the histological condition of the pulp. *Dent. Practit. dent. Rec.*, **20**, 333–336.
Vargas, F. and Vidaldi, L. (1959) Correlation between nervous accommodation, symptomatology, and histology of normal and pathologic tooth pulp: its application to electrodiagnosis. *J. dent. Res.*, **38**, 866–880.
Weast, R. C. (1972) (ed.) *Handbook of Chemistry and Physics*, 53rd ed., p. F98. Cleveland: The Chemical Rubber Company.

# 12

# Pain from the periodontal tissues

Perhaps the fault lies in early clinical teaching, but it seems to be widely thought that pulp disease and periapical disease are entities more separate than they really are. This attitude expresses itself in the diagnostic dictum that pain on applying heat to a tooth indicates pulp disease, whereas pain on percussion indicates periapical disease. This is only approximately correct, and part of the object of this chapter is to correct these oversimplifications.

## ACUTE PERIAPICAL PERIODONTITIS

Once the dental pulp becomes acutely inflamed toxins are able to pass through the pulp canal to the periapical tissues. Later, micro-organisms pass through together with the chemical products of tissue disintegration, so it is to be expected that acute pulpitis and acute periapical periodontitis can be present at the same time. Whether they are coincident or not depends on factors such as the virulence of the micro-organisms concerned, any outward drainage, and the stage of development of the disease. These factors account for the variability of the histories given by different patients.

Once acute inflammation starts in the periapical tissues it develops as it does elsewhere, the blood vessels dilate and the periodontal membrane may become sufficiently engorged for the tooth to be slightly extruded from its socket. At this stage the patient may feel that he bites on the tooth concerned before the remaining teeth occlude, and this is associated with a mild level of pain which passes off if the patient continues to bite on the tooth. It has been suggested that biting on the tooth is effective in stopping pain because it drives blood out of the vessels, and perhaps it does, but it could be that pain stops because adaptation occurs, and adaptation has been shown to occur at similar low pain intensities arising from pulpal stimulation (Mumford, 1965). Another possibility is that stimulation of larger nerve fibres might close the 'gate' in the central nervous system (as suggested in Chapter 4).

As the acute inflammation develops stasis occurs in some vessels and it has been suggested that pressure on the tooth causes pain because blood cannot be driven out of them. This seems unlikely because even if blood could be driven out it would go too slowly to cushion the applied pressure. Of course, such pressure does cause pain, or an intensification of pain already present, the reason being that nerve endings have been sensitised by algogens, such as 5-hydroxytryptamine, so that excitation occurs with lower stimulus intensities than normal. (The endogenous pain-producing substances have already been considered in Chapter 10.)

In about two-thirds of cases pain is described as localised rather than diffuse and is accurately localised to the tooth eventually found to be the site of the disease responsible. In about a seventh of cases pain is diffuse, and occasionally pain is radiating, the latter being in cases of severe intensity. If asked to state in which part of the tooth or surrounding tissues they feel the pain patients usually think it is in and about the root, but some localise it in the crown or even at the incisal edge.

Most patients have had pain for a day to a week by the time they are seen, but many report some slight pain or awareness of the tooth for months or years before. The latter cases are acute exacerbations of previous chronic conditions and are likely to have periapical bone rarefactions (see later).

In almost all cases pain occurs spontaneously (i.e. without any recognisable external stimulus) and also pain frequently occurs on biting. In a series of 34 cases 28 patients reported that pain occurred spontaneously, and this was the chief cause in 27 of them. Biting caused pain in 23 cases and was the chief cause in 9 instances; the second cause in 12 instances. It may be supposed that biting comes second to spontaneously because biting is largely under the patient's control, and this presumably accounts for biting not been mentioned even more often.

It may seem confusing but pain occurred from heat in 9 cases and from cold in 6 cases. Such cases might be accounted for by mistaken diagnosis, but the final diagnosis of the cases considered here was based not only on initial clinical methods but also on information derived from operative treatment and from histological methods where possible. Some cases where pain occurs from hot and cold stimuli might be due to the dentist seeing the patient at an early stage when the pulp, though moribund, is not completely dead. In fact, the clinical picture does sometimes change from one day to the next, and this is to be expected as the pulp finally succumbs. In other cases application of heat causes fluid within the pulp space (liquid and gas) to expand through the apical foramen and press on the sensitive periapical tissues.

When pain arises spontaneously it is usually a dull ache which lasts for hours, perhaps days. In some cases it is a throbbing pain which is due to the momentary increase in pressure with the arrival of each arterial pulse. Patients asked to represent such pain as a graph do so as shown in Fig. 11.4, B, though only about 50 per cent of patients represent throbbing as the wavy line illustrated. It has been shown that a tooth can move rhythmically in its socket in synchrony with the heart beat (Picton, 1969).

When hot or cold stimuli provoke the pain it is more likely to be described as sharp pain which lasts for a short time, fading to a dull ache of lower intensity. Patients asked to make a graph of such pain represent it similarly to that shown in Fig. 9.19.

*Intensity of pain.* This is usually moderate or severe but in some cases it is described as unbearable, the patient looking pale and feeling sick. He may have been walking up and down the bedroom for much of the night or walking about the house for something to distract him. He may have wanted to bang his head on the wall to create an alternative unpleasant sensation which would be more tolerable, and may even have done so.

In most cases there is pain on percussion but no pain from applying hot or cold stimuli. Electrical stimulation yields no response, and this fits with the fact that there is usually no pulp tissue found when embarking on pulp canal treatment. When the pulp canal is opened there may be a serous discharge, perhaps tinged with blood. There may be pus which sometimes wells out, but it may only ooze out and even this may need gentle pressure to be applied to the mucosa over the apical area. Sometimes there is a grey liquid, slightly gelatinous, with an unpleasant odour, possibly occupying only the apical portion of the pulp space; the crown in such cases is usually a grey colour, and this means that the pulp has died of gangrene.

*Relief of pain.* Pain is sometimes eased by application of heat, perhaps because of its pleasant stimulation of associated nerve fibres, and this is in conformity with the gate control theory and its modern development. Also, it is sometimes eased by cold, perhaps by diminishing blood flow to the area.

Pain also ceases or diminishes if drainage occurs naturally or is obtained by extraction or endodontic treatment, as described below.

**Acute purulent periapical periodontitis**

As can be expected from the severity of pain, patients suffering from acute inflammation of the periapical tissues are likely to demand early attention, but the disease may be allowed to develop untreated, and pain in such cases may cease in the manner described below. As the disease progresses there is an outflow of fluid from the blood vessels together with polymorphonuclear leucocytes, many of which die, along with numerous micro-organisms, giving rise to pus. There is insufficient space available in bone to accommodate the pus without an increase in pressure so pain is severe, and there may be general symptoms of malaise and a raised temperature. This is an acute apical abscess, or purulent periapical periodontitis, but it cannot be said that pain is greater than when there is no pus. At this stage there may be a slight swelling and erythema of the overlying mucosa. If finger pressure is applied to the mucosa over the apex of the affected tooth it causes pain; in other words there is tenderness. The same effect may also occur from pressing on the skin over the area. This tenderness is a valuable diagnostic point. In fact, the patient may even complain that pressing on the tooth with his tongue causes pain.

In the upper anterior region the nasolabial fold is obliterated, cellulitis develops and spreads to the lower eyelid which may accommodate so much fluid that it swells to close the palpebral fissure. The result is that the patient cannot see from this eye and may be frightened. This is natural, especially since the patient will have suffered a great deal by this time and will be distressed already.

In the lower anterior region the groove below the lower lip is diminished or obliterated and tension may be so great that the area feels numb, as though a local anaesthetic solution had been injected. This paraesthesia may also affect the teeth so that the patient complains that the 'teeth feel peculiar'.

In the lower molar region swelling may cause difficulty in swallowing.

**Lymphadenitis**

When an acute infection is present the related lymph nodes are likely to be affected and this results from other conditions as well as acute periapical disease. As a rule the submandibular lymph glands are affected, the area becoming swollen, and the lymph glands are tender on palpation.

**Drainage of pus**

In considering the direction taken by pus it is important to realise that the ability of pus to track through the tissues implies some release of pressure because a greater volume of tissue is becoming involved. This means that pain is likely to be less than it would otherwise have been. Moreover, there is also a range from acute conditions to chronic conditions.

Pus may track through the bone in one of several directions before it reaches the soft tissues. The most frequent direction taken is through the outer alveolar bone, and pain ceases as this is penetrated, pus gathering as a submucosal abscess, the classical gumboil, which is not painful (Fig. 12.1) — see below. The wall of this abscess breaks down so that pus is discharged into the mouth and any lingering mild pain ceases altogether. There is thus a track from the periapical abscess through the bone to the surface of the oral mucosa — a pathological sinus or fistula. The sinus frequently closes and pain can recur if pressure builds up, but not to any intense level because before this can happen the sinus opens again, discharging pus and thus relieving any pressure (Fig. 12.2). Pressure on the area around the sinus at this stage usually causes a small quantity of pus to be discharged. At other times there is no pus but there is a noticeable epithelial nodule which develops around the sinus in long standing cases, and this may be a valuable clue in diagnosing the cause of a vague pain. If any doubt persists a probe can be eased into the sinus (Fig. 12.3) and this action is only slightly painful or not painful at all.

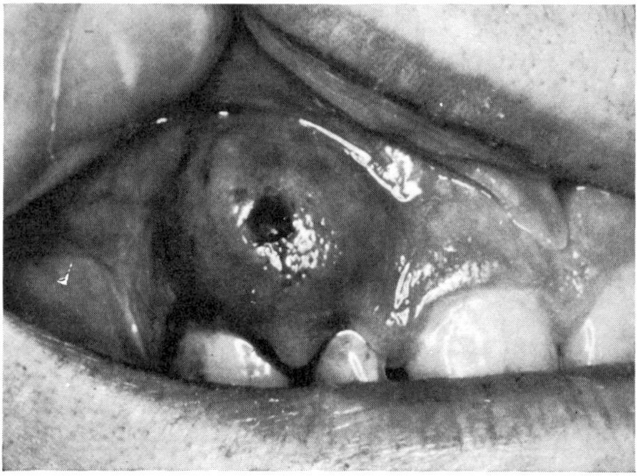

**Fig. 12.1.** Submucosal abscess (gumboil) associated with the right upper lateral incisor.

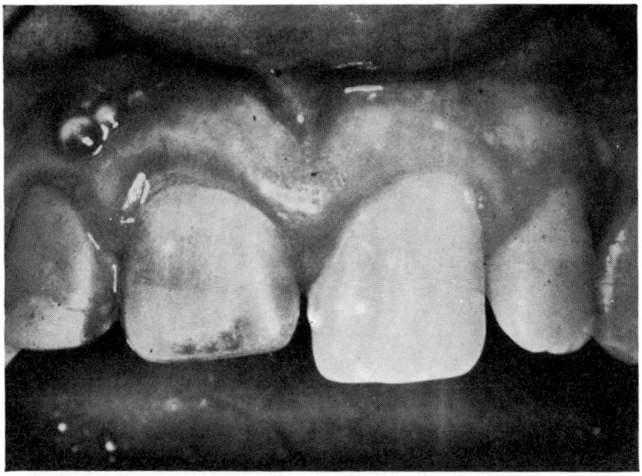

**Fig. 12.2.** Orifice of a pathological sinus leading from the periapical area of the right upper lateral incisor.

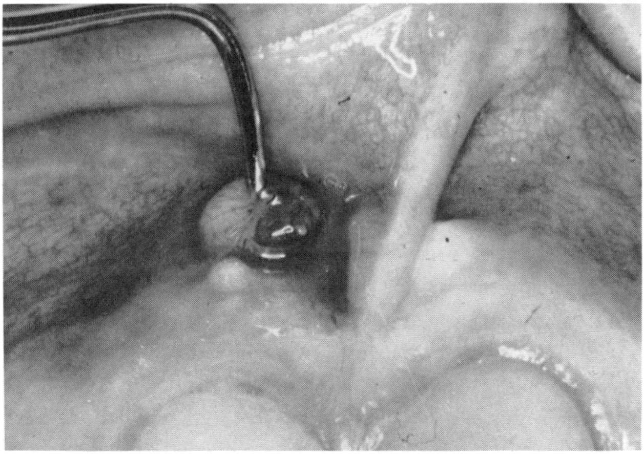

**Fig. 12.3.** Probe in sinus.

A periapical abscess associated with a deciduous tooth is less painful than a similar abscess on a permanent tooth because the affected area is nearer to the surface; the thinner alveolar bone is more readily penetrated, so drainage occurs earlier and the condition becomes chronic. The submucosal abscess that results may be found incidentally during a routine inspection.

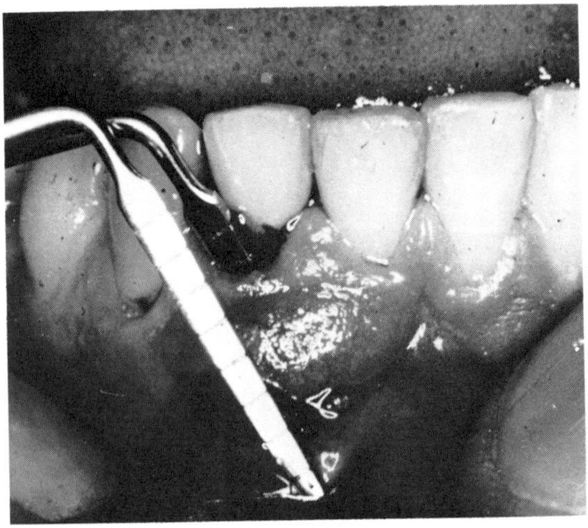

**Fig. 12.4.** Drainage along the periodontal membrane. A periodontal measuring probe has been placed on the outer surface of the gingiva as well as in the drainage track to show the depth.

There may also be drainage along the periodontal membrane to the gingival margin (Fig. 12.4). When pus escapes in this way the appearance may resemble that of a lateral periodontal abscess (parodontal abscess) and this may not matter if the tooth is to be extracted, but differential diagnosis must be made if the tooth is to be treated conservatively since the treatment is different for each case.

Sometimes pus escapes into the nose or the maxillary sinus and is not noticed, although pain ceases. It follows that when pain ceases abruptly without obvious drainage these two escape routes should be considered. Subsequent inflammation of the maxillary sinus may supervene and cause further pain.

Pus from an acute apical abscess associated with an upper tooth, especially a lateral incisor, may drain towards the palate, and possibly along the periodontal membrane at the same time (Fig. 12.5). Sometimes it tracks along the hard palate to form a submucosal abscess more posteriorly than would usually be expected. At other times pus is contained by the soft tissues and does not evacuate naturally so that pain continues and the abscess becomes larger (Fig. 12.6).

Pus may also track to the face, infratemporal fossa, pterygomandibular space, the side of the pharynx and the retropharyngeal space. It may even extend to the mediastinum causing pneu-

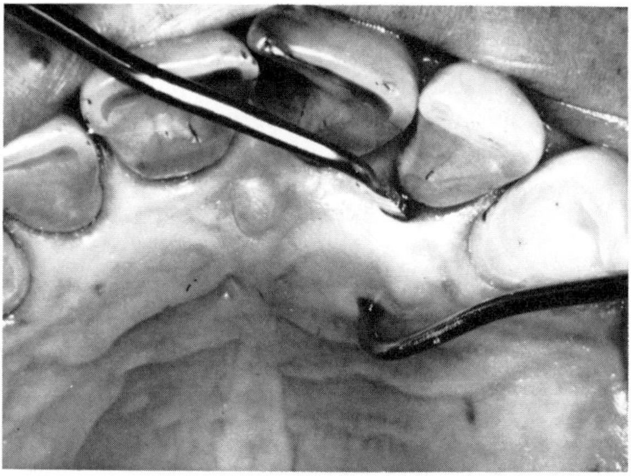

**Fig. 12.5.** Drainage through the palate and the lingual side of the periodontal membrane.

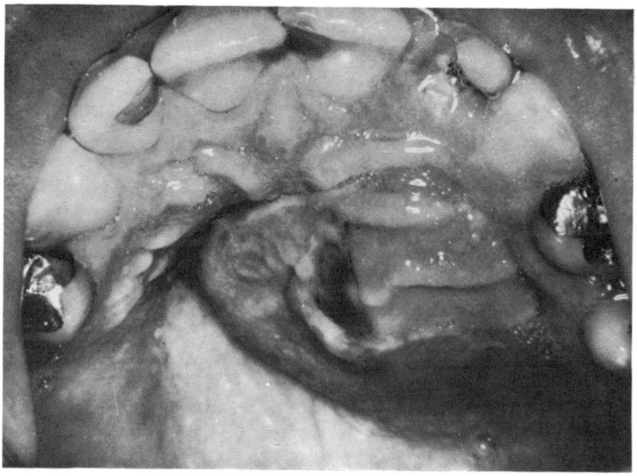

**Fig. 12.6.** Large palatal abscess derived from a periapical abscess over the upper left lateral incisor.

mothorax and death (Hendler and Quinn, 1978). Death may also occur from cavernous sinus thrombosis, and a cerebral abscess is occasionally reported (Hollin, Hayashi and Gross, 1967; Henig et al, 1978).

## Treatment of acute periapical periodontitis

In simple cases the best treatment is root canal therapy. This eliminates the remnants of diseased pulp and provides a drainage channel for inflammatory exudate. Local anaesthesia may be used and this stops the pain in the first instance which helps the patient to relax and often makes the dentist feel happier too. However, it is considered desirable to avoid injecting into diseased areas if possible and it is not essential to use a local anaesthetic, especially with sensible cooperative patients. This is because the pulp is dead so the dentine is no longer innervated and can be drilled with no pain from this source. However, application of pressure when drilling is likely to be painful, especially when first applied because of the hyperalgesic periodontal tissues, so the drill is applied carefully with light pressure and *maintained steadily*; not putting the drill on and off. Also a diamond bur is less likely to jar than a tungsten carbide bur. Obviously, this requires the high speed water cooled turbine; the slower engines are not recommended. Working without a local anaesthetic in this way provides a dramatic aspect of dentistry because once the drainage is established the severe pain is relieved in just 2 or 3 minutes and the patient visibly relaxes, although a milder background pain may continue for some time.

When working on such a tooth, endodontic instruments must be eased into the root canal because if one is pushed in too quickly it acts as a plunger, forcing fluid through the apical foramen onto the damaged and sensitive tissues. Moreover, the instruments must not be pushed through the apical foramen for this would add trauma, perhaps chemicals and even additional microorganisms to the already damaged zone. However, there is one situation where the endodontic instrument may be pushed through the foramen and that is to secure drainage if this has not been obtained already. Having secured drainage the canal may be left as it is or it may be widened, but in either case it must be left open for the first few days to maintain drainage.

It is also desirable to relieve the incisal or occlusal surface so that the tooth no longer occludes with the opposing teeth. If this is not done normal occlusal stimuli will cause pain by pressure on the still-hyperalgesic periapical tissues. Since there is likely to be some residual pain analgesics are prescribed, the first choice being soluble aspirin 500 mg 1 or 2 tablets up to 6 times a day, but paracetamol 500 mg 1 or 2 tablets up to 6 times a day is also appropriate, as are various other preparations.

More severe cases will require antibiotic treatment, given systemically, the first choice being penicillin. This has the additional merit of reducing pain by helping to bring the disease under control. In such a case it is desirable to consider the possibility of penicillin resistance, to test the microorganisms and to be prepared to change to another antibiotic. This is even more important in the most severe cases where the disease is spreading and the patient is toxic. Such a case should be hospitalised, and it may be necessary to extract the tooth or teeth involved. Extraction is also appropriate with poor dentitions. After all, extraction gives the best drainage as well as removing most of the diseased tissue.

Throughout the treatment it is important to provide reassurance whenever required e.g. when oedema has spread to the lower eyelid and closed the eye the patient may be frightened and must be told that the eye itself is perfectly alright. This is almost always true but, occasionally, spread of infection to the orbit can protrude the eyeball and this requires immediate attention (Pellegrino, 1980).

## CHRONIC PERIAPICAL PERIODONTITIS

Depending on the amount of natural drainage and the virulence of the micro-organisms concerned a chronic periapical periodontitis may arise. This may also develop from an inadequately treated case or an untreated case which has drained naturally. Radiographic examination reveals periapical rarefaction which is not seen in cases

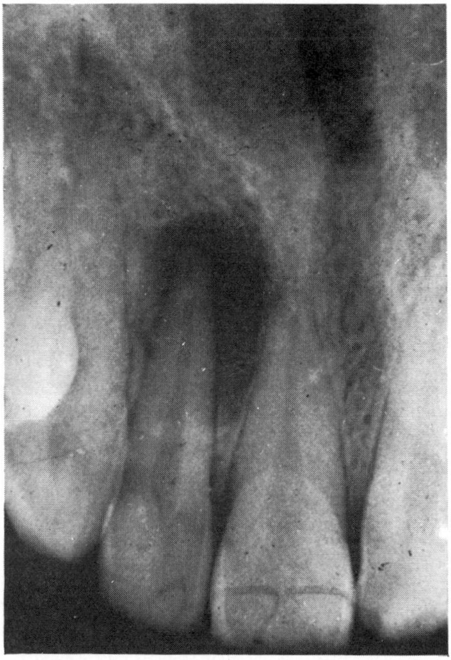

**Fig. 12.7.** Chronic periapical periodontitis.

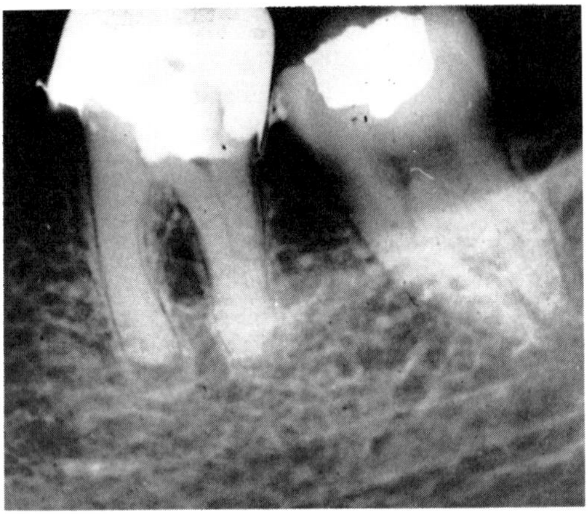

**Fig. 12.8**. A granuloma at the apex of the mesial root of the lower first molar. The area appears more radiolucent than the surrounding bone.

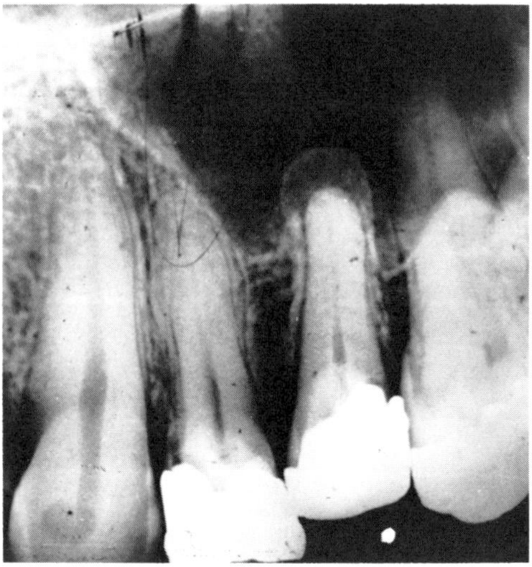

**Fig. 12.9**. A granuloma at the apex of the upper second premolar. The area appears more radio-opaque than the maxillary sinus.

of acute inflammation unless this has occurred as an exacerbation of a chronic condition. There is a wide range in the amount of bone loss and this resorptive process tends to increase, so the amount of bone loss influences treatment planning. The periapical condition may be a chronic periodontitis (Fig. 12.7), a granuloma (Figs. 12.8, 12.9) or a dental cyst (Fig. 12.10), and these are not

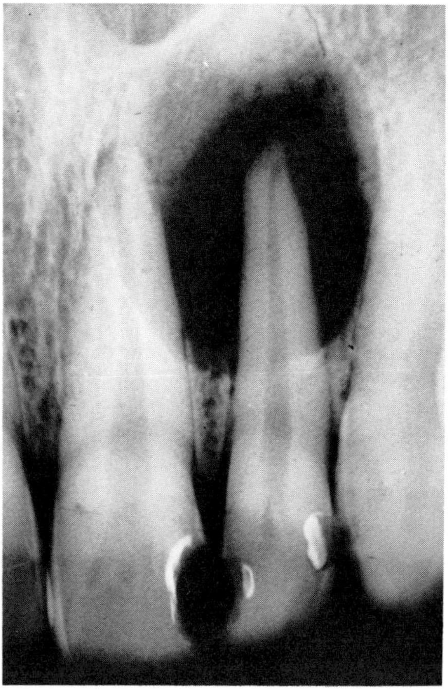

**Fig. 12.10**. Dental cyst.

usually painful although acute inflammation can supervene at almost any time with recurrence of pain. Attention may only be drawn to such lesions when investigating extensively carious, fractured or discoloured crowns.

## ACUTE AND CHRONIC PERIODONTITIS

Both dentists and patients are sometimes tempted to leave quiescent chronic periapical disease untreated, on the 'leave well alone' principle, and this is understandable because treatment produces at least a temporary disturbance which can be sufficient in itself to cause an acute exacerbation. However, periapical disease should be treated because a cyst may form or become larger, or an acute exacerbation may occur at any time, perhaps after many years. When it does occur it is most likely to be when the patient's resistance is lowered by other disease such an influenza, in which circumstances he can least afford to have an acute abscess in bone.

When an acute periapical inflammation is superimposed on previous chronic inflammation the pain and general character of the

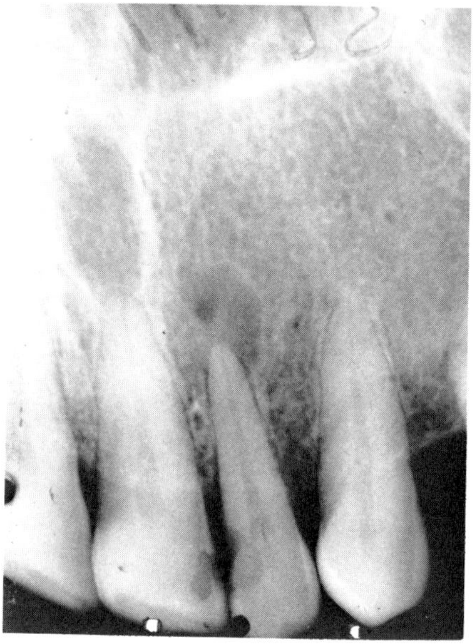

**Fig. 12.11.** Acute exacerbation of chronic periapical periodontitis over the lateral incisor. Within this radiolucent area the darker spot is a perforation through the alveolar plate. The radiolucent area over the central incisor is normal — the incisive fossa.

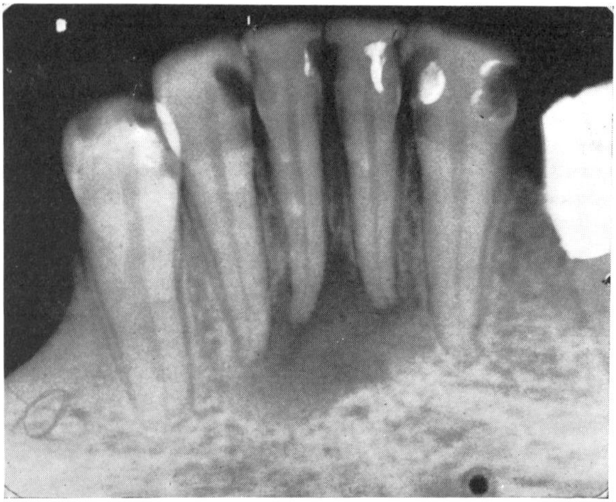

**Fig. 12.12.** Acute exacerbation of a chronic periapical periodontitis of the right central incisor which has spread to involve adjacent teeth. The other teeth gave normal readings on electrical stimulation.

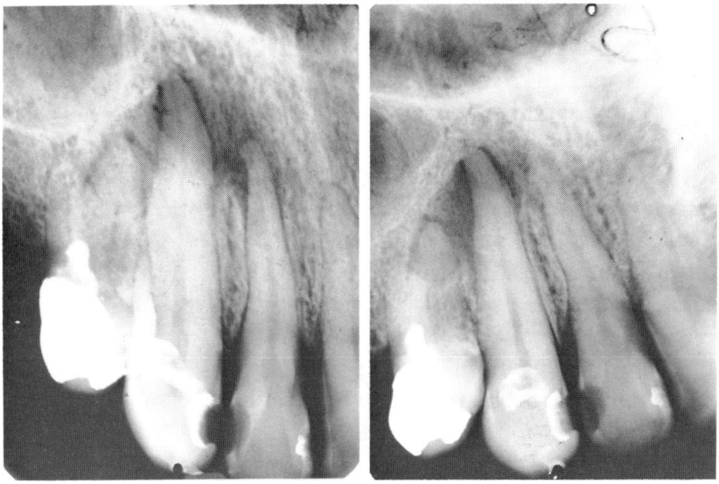

**Fig. 12.13.** Acute exacerbation of a chronic periapical periodontitis. Left, the periapical radiolucence is mainly over the lateral incisor but, right, the premolar was responsible. Both lateral incisor and canine teeth gave normal readings on electrical stimulation, which may seem surprising, but extraction of the premolar was followed by resolution of the bone lesion.

case is the same as in an acute inflammation arising in the first instance, with the exception that a case which was previously chronic will demonstrate periapical rarefaction on radiographic examination (Fig. 12.11). This may have had time to spread beyond the tooth responsible to involve the apices of other teeth, and this could be misleading, but electrical stimulation will reveal which pulps are vital and which are not (Fig. 12.12). This diagnostic method is specially valuable when the rarefaction 'involves the wrong tooth' (Fig. 12.13).

*Treatment*

Any pain that occurs with chronic periapical conditions is usually controlled by analgesics, and is effectively stopped when the case is treated by conventional endodontic and surgical procedures. When treated at the right time treatment may be more conservative than was once thought possible (Mumford and Melville, 1970).

## PAIN DURING ENDODONTIC TREATMENT

During the course of pulp canal treatment pain can occur in several ways. Where a chronic periapical condition exists there is an approximate balance between the disease-producing agents and the body's defensive mechanisms. The object of treatment is to aid defence but sometimes the balance is adversely affected, and merely drilling into the pulp canal can alter the environment, possibly aiding aerobic micro-organisms. Passing reamers or other instruments into the pulp canal can force infected debris through the apical foramen into the periapical tissues and lead, after the lapse of some hours, to acute exacerbation and pain.

Even if the pulp canal has been cleared of debris there may be exudate in the canal which can be forced back into the periapical area by the plunger action of endodontic instruments, and this may cause immediate pain, unless the periapical tissues are too diseased for the fluid pressure to reach nerves. Pain is worst in the presence of acute inflammation where the nerve endings have been sensitised by endogenous algogenic agents.

It is evident that endodontic instruments should be eased into the pulp canal rather than pushed in rapidly, so that the plunger effect can be minimised, but even then there may be pain and it is not easy to know exactly why. However, it is possible that a pulp which is apparently dead is not completely so, and histological examination has revealed vital pulpal remnants in some teeth where the pulp was extensively diseased (Chapter 11). A similar result can arise from incomplete removal of the pulp during pulpectomy, and the author has experienced this on a number of occasions, even after it was thought that the root canal had been meticulously filed and reamed. It is supposed that some living nerve fibres remain but it is difficult to prove this. Perhaps for this reason, pain from this cause is regarded by some clinicians as less likely than pain due to the plunger effect mentioned above (Mullaney, Howell and Petrich, 1970).

With suitable patients pain is not so severe as to prevent a competent operator from passing in a barbed broach and expeditiously removing the remaining tissue, but such treatment is somewhat heroic and student operators must not attempt it.

In the above group of pain cases may be considered a patient to whom the author's attention was directed. A student operator was attempting to prepare a pulp canal on a lady who was screwed up in the dental chair, hands clenched on the knobs of the arm rest, knuckles blanched, gasping for breath, brow wrinkled and tears streaming down her face. On being firmly told to relax she did so and stayed relaxed with the help of a stream of murmured reassurance. There was no sign of pain on passing instruments right up the pulp canal, and the total painful appearance described above was ascribed to a combination of apprehension and histrionics.

Another possible cause of pain during endodontic treatment is passage of instruments through the apical foramen (Fig. 12.14). Such apical perforations can be avoided by using instruments of predetermined length together with stops which prevent the instruments from going too far. However, it is sometimes necessary to deliberately pass instruments through the apical foramen into the periapical tissues to secure drainage of an acute abscess, thereby relieving pain. Rarely, apical perforation damages the inferior dental nerve, resulting in a sense of numbness of the lower lip on the affected side.

It is obviously undesirable to produce a lateral perforation (Fig. 12.15) or perforation of the bifurcation, both of which cause immediate pain from the trauma (if not anaesthetised), as well as later pain from the acute traumatic periodontitis that is likely to follow. It is even worse to follow up with a root filling (Figs. 12.16, 12.17).

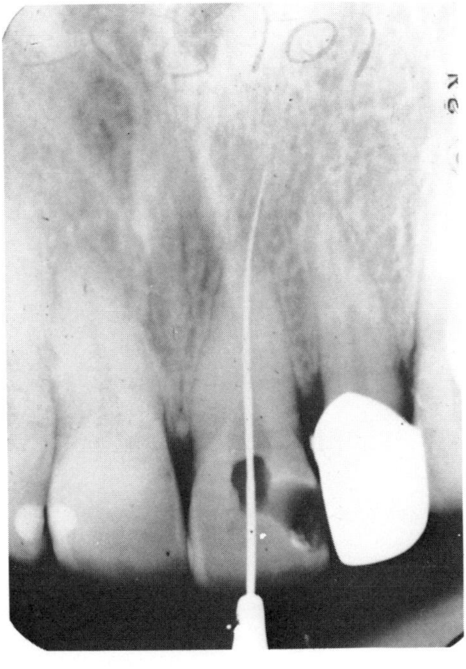

**Fig. 12.14.** Apical perforation by a reamer.

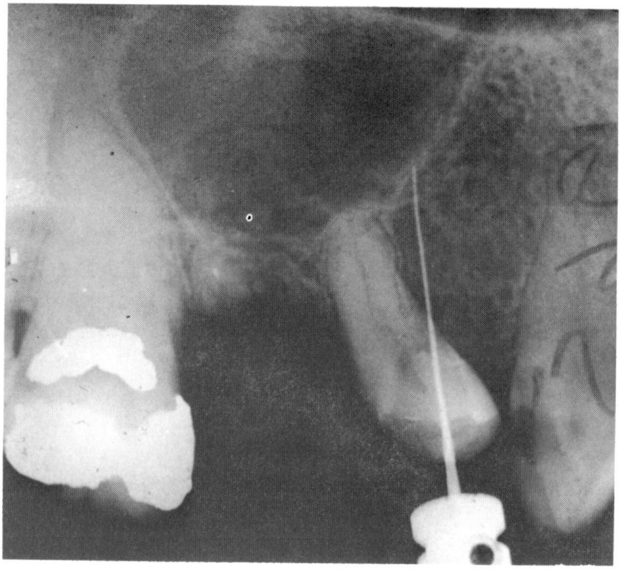

**Fig. 12.15.** Lateral perforation by a reamer.

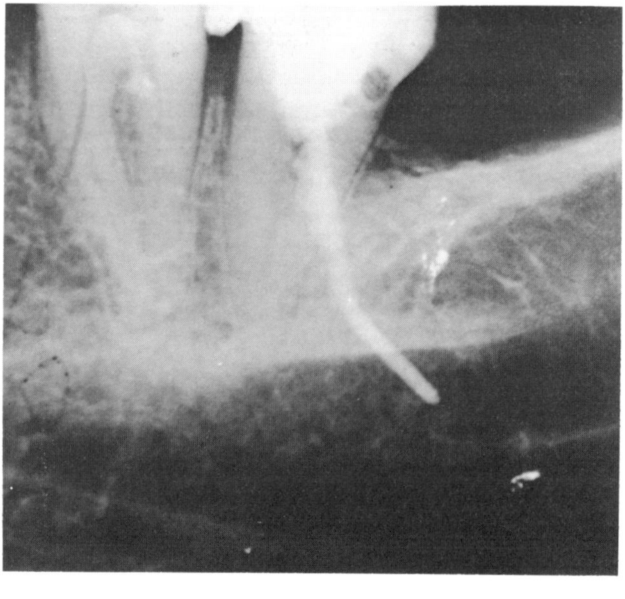

**Fig. 12.16.** A patient complained of pain from a 'needle' sticking in his tongue. The 'needle' was found to be a gutta percha root filling penetrating from the tooth, through the lingual cortical bone of the mandible and out through the mucosa.

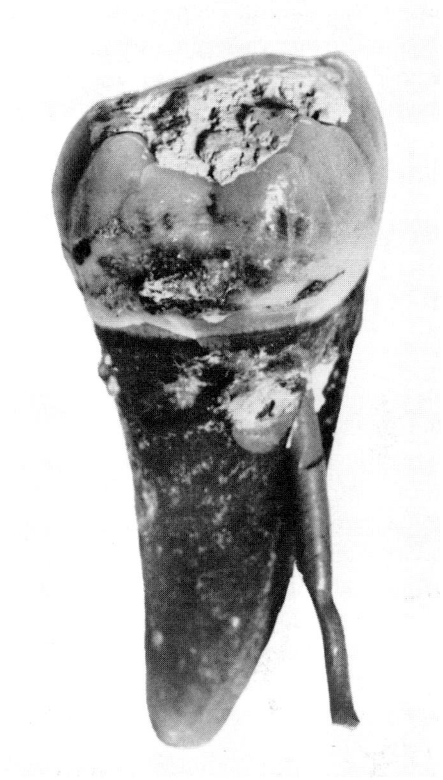

**Fig. 12.17**. The tooth and gutta percha point illustrated in Fig. 12.16.

*Treatment*

Pain due to these problems is best avoided by following the standard procedures of endodontic treatment. If any perforation is obtained laterally or at the bifurcation it should be quickly recognised, not repeated and filled as soon as possible. Apical perforation is avoided by correct setting of instruments and is less troublesome than the other two forms of perforation. If pain occurs when reaming or filing the root canal this may be due to living nerve remnants left in the canal, and a further local anaesthetic is needed to control the pain.

**Chemical periodontitis**

Trauma from endodontic instruments may be associated in some cases with infection and chemical irritation. Chemicals are usually applied on paper points which are manufactured fairly stiff so that they can penetrate deep into the pulp canals. Unfortunately a paper point may penetrate further than intended or be pushed further in attempts to remove it at a later visit, carrying chemicals with it. In some cases, such as where the crown has been lost, a paper point may be too long. To avoid the above problem it should be shortened before insertion. The paper point does not have to be in contact with the canal wall because it is the antiseptic vapour that matters, so some dentists prefer to apply antiseptic on a pledget of cotton wool placed in the pulp chamber.

**Barodontalgia**

This is the phenomenon of pain occurring in a tooth in association with the reduced pressure that might arise in aviation. It is sometimes suggested that air may be trapped beneath a newly placed filling or cement lining and that this could expand as the aircraft ascends, thus causing pain. The author has not knowingly seen such a case, and a more likely explanation is that the reduced pressure produces engorgement of the nose and maxillary sinuses and this gives rise to neural impulses which, considered alone, might be below the level of perception; but if there were some residual mild inflammation in the pulp deep to the new restoration and this was also giving rise to subthreshold neural impulses the two groups of impulses could summate as a result of neural convergence thereby giving rise to pain.

A patient undergoing endodontic treatment had the pulp of an upper premolar removed and the pulp space sealed. There was no pain for several days, but when he made an air journey pain occurred in the tooth which became tender on biting pressure. Pain ceased within 24 hours and there was no further pain for 2 weeks. Pain recurred on the return journey but ceased in a few hours and the tooth remained quiescent for several days after which it was successfully root-filled, with no further pain even during subsequent flights.

Another patient (an airline pilot) had a mild background pain in an upper premolar when he was at ground level. There was no change on flying at 12 000 feet but pain became more severe when flying at 30 000 feet. The tooth was already root filled but it was found to have a lateral perforation. The same explanation is given although the ground level pain was just suprathreshold and the effect of convergence was to 'top it up' to the more severe intensity.

Barodontalgia can also occur in skin divers and cause some anxiety because of the diver's vulnerable situation, but they can be reassured that the pain is not threatening.

It must be supposed that teeth with untreated dead pulps could react to pressure changes in a similar way.

**Chronic gingivitis**

Chronic gingivitis does not give rise to pain, except occasionally when there is transient pain due to trauma from a bone or other hard substance in food. This is perhaps unfortunate because pain might motivate people to seek treatment earlier. A piece of calculus may break away from the tooth and be pushed into the tissues, in which case a gingival abscess can occur. Pain from this does not become severe because it is so near the surface that it drains rapidly, and pain of a mild character may last for only a few hours to a day.

If chronic gingivitis is untreated, inflammation of the periodontal membrane follows and there may be a purulent discharge (hence the old name pyorrhoea) and as long as pus discharges freely the condition does not cause pain, but if drainage is prevented an acute exacerbation occurs.

**Lateral periodontal abscess**

If drainage of pus becomes blocked a lateral periodontal abscess occurs (parodontal abscess), and this can involve the bifurcation.

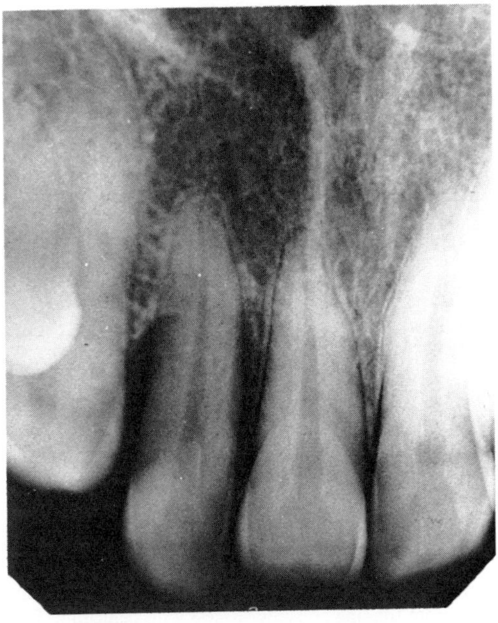

**Fig. 12.18.** Lateral periodontal abscess associated with the upper lateral incisor.

As a rule it is not as painful as an acute periapical abscess, presumably because the pressure cannot build up quite so much, the lateral periodontal abscess being nearer to the surface and thus more likely to drain (Fig. 12.18) but patients have been seen in whom the pain was very severe.

A tooth with a lateral periodontal abscess is usually less sensitive

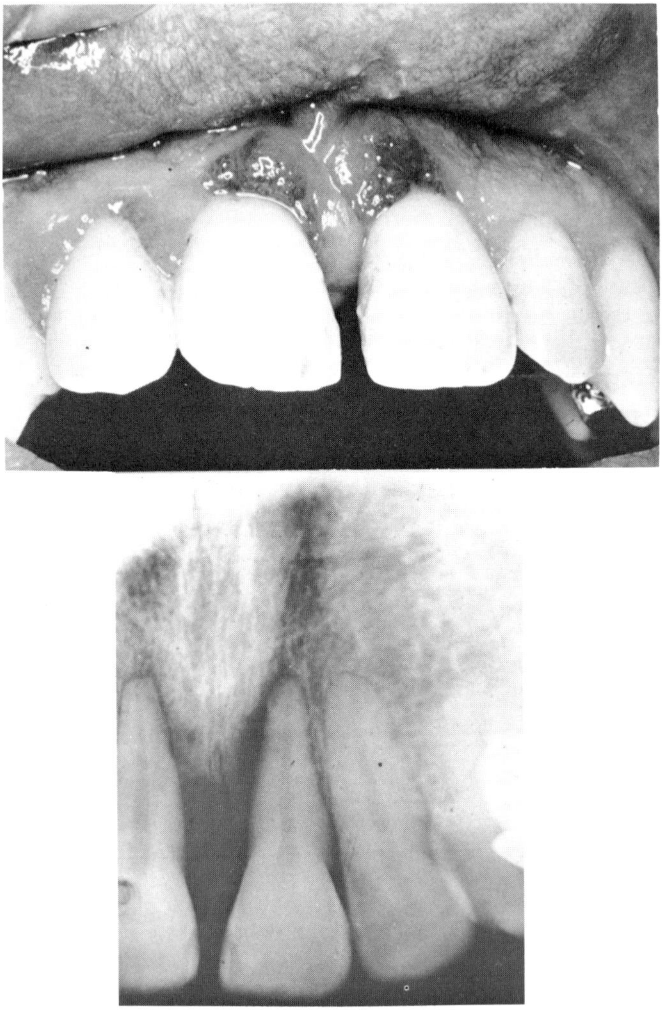

**Fig. 12.19**. Localised gingival disease in an otherwise healthy mouth, associated with the deep lateral periodontal abscess seen on the radiograph. This chronic condition resulted from treating an acute abscess with penicillin. The teeth had vital pulps.

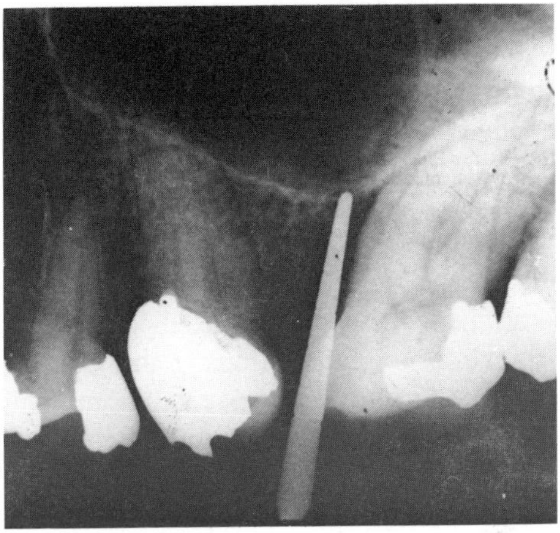

**Fig. 12.20**. Deep lateral periodontal abscess with probe to show depth.

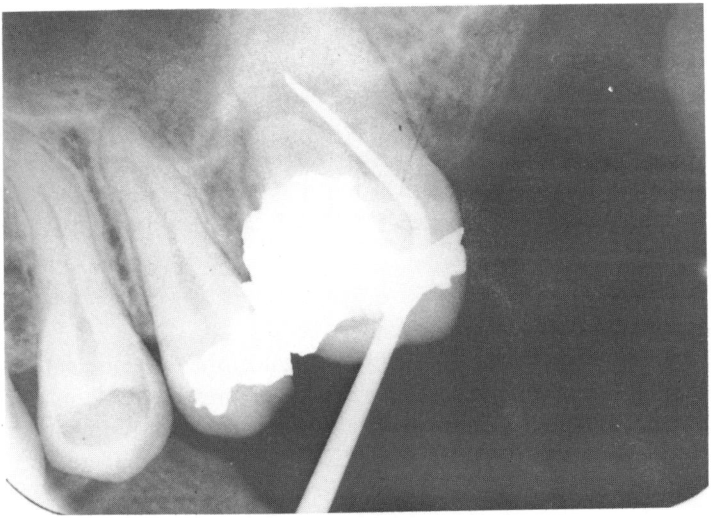

**Fig. 12.21**. Straight probe eased into a sinus to reveal the origin of inflammation at the root trifurcation.

to percussion than one with a periapical abscess, but sometimes it is very sensitive. It is sometimes claimed that the direction of percussion makes a difference in pain experienced, but the author has found little difference in response to directional percussion between cases of lateral and apical periodontal abscesses.

The condition of the gingiva in the rest of the mouth is important, being usually worst in cases of lateral periodontal abscess, but sometimes the condition is quite localised, perhaps because the occlusal arrangement is abnormal, but not necessarily so (Fig. 12.19). Periodontal measuring probes should be used to measure the depths of pockets (Fig. 12.20), or simple probes to see where a sinus originates (Fig. 12.21). Radiographic examination is important as shown by the illustrations to this chapter, and testing the vitality of the pulp may be the most significant factor. Electrical stimuli are better than thermal ones because lack of a response with the latter is not proof that the pulp is dead; also a response can occur even when the pulp is dead if application of heat causes expansion of fluids from the pulp space on to sensitised periodontal pain receptors (Mumford, 1964a, 1967a).

*Treatment*

It is not always easy to make a correct diagnosis especially for posterior teeth which may have both large restorations and lateral periodontal disease. If the tooth is to be extracted the precise diagnosis might not matter, but if the tooth is to be retained it does matter because the treatment is different, lateral periodontal abscess being healed by correct periodontal treatment, whereas periodontal treatment alone will fail if the disease arises from the pulp, possibly via an accessory root canal; in such a case pulp canal treatment is essential.

**Combined lateral and periapical abscesses**

Gingival recession would normally act against the development of a lateral abscess because any pocket is progressively eliminated. However, if one does form the distance to the apex is so much less than usual that the apical area may be involved. It is difficult to be sure whether such an abscess has arisen from the pulp or the gingival margin, but electrical stimulation of the tooth may show that the pulp is vital. However, the pulp could be partly vital in one or two root canals but necrotic in the third. The problem, of course, is academic in the vast majority of cases because such a tooth will be extracted.

Occasionally a similar problem arises when an abscess develops from the pulp via a lateral pulp canal.

## TRAUMATIC PERIODONTITIS

### Accidental trauma

Accidental trauma causes injury of the teeth and periodontal tissues and this is, of course, painful, but when the patient is seen there is less pain than might have been expected. This is partly because nerves may be damaged and have ceased to conduct, and partly because exudate is accommodated in the soft tissue with little increase in pressure. The lips may be swollen and often the patient complains of numbness rather than pain. The gingiva may also be swollen, torn and bleeding.

Teeth may be lost and fluids can escape from the sockets. If not lost, the teeth may be dislocated and in the abnormal position are subject to premature contact with opposing teeth. This is painful and extraction or repositioning is necessary with appropriate splinting. In some cases occlusal or incisal grinding is helpful in preventing premature contact and thus reducing pain.

Teeth may be fractured in various positions as described in earlier chapters. If fractured within the bone the two parts may be separated so that fluids are accommodated in the fracture zone and

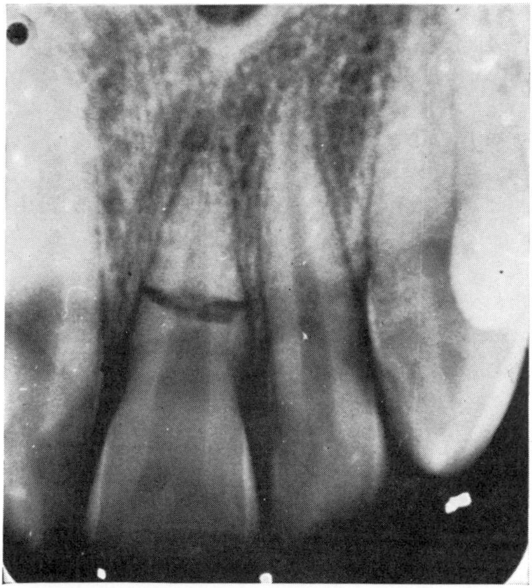

**Fig. 12.22.** Fractured incisor in a boy of 14 years. It was not treated but the pulp was still vital and the colour normal 4 years later.

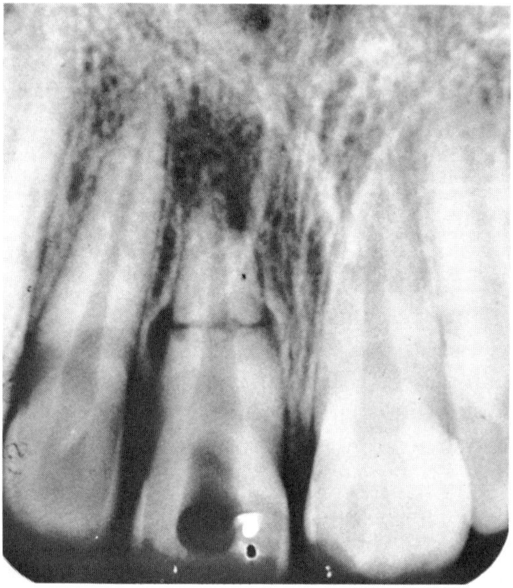

**Fig. 12.23.** Following a root fracture there has been lateral inflammation in the periodontal tissues as well as apical resorption.

the periodontal membrane. Pain is then less than might be expected and the condition sometimes heals without treatment (Fig. 12.22). However, infection can occur (Fig. 12.23) perhaps as a result of pulp canal treatment and this leads to pain which is difficult to stop except by extraction or apicectomy. When bone fractures are present it is safer to extract the fractured teeth rather than to attempt conservative treatment.

**New restorations**

A newly placed restoration can cause severe pain if it is not properly contoured and is left 'too high'. A gross fault is so obtrusive that it cannot be tolerated, and the restoration is reduced before the patient leaves the surgery, but smaller faults may not be noticed, especially if there is local anaesthesia present at the time. The fault is noticed at the end of anaesthesia at which stage it is only a pain evoked by the biting stimulus. Continuous pain may not arise for some hours because inflammation of the periodontal membrane takes time to develop.

There are two kinds of pain which tend to occur together, the more significant, diagnostically, being a sharp pain which occurs on biting and lasts about a second. This is well localised to the tooth concerned which is seen to have a newly placed restoration with a high spot clearly indicated by a smooth shining facet. Sometimes there are several facets. After the sharp pain has occurred a few times a diffuse dull ache also develops, indicating that periodontitis is now present. This may continue at a mild or moderate intensity for many minutes to several hours. Superimposed on this is the sharp pain caused by biting on the tooth.

In addition to pain on biting, some patients say that pain occurs spontaneously, and this is the diffuse dull ache. They may also say that there is pain on application of heat and cold, and this might be because hyperaemia in the periodontal membrane has spread to cause pulpal hyperaemia. It can also be because of convergence of neural input along nerve fibres from both periodontal membrane and the pulp; the greater number of impulses from the periodontal membrane requires only a few additional impulses from the pulp to reach the pain perception threshold. However, it should be recognised that a newly restored tooth is sometimes sensitive to thermal change because of removal of dentine or perhaps failure to place an adequate lining.

Another source of confusion arises from the fact that the opposing tooth is also subject to the excessive biting force and may also be painful. This accounts for some patients giving histories which are not always clear — 'at first I thought it was in the upper jaw; then in both'.

In cases of pain due to acute traumatic periodontitis a certain amount of pressure is needed, unlike those due to electrolytic activity between dissimilar metal fillings; the latter also occur with newly placed restorations but mere contact is sufficient to allow the electrical stimulus to pass, no pressure being needed (Chapter 9).

In addition to this localised pain a 'high' restoration can cause painful dysfunction of the masticatory system (Chapter 14). Such restorations may be of amalgam, gold or other material, and the problem can also occur on placing a partial denture.

*Treatment*

Removing a small amount of metal at and about the facet avoids occlusal contact and this prevents pain on biting, but if periodontitis has developed the dull ache might not cease immediately since the inflammation may require a day or so to resolve. In some cases the condition eases of its own accord, the facets forming into the correct occlusal relationship so that pain ceases.

## Operative procedures

Pain associated with endodontic instrumentation has been described in an earlier section and this can be severe because of the enclosed state of the affected tissues. In comparison, peripheral damage is less painful but care is nevertheless needed in using burs, chisels, bands or other instruments. Although patients seem to accept this degree of postoperative pain without complaint such damage is easily avoided by careful operating and a little forethought.

Periodontal surgery may lead to pain in several ways. After gingivectomy the teeth are no longer as well insulated against thermal change, the cervical dentine being more exposed to stimuli, and this may allow pain which is severe (Fig. 12, 24). Such pain has been known to last for half an hour after imbibing hot liquids, apparently indicating pulpitis, but that would be an incorrect diagnosis.

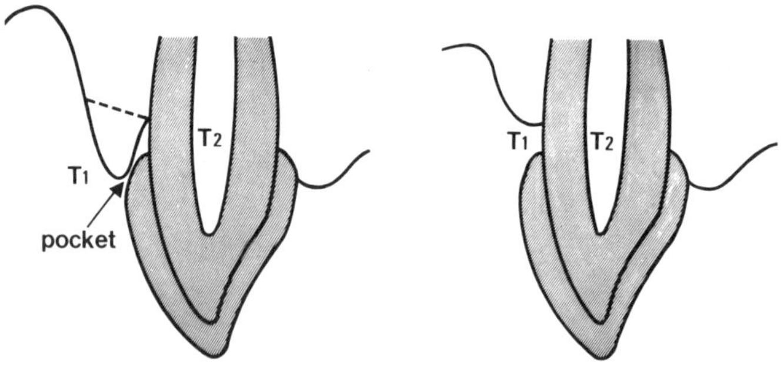


**Fig. 12.24.** *Left.* Before gingivectomy the gingiva gives some protection against thermal change; *Right.* After gingivectomy this protection is lost and there may be considerable pain.

When recontouring the gingiva and bone (gingivoplasty and osteoplasty) there is a risk of the cutting instruments removing part of the tooth surface. Though such damage is small it can lead to considerable pain as described in Chapters 7 and 9.

## Chronic traumatic periodontitis

Though there may not be any pain, unsatisfactory occlusal relationships may give rise to periapical changes as well as to damage nearer the gingival margin, and may cause resorption of the periapical tissues. When this occurs it is important to have proper information about the condition of the pulp because the radiographic appearance is similar to chronic periapical periodontitis aris-

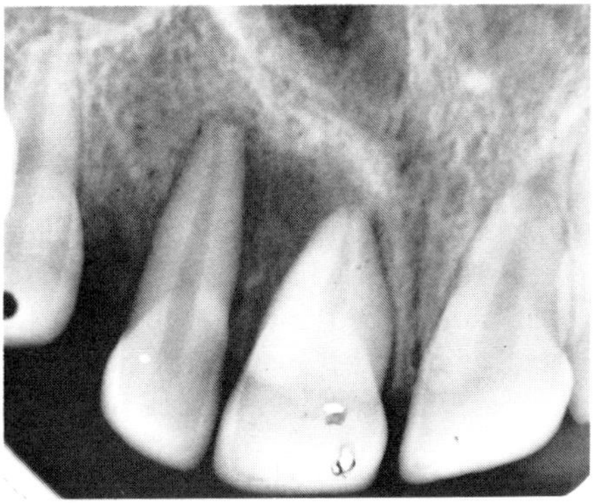

**Fig. 12.25**. Loss of bone following orthodontic movement of upper incisors. Both pulps were found to be vital on electrical stimulation.

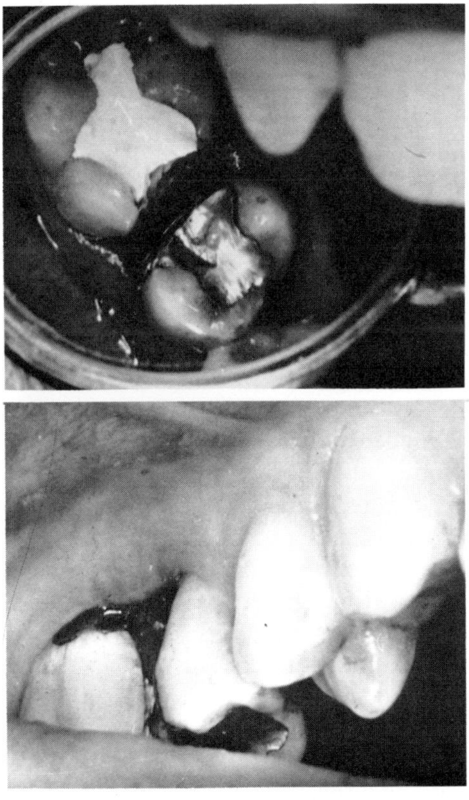

**Fig. 12.26**. Interproximal damage caused by food packing.

ing after pulp death. In the case of occlusal trauma electrical stimulation of the pulp produces a response from the patient. Conditions of this nature have also been seen following orthodontic treatment (Fig. 12.25).

Interdental spaces which are present all the time or which occur by plunger cusp action lead to periodontal damage by food being jammed into the space and held there. This causes a mild continuous pain which is described as irritating rather than pain; interdental stimulators remove the food and the sense of irritation. Sometimes a small 'socket' may develop as a result of chronic irritation but even this is not painful except as just described (Fig. 12.26).

*Treatment*

In cases of occlusal trauma the intolerable occlusal forces must be removed and the tissues rested.

Damaged interdental spaces are treated by periodontal procedures including recontouring the gingiva and alveolar bone. The teeth are restored, paying special attention to the proximal surfaces so that the contact area is well placed and properly formed.

## PAIN ON PERCUSSION

If a perfectly normal tooth set in a normal periodontium is percussed with too much force there is pain, so proper care is needed when using this diagnostic method. One way of controlling it is by percussing apparently normal teeth before the suspected tooth, after which the patient indicates which tooth was associated with the greatest intensity of sensation. In many cases the patient's reaction to percussing the suspected tooth is only too obvious, and further examination is hindered while the patient exhibits the various features of a person in severe pain — groaning or other vocalisation, muscular activity extending perhaps all over the body so that he may become rigid in the chair, and nursing the affected side of his face. It must be stressed that only a light tap should be used at first, and increased if necessary. It is also a good idea to disguise which tooth is being percussed, especially for patients who may not be giving accurate information for any reason.

There can be no doubt that acute periapical periodontitis is associated with pain on percussion. However, it has already been explained how percussing a loose restoration can force fluid through dentine and thereby cause pain, perhaps even with an underlying pulp which is normal (Chapter 9), and such a possibility

**Table 12.1** Histological Appearance of the Pulp in Teeth which were Painful on Percussion (after Tyldesley and Mumford, 1970)

| Patient's description of pain | Pain only on percussion | | Pain on percussion and from heat | | Pain on percussion and from cold | | Pain on percussion and from both heat and cold | |
|---|---|---|---|---|---|---|---|---|
| Intermittent mild | Normal pulp | 1 | | | | | Normal pulp | 1 |
| | Acute pulpitis | 1 | | | Acute pulpitis | 1 | | |
| | Chronic pulpitis | 2 | | | Chronic pulpitis | 2 | Chronic pulpitis | 1 |
| | Degeneration | 2 | | | Degeneration | 1 | | |
| | Necrosis | 1 | | | Necrosis | 1 | Necrosis | 1 |
| Intermittent severe | | | | | | | Normal pulp | 2 |
| | | | Localised acute pulpitis | 2 | | | Localised acute pulpitis | 5 |
| | | | Acute pulpitis | 1 | Acute pulpitis | 2 | Acute pulpitis | 4 |
| | Acute with chronic pulpitis | 1 | | | Acute with chronic pulpitis | 2 | Acute with chronic pulpitis | 5 |
| | Chronic pulpitis | 1 | | | Chronic pulpitis | 2 | Chronic pulpitis | 1 |
| | | | | | Necrosis | 1 | Necrosis | 1 |
| Constant mild | Normal pulp | 1 | | | | | | |
| | Localised acute pulpitis | 1 | | | Localised acute pulpitis | 1 | Localised acute pulpitis | 1 |
| | Necrosis | 2 | | | | | | |
| Constant severe | | | | | | | Normal pulp | 1 |
| | | | | | | | Localised acute pulpitis | 3 |
| | Acute pulpitis | 2 | | | | | Acute pulpitis | 9 |
| | | | | | | | Acute with chronic pulpitis | 1 |
| | Chronic pulpitis | 2 | | | | | Chronic pulpitis | 1 |
| | | | Degeneration | 1 | Degeneration | 1 | Degeneration | 1 |
| | Necrosis | 2 | | | | | Necrosis | 1 |

needs to be considered. Even after eliminating this factor pain caused by percussion cannot be regarded in too simple a manner as indicated by Table 12.1, derived from Tyldesley and Mumford (1970). Unfortunately it is usually not possible to obtain a good sample of the periodontal tissues along with extracted teeth. If such a sample had been obtained for each of the teeth in Table 12.1 it is conceivable that everyone might have shown a histological appearance of acute periodontitis. In the circumstances it can only be said that in a number of teeth the histological appearance was such that periodontitis would not have been expected.

Percussion increases the number of neural impulses going to the brain along periodontal nerve fibres. It is important to realise that the effect of these impulses can be enhanced by any increase in neural activity from the pulp such as occurs in acute inflammation even if the latter is only slight. In other words there is convergent input of neural impulses so it is possible to have pain on percussion because of pulpal inflammation without periapical inflammation.

**Localisation of pain due to periodontal disease**

It is said that localisation of pain from the pulp is poor whereas localisation of pain from periodontal disease is good. Experimental subjects certainly find it difficult to localise pulpal pain produced by electrical stimulation (Friend and Glenwright, 1968; Mumford and Newton, 1971), and numerous cases have been seen where pain from periodontal disease does seem to be better localised, but this is not simply an expression of the central nervous system recognising the origin of neural impulses. It is partly also a matter of the person knowing where a stimulus has been applied. In daily life hot and cold stimuli reach several teeth at a time whereas biting and tapping on a tooth are more restricted.

A difference in localisation of pain from the pulp and periapical tissues might depend on several neurological factors. The periodontium has mechanoreceptive fibres which pass to the principal nucleus and nucleus oralis of the trigeminal system. Here there are synapses which offer a high degree of synaptic security, and the secondary neurones carry the information to the ventroposterior nucleus of the thalamus where the fibres are arranged in a somatotopic manner. Tertiary fibres convey the information to the sensory part of the cerebral cortex where there is again somatotopic representation. In other words the system allows recognition of the place of origin of the neuronal information. On the other hand, neural impulses from the pulp go to the spinal nucleus of the trigeminal nerve and thence to the reticular system. Here there is opportunity for the neural impulses to spread more widely in the brain stem so that the person is only able to form a more generalised idea of the place of origin. (Chapter 3).

## ELECTRICAL STIMULATION OF PERIODONTAL TISSUES

Electric currents are passed through human teeth mainly to determine pulp vitality. They have also been used to medicate the periodontal tissues at the apex of a tooth by carrying electrically charged radicles from the pulp chamber through the pulp canal (electrophoresis). They can also be used to measure the electrical resistance of the calcified dental tissues which gives some indication of the depth of caries, the presence of pulp exposures (Mumford, 1956) or the effectiveness of fissure sealants. For these reasons it is of interest to know if pain occurs in the periodontal tissues as a result of these procedures.

In 1917 Crane obtained a response from his patient on passing a current of one milliamp. Leist (1926) produced what he called a 'periosteal reaction' on using currents of 4·5–6·0 milliamps. These are huge currents compared with which pain from pulpal excitation occurs at values a thousand times smaller. At more reasonable current amplitudes, Nünlist (1931) obtained a response at 150 microamps, and Ziskin and Zegarelli (1945) at 70 microamps. The very wide range of current amplitudes is partly an expression of the inadequate electrical control used by earlier investigators. A direct current pulse of precise duration and fixed frequency has been used to stimulate the periodontal and gingival tissues at the gingival crevice (Mumford, 1967b) and the pain perception threshold occurred at currents ranging from 55–150 microamps (46 readings). These values are higher than those obtained when stimulating the pulp, not necessarily because of any difference in sensitivity of neural receptors in the two situations, but because of current density. In the pulp the electric current is largely confined by the calcified dentine, whereas the current reaching the gingiva and periodontal membrane can spread throughout the tissues.

It would be expected that current density would be an important factor at the apex of a tooth. Outside the apex, in the bone, current could spread widely thus producing a low current density, but just as current emerged from the narrow pulp canal current density would be relatively high and might more readily produce nerve excitation. However, numerous teeth with dead pulps have been tested by a method which involves current passing through the periapical tissues (Mumford, 1964b, 1967b) and in no cases did the patient indicate pain even though the current reached 250 microamps in some cases. A more accurate investigation by Cunningham and Mumford (1976) found lower values with a mean pain perception threshold of 135 microamps, the range being 9–250 microamps. The explanation of this is probably that the current is never limited to the pulp canal but spreads through the dentine of the root. The actual current passing through the pulp canal is less than that shown on the meter.

It seems possible that the idea of the patient perceiving pain from the periapical tissues could have arisen from a few cases in which the pulp has been almost completely necrotic whilst still retaining living nerve fibres in the most apical portion of the pulp canal, as described earlier. However, this would occur in few cases (Mullaney, Howell and Petrich, 1970).

## REFERENCES


Crane, A. B. (1917) A call for standardization in root canal treatment. *Dent. Cosm.*, **59**, 777–788.

Cunningham, J. and Mumford, J. M. (1976) Pain perception to electrical stimulation of the periapical tissues in human subjects and the possible influence of disease. *Archs. oral Biol.*, **21**, 95–97.

Friend, L. A. and Glenwright, H. D. (1968) An experimental investigation into the localization of pain from the dental pulp. *Oral Surg.*, **25**, 765–774.

Hendler, B. H. and Quinn, P. D. (1978) Fatal mediastinitis secondary to odontogenic infection, *J. oral Surg.*, 36, 308–310.

Henig, E. F., Derschowitz, T., Shalit, M. and Toledo, E. (1978) Brain abscess following dental infection. *Oral Surg.*, **45**, 955–958.

Hollin, S. A., Hayashi, H. and Gross, S. W. (1967) Intracranial abscesses of odontogenic origin. *Oral Surg.*, **23**, 277–292.

Leist, M. (1926) Über die Vitalität pulpenamputierter Zähne. *Z. für. Stom.*, **24**, 533–541.

Mullaney, T. P., Howell, R. M. and Petrich, J. D. (1970) Resistance of nerve fibres to pulpal necrosis. *Oral Surg.*, **30**, 690–693.

Mumford, J. M. (1956) Relationship between the electrical resistance of human teeth and the presence and extent of dental caries. *Brit. dent. J.*, **100**, 239–244.

Mumford, J. M. (1964a) Evaluation of gutta percha and ethyl chloride in pulp testing. *Brit. dent. J.*, **116**, 338–342.

Mumford, J. M. (1964b) Electric vitality tester; an aid in diagnosis of periapical lesions. *Dent. Radiogr.*, **37**, 75–80.

Mumford, J. M. (1965) Pain perception threshold and adaptation of normal human teeth. *Archs. oral Biol.*, **10**, 957–968.

Mumford, J. M. (1967a) Thermal and electrical stimulation of teeth in the diagnosis of pulpal and periapical disease. *Proc. Roy. Soc. Med.*, **60**, 197–200.

Mumford, J. M. (1967b) Pain perception threshold on stimulating human teeth and the histological condition of the pulp. *Brit. dent. J.*, **123**, 427–433.

Mumford, J. M. and Melville, T. H. (1970) Conservative treatment of periapical lesions. *J. Brit. Endo. Soc.*, **4**, 23–27.

Mumford, J. M. and Newton, A. V. (1971) Convergence in the trigeminal system following stimulation of human teeth. *Archs. oral Biol.*, **16**, 1089–1097.

Nünlist, A. (1931) Bemerkungen zur Vitalitätsprüfung der Pulpa nach Schröder. *Schweiz. Mschr. Zahnheilk.*, **41**, 784–788.

Pellegrino, S. V. (1980) Extension of dental abscess to the orbit. *J. Amer. dent. Ass.*, **100**, 873–875.

Picton, D. C. A. (1969) The effect of external forces on the periodontium. In *Biology of the Periodontium*, ed. Melcher, A. H. and Bowen, W. H., pp. 363–419. London: Academic Press.

Tyldesley, W. R. and Mumford, J. M. (1970) Dental pain and the histological condition of the pulp. *Dent. Practit. dent. Rec.*, **20**, 333–336.

Ziskin, D. E. and Zegarelli, E. C. (1945) The pulp testing problem: the stimulus threshold of the dental pulp and the peridental membrane as indicated by electrical means. *J. Amer. dent. Ass.*, **32**, 1439–1449.

# 13

# Pain due to factors within the bones

## INFLAMMATORY CONDITIONS

Amongst the most frequent and important conditions within the bone which cause pain are the periapical and lateral periodontal abscesses already described. One way in which the periapical abscess develops is by spread through the spaces within the cancellous bone so, in a way, this could already be called osteomyelitis — inflammation of the bone marrow — but a distinction is usually made between the two conditions.

### Osteomyelitis

In osteomyelitis damage becomes so great that the blood supply is cut off, both from the adjacent cancellous bone and from the overlying periosteum. As a result the affected bone undergoes necrosis,

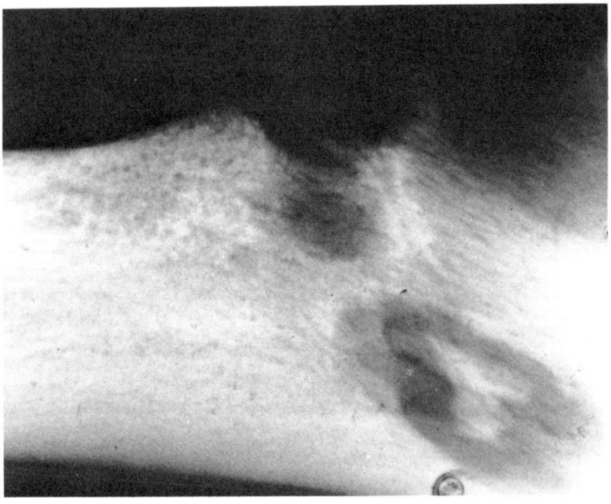

**Fig. 13.1.** Osteomyelitis. There was a hard swelling over the area, together with swelling in both the submandibular and submental areas. The patient had suffered pain for 3 days together with numbness of the left side of the lower lip for 2 days. A sequestrum can be seen in the lower radiolucent area.

and this dead tissue is separated off by osteoclastic resorption which necessarily takes place in the surrounding living bone. Once the dead bone has separated it is called a sequestrum and is eventually shed. Meanwhile, it remains radiopaque (Fig. 13.1).

The disease is serious and there is pyrexia, halitosis and trismus as well as severe pain. The associated teeth are sensitive on percussion and may loosen. The overlying tissues are tender, and nerve involvement may lead to paraesthesia or numbness in the skin area of the terminal fibres. Drainage allows foul smelling pus to escape, possibly under pressure, and antibiotic therapy is essential. Both drainage and antibiotic treatment diminish pain.

## Sinusitis

Inflammation of the nasal sinuses is most likely to occur in association with a common cold and this partly explains the uncomfortable sense of fulness that may be felt in the area in mild or subacute forms. It also partly explains the tendency for more than one sinus to be affected at the same time.

### *Maxillary sinusitis*

Maxillary sinusitis is usually of nasal origin but it can also occur, in about a fifth of cases, from infection of dental origin, especially if roots, fractured during extraction, are accidentally pushed into the sinus. As a part of the acute sinusitis the mucosa over the middle turbinate bone is inflamed and as it swells the ostium of the sinus becomes blocked so that drainage is impaired, pressure in the sinus increases and pain becomes worse. It is aching in character, lasts for several days, and is experienced mainly in the cheek area represented in Fig. 13.2, left. This area is tender, is slightly pinker than

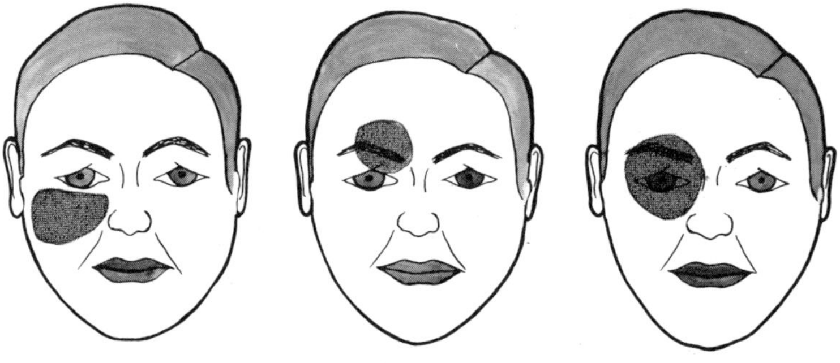

**Fig. 13.2**. Area of pain in maxillary sinusitis (left), frontal sinusitis (middle) and ethmoidal sinusitis (right).

normal and has a slight diffuse swelling (puffiness under the eye). The maxillary cheek teeth are tender on pressure and sensitive to percussion, whilst the gingiva are also tender, such as when the tongue is pressed against them. Some patients can carry on quite well but others feel too sick to work.

The infraorbital nerve can be affected for the patient may complain of a sense of numbness or a bruised feeling in the area of the infraorbital foramen — paraesthesia. There may also be headache, as with disease of the other sinuses.

It has been said that if pain occurs upon jumping and landing on the heels it suggests maxillary sinusitis; this is a reasonable view, but it is only an outlandish way of percussing the teeth, and pain induced in this manner has been noted in patients with simple periapical disease of both upper and lower molars; in other words it only indicates that there is sensitivity of the periapical tissues.

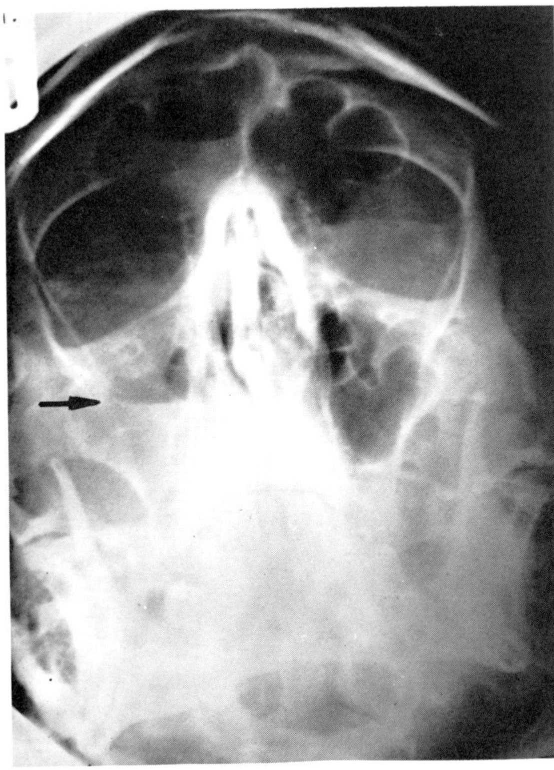

**Fig. 13.3**. Acute maxillary sinusitis. The patient complained of a dull ache on one side, and nasal discharge. There is a fluid level in both the maxillary and frontal sinuses.

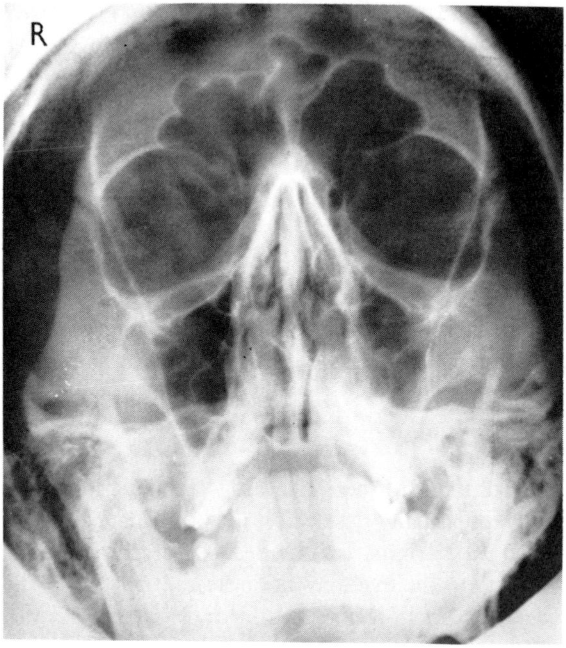


**Fig. 13.4**. Opacity in the left maxillary sinus. There was a background numbness from the area of the infraorbital foramen up into the orbit. Pain started in ⌈5; then to ⌊2; then alternating from ⌈5 to ⌊2. Spontaneous onset, and also with heat. Described as a severe sharp pain fading to a mild, dull ache. ⌈5 was cariously exposed and incidental to the main condition.

Pain gradually diminishes when the patient lies down with the diseased side uppermost (to permit drainage), approximately 30 minutes being needed for relief to occur (Wolff, 1963). There may also be some relief on nose-blowing.

Radiological investigation is important but there is usually no obvious radiographic change in acute sinusitis even when a purulent discharge is present. However, there may be a fluid level in some cases (Fig. 13.3). In other cases there may be a more general opacity which suggests an exacerbation of a pre-existing chronic state (Fig. 13.4). From an investigation of 416 patients Axelsson and Chidekel (1972) found that the amount of pain, headache and degree of olfaction were not obviously related to the extent of radiological change, though purulent or mucous discharge was more frequent when there was less opacity, being present in 83 per cent of such cases.

Pain from the maxillary sinus can occur in the absence of infection if the person is subjected to pressure changes, e.g. a young man complained of pain on skin-diving. In the potentially dangerous situation of being under water it worried him, but he was satisfied with an explanation and reassurance. Such pain ceases when the ostium opens to equalise the pressure on both sides.

*Frontal sinusitis*

The area of pain in frontal sinusitis lies over the sinus as shown in Fig. 13.2, middle, and the patient may complain of a frontal headache. A fluid level may show if radiographic examination is made (Fig. 13.3). If the microorganisms are virulent there is a risk of meningitis or frontal cerebral abscess with nausea, vomiting and possibly confusion from interfering with function of the frontal lobe of the brain.

*Ethmoidal sinusitis*

This is more difficult to recognise because the patient is less able to localise the pain, usually describing it as a headache. The area indicated in Fig. 13.2, right, is intended to be only approximate and the area medial to the eye may be indicated instead, or the patient may locate the pain in the eye. Infection may spread through the lateral wall of the ethmoidal sinus and this may relieve pain by reducing the pressure, but pain may then develop from orbital cellulitis which may produce protrusion of the eyeball and pain on eye movements.

*Sphenoidal sinusitis*

Localisation of this pain is very poor. It may be experienced deep behind the eyes, at the vertex, the occiput, the temple or even in the teeth. On one occasion, whilst an otorhinolaryngologist was performing an operation for pituitary ablation, the patient complained of pain in the teeth as the needle was tapped into the sphenoidal sinus. Unfortunately, the sedated patient was unable to say which teeth.

*Treatment of sinusitis*

In the mild cases of sinusitis associated with a common cold analgesics and reassurance may be sufficient. More severe cases may be advised to rest, and antibiotics can also be prescribed. If even more severe, surgical drainage, rest, analgesics and antibiotics are combined. In the special case when ethmoidal sinusitis spreads to the orbit there may be pressure on the central artery of the retina, threatening blindness, so emergency surgery is needed since antibiotics do not work fast enough.

**Infected cysts**

The most likely cause of pain is of a dental cyst that becomes infected, in which case an acute abscess may develop causing pain as described in Chapter 12. However, a less severe pain may occur occasionally during a period of months or even years, in which case it is usually a dull ache lasting for hours, perhaps all day, followed by apparent remission. But the cyst continues to grow and the patient or the dentist notices a smooth bone 'expansion' which is felt in the buccal sulcus, or perhaps via the skin. There may be paraesthesia in the overlying skin and possibly even anaesthesia.

Sometimes the simple cystic appearance seen on the radiograph is confusing (Fig. 13.5).

Other cysts may become infected and cause pain.

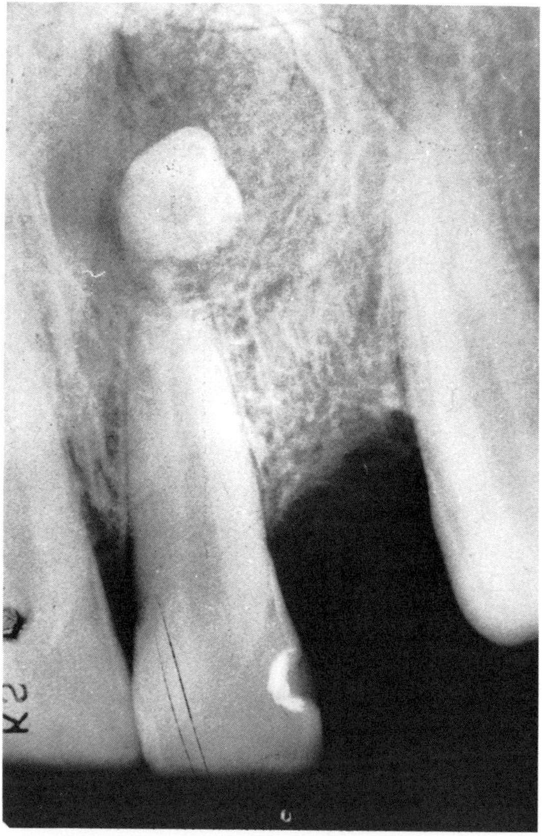

**Fig. 13.5.** Infected dental cyst with a deciduous canine or supernumerary tooth. The complaint was of pain and a small hard swelling lateral to the wing of the nose; there was no pain in any teeth.

**Normal radiolucent areas**

On the radiograph the maxillary sinus or inferior dental canal may be superimposed on teeth and this should not be confusing, but cases such as that shown in Fig. 13.6 might be if attention is drawn to the area by a patient complaining of pain. Loss of the first molar and drift of the second molar has changed the stress pattern, reducing the number of bone trabeculae needed and resulting in the apparent 'disease' illustrated. It was reassuring to determine the pain perception thresholds of the teeth adjacent to the radiolucence and to find that they were within the normal range.

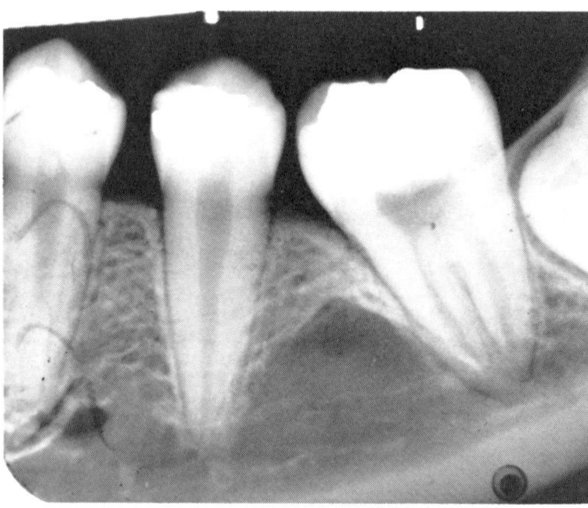

**Fig. 13.6.** The condition is normal (see text).

## PAIN DUE TO TEETHING

That a person is in pain is often recognisable by his outward appearance and behaviours, but mostly the clinician knows about the patient's pain by what he is told. However, babies cannot talk so it is not possible to obtain verbal evidence of the pain or discomfort they suffer due to teething. Teething in babies has been held responsible for numerous conditions including convulsions, bronchitis, fevers and intestinal disturbances, but nowadays this relationship is not accepted. This changing opinion could throw doubt on whether teething in babies is associated with pain, but it is reasonable to suppose that discomfort and pain do occur if only because children and older people certainly suffer discomfort and pain during tooth eruption.

There is also some more direct evidence that pain occurs. Seward (1969) conducted a double blind clinical trial of a teething solution on 291 babies aged 5–31 months, 136 of them being included as a control group. The teething solution, which contained a local anaesthetic agent, was applied by the mother to the baby's gingiva over an erupting tooth, and she estimated its effectiveness in eliminating irritability, crying, etc. A control solution was used but the one containing a local anaesthetic was more effective which suggests, of course, that painful stimulation of nerves had really been present in the affected area.

The possibility of some other disease should also be recognised. A baby who persistently cries and rubs its ear and cheek could be suffering from otitis media.

Even when teeth are erupting normally older children may complain — 'I've got a lump in my mouth which is annoying me; it's like a little mountain. It's like having an itch; you keep wanting to scratch it, not so much because it hurts, but it does hurt if you press hard.'

There may also be some irritation when a deciduous tooth is about to be shed, and this may be associated with pain. However most people deliberately manipulate such teeth with fingers and/or tongue and almost enjoy the mild pain caused (metaesthesia). At such a stage the patient may complain that the tooth feels 'higher' than the other teeth when he closes his mouth.

As the successional teeth erupt, resorption of the deciduous teeth progresses and this does not usually cause pain, but resorption is often greater than the radiographic appearance suggests and infection from the mouth might reach the resorbed area and cause acute inflammation with pain.

In young adults the sensation may also be described as uncomfortable and nagging rather than as painful, but pain frequently occurs when third molars are erupting. Usually it is described as a dull ache which starts of its own accord and lasts for hours. It is of mild or moderate intensity at a steady level and is not clearly localised but more diffuse in the affected area. Radiographic examination shows the erupting teeth with no obvious abnormality.

**Buried roots**

Buried roots do not necessarily cause pain but are likely to do so if associated with infection. Also, as they try to erupt they press on the gingiva from within; additional pressure during eating then causes pain. Most cases are revealed on radiological examination and expeditiously dealt with, but some are missed for various reasons and can contribute to causing pain. This may be sufficiently severe for idiopathic trigeminal neuralgia to be suspected (Chapter 16), or the pain may be more persistent and vague so that it is thought of as atypical facial pain (Chapter 19). When such problems arise there must be a careful search for buried roots: if found they are removed.

**Impacted teeth**

The pain from an impacted tooth is a diffuse dull ache, spreading beyond the area of the tooth responsible, and lasting for days (unless controlled by analgesics). It occurs spontaneously and also on biting. It is not affected by thermal stimuli but there is pain on percussing the adjacent tooth against which it is impacted (Figs. 13.7, 13.8). It can be confused with pain resulting from the masticatory dysfunction syndrome (Chapter 14), especially since the site of the ache depends partly on the tooth which is impacted (Fig. 13.9). Pain stops when the pressure is relieved by extracting the impacted tooth itself or the tooth against which it is impacted.

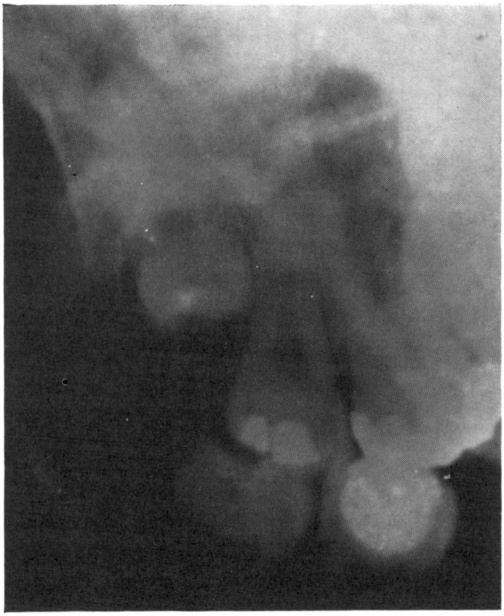

**Fig. 13.7**. The patient, aged 22 years, complained of 3 days of dull diffuse pain located mainly in the ear but also in the neck (Fig. 13.9, left).

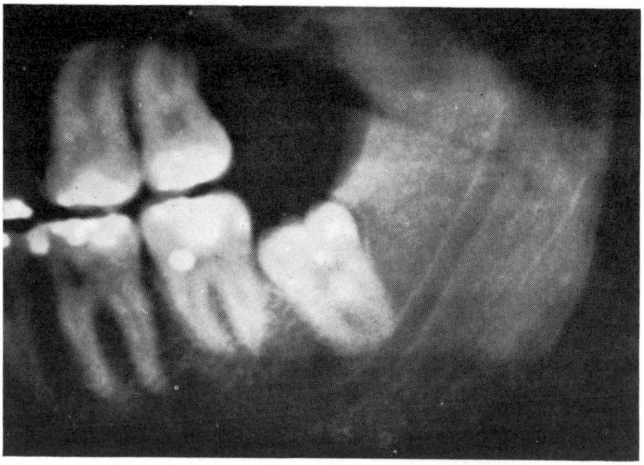

**Fig. 13.8**. Impacted third molar. This is part of a pantomograph, and the image is less sharply defined than in the usual lateral oblique radiograph.

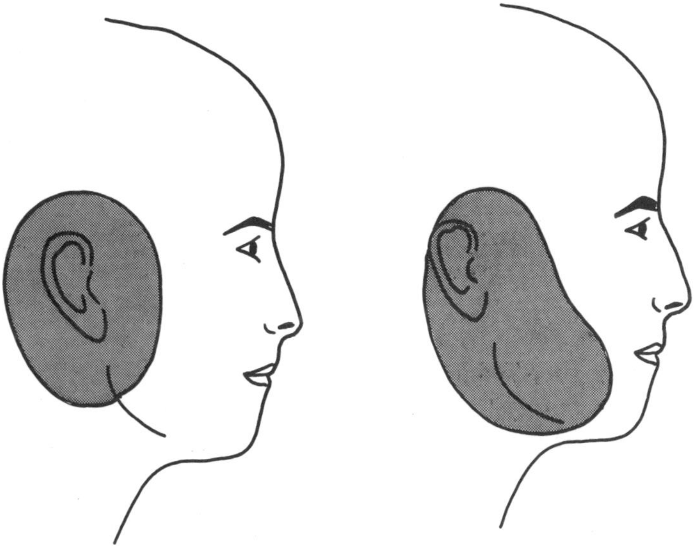

**Fig. 13.9**. Distribution of pain in patients suffering from impacted third molars. Left, area involved from an upper molar. Right, area involved from a lower molar.

Pressure from the crown of the impacted tooth can cause resorption of the adjacent roots and the pulp may be exposed with ensuing pain (Fig. 13.10).

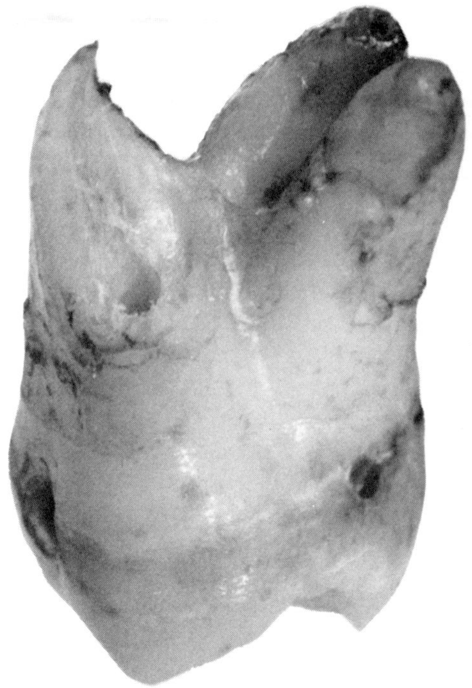

**Fig. 13.10**. The distal aspect of the buccal root has been resorbed and the pulp exposed by pressure from the impacted tooth.

## Cyst of eruption

When an erupting tooth approaches the mucosal surface it is sometimes observed that there is a cyst over it which is usually a greyish blue colour. It is sore when bitten on, or if it becomes infected, but pain is seldom severe because proximity to the surface allows drainage to occur, and a sinus may be found (Fig. 13.11).

## Pericoronitis

As the tooth continues to erupt the overlying gingiva may recede rapidly but in some cases it remains over the erupting tooth where it is bitten, resulting in pain, and may also become infected. The ensuing pericoronitis can cause pain of various intensities depending upon the severity of the infection, the extent of drainage and the frequency with which the area is traumatised.

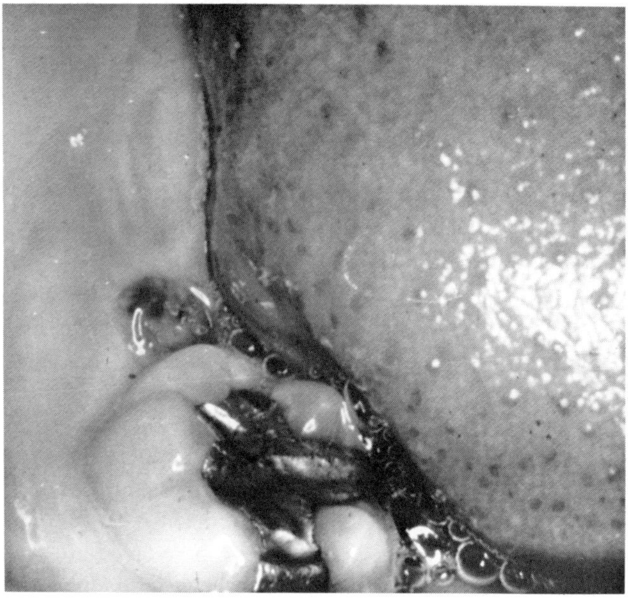

**Fig. 13.11**. Sinus over an unerupted lower second molar.

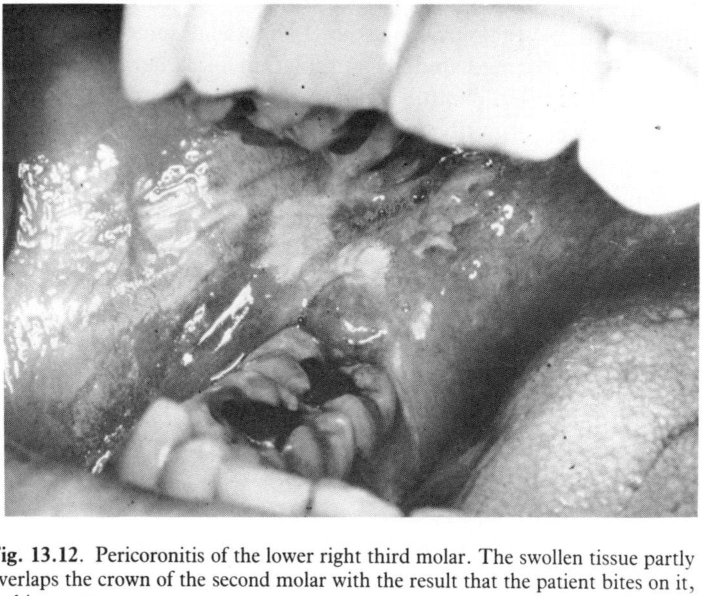

**Fig. 13.12**. Pericoronitis of the lower right third molar. The swollen tissue partly overlaps the crown of the second molar with the result that the patient bites on it, making matters worse.

Usually there is a dull ache, aggravated when the patient bites on the area. This is likely to be worse at the first meal of the day, presumably because pressure rises as a result of inflammatory fluids accumulating overnight.

In chronic cases pain is less severe and may only be present intermittenly.

In acute cases pain is much more severe and is exacerbated not only by biting on the area but even by the arterial pulse; in other words there may be throbbing pain. In such a case there is swelling, which may be obvious extraorally, and which causes both trismus and difficulty in swallowing. The mucosa in the area is reddened and possibly ulcerated. It is also swollen and so may show indentations produced by the cusps of the opposing tooth. In some cases pus may be seen exuding from beneath the flap, or can be caused to do so by gentle finger pressure. In such a severe case the patient really looks a sick person, has pyrexia and cervical lymphadenitis.

In young adults the most likely teeth to be ivolved are the third molars (Fig. 13.12) whereas, in children, the first molars are the teeth affected.

**Treatment of pain due to teething**

In normal teething babies seem to get some help from biting on hard objects such as teething rings or special biscuits. The effect might be the psychological one of giving them something to do, and/or it may be mediated by stimulation of larger nerve fibres which modulate the 'painful' neural input (Chapter 4). A teething ointment can be prescribed containing a local anaesthetic, and the mother rubs this on the gum in the affected area. It contains 7·3 g benzocaine, 1·8 g chlorbutol, 3·0 g tragacanth, 10·0 ml glycerin, peppermint oil q.s., in distilled water to make 100 ml (Birch, 1980). It may be necessary to reassure the mother and it is a good idea to deprecate the use of sugary syrups in pacifiers because of the risk of gross dental caries. 'Tender loving care' should be encouraged.

Older children can manage what is usually a small amount of pain but children's size aspirin may be taken. Removal of teeth about to be shed or which should be shed helps. Tender loving care also helps. Young adults may be satisfied with an explanation but they can also take aspirin as needed. The most likely teeth to be affected are the third molars and these 'wisdom teeth' may be removed if this is considered appropriate.

Pericoronitis is treated by irrigation with mild antiseptics, but if the opposing tooth is traumatising the infected area it is reduced by occlusal grinding or even extracted. If the unerupted tooth has to be removed the pericoronitis must be reduced first. Systemic antibiotics may be needed to achieve this. As an alternative to antibiotics metranidazole may be considered; the dose is 200 mg four times a day for five days (McGowan, Murphy and Sheiham, 1977). In severe cases the patient may be toxic and hospitalisation is indicated.

## PAIN DUE TO TRAUMA

### Accident trauma

Fractures of the facial bones are associated with pain in various ways. In addition to pain at the time of injury there may be pain associated with the fracture. However, both the incidence and intensity of pain are less than might have been expected. One reason is that there are so many spaces in and about the facial bones that fluids can be accommodated without build up of pressure. Another reason is lack of movement between the fractured parts. If there is movement then pain is more likely to be experienced especially if a nerve runs through the fracture. In such a case the patient avoids unnecessary movement, thus keeping pain to a minimum. However, the nerve may be damaged, with the result that paraesthesia or anaesthesia occur in the area supplied by the nerve terminals.

In the surrounding areas inflammation of the periosteum leaves it tender on pressure. There may also be pain associated with damage of the temporomandibular joint, and there is a risk of osteomyelitis with its accompanying pain.

In these cases of accidental trauma deranged occlusion, asymmetry, and unnatural mobility are important features, and radiographic examination is essential.

*Treatment*

This falls in the realm of maxillofacial surgery. The patient needs reassurance about appearance and recovery of normal sensation.

### Operating trauma

Pain due to root perforation during endodontic treatment has been described in Chapter 12.

Some trauma is inevitable during routine extractions and may be greater when surgical removal is necessary. Unintended damage to adjacent teeth may occur (Figs. 13.13, 13.14) and result in pain the cause of which may become apparent only after further extraction.

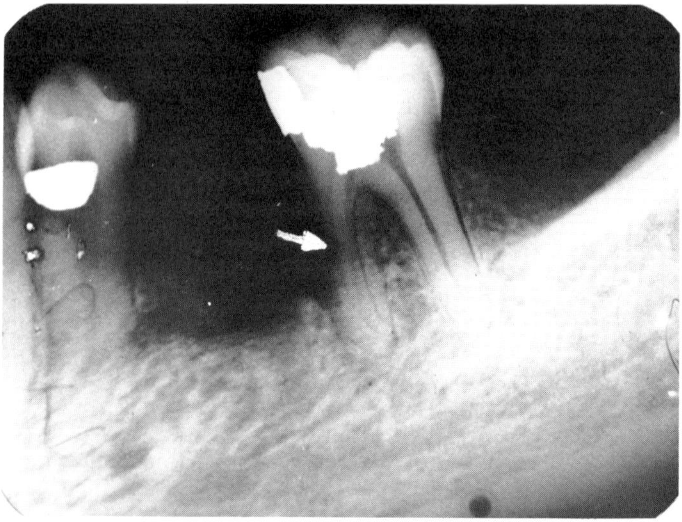

**Fig. 13.13**. Operating trauma to the mesial root of the lower first molar. There is a notch in the middle third of the mesial surface.

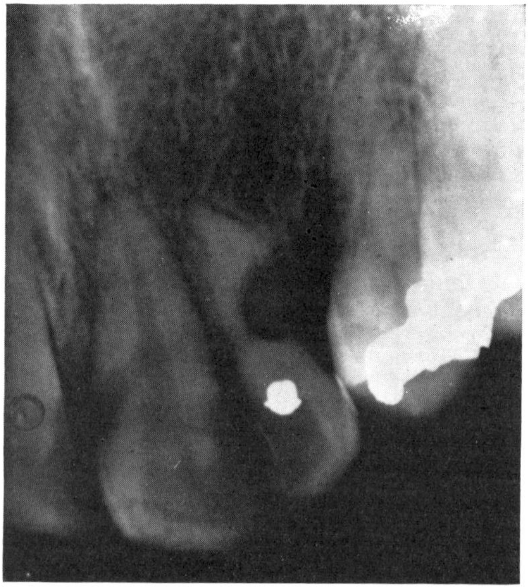

**Fig. 13.14**. The left upper canine tooth was extracted, partly to protect the lateral incisor, the apex of which was becoming resorbed. After the operation thermal stimuli caused a sharp pain in the lateral incisor which was found to have been damaged during the operation.

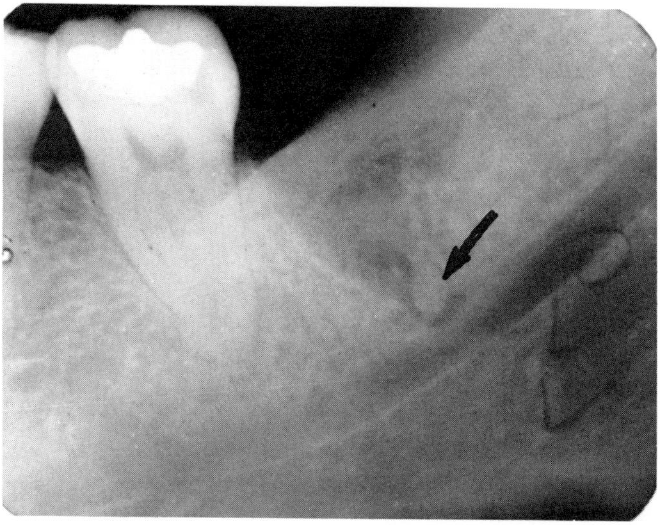

**Fig. 13.15.** Retained root fragment with sclerosing osteitis. The patient suffered pain and also paraesthesia of the left side of the lower lip. There was also paraesthesia of the overlying skin including the adjacent part of the neck.

Damage to the floor of the maxillary sinus may occur. Apices may be left during extractions or even after an apicectomy operation, and lead to a continuation of inflammatory process, though pain need not necessarily follow if the inflammation is of the chronic variety. Most roots left after an operation are obvious radiographically but some fragments are not (Fig. 13.15).

**Dry socket**

The condition is a localised osteitis which arises because the blood clot breaks down following extraction, possibly because of too vigorous rinsing or of the patient sucking on the wound. Larger than usual doses of local anaesthetic with vasoconstrictor may also be a factor in reducing the volume of clot originally formed. Pain presumably occurs because nerve endings have been sensitised by endogenous algogenic agents such as 5-hydroxytryptamine (Chapter 10). Birn (1972) has shown that kinins are present in concentrations sufficient to explain the severe pain.

The pain of dry socket characteristically occurs 2 days after a tooth has been extracted since this time is required for the blood clot to break down. The patient reports some time after this so pain is described as lasting for hours or days. It is a moderate to severe,

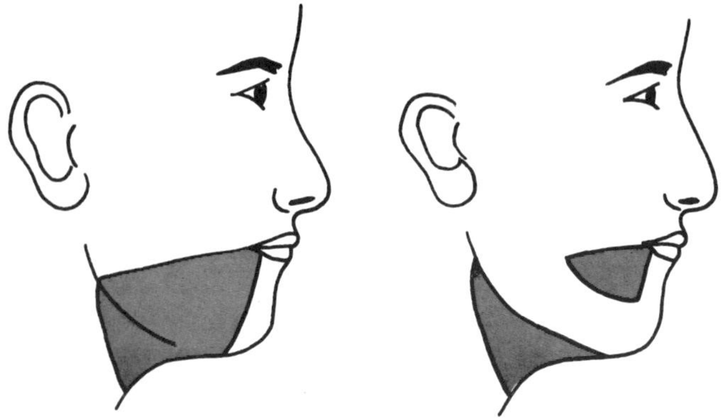

**Fig. 13.16**. *Left*. Area of pain in a case of dry socket of the lower right second premolar.
*Right*. Some discerning patients separate the pain into that of the dry socket itself and also the tenderness in the area of submandibular lymphadenitis.

constant, diffuse pain (Fig. 13.16), occurring of its own accord without the application of external stimuli. It is usually a dull ache made much worse by mechanical treatment of the area; pressure on the surrounding gingiva does this, and probing or pressing into the socket can produce a very severe pain. In some cases pain is throbbing and there may be earache from a lower molar dry socket.

Radiographic examination shows no abnormality but, clinically, there is an obvious socket, devoid of blood clot, and foul smelling due to debris. Associated there is a foul taste. There is swelling and lymphadenitis but no pus. The appearance and time since extraction make the diagnosis easy in most cases. However, sometimes the condition is less acute and the socket is partly healed. A partly healed, partly covered dry socket can continue untreated for months causing pain occasionally which lasts for several hours as a dull ache. Sometimes no socket is obvious but a 'closed dry socket' may be postulated and after the area is surgically opened the pain ceases.

*Treatment*

The socket is gently sprayed to remove food debris, care being needed because this can be painful in itself. The socket is gently dried, and packed with a ribbon gauze impregnated with Whitehead's varnish (based on iodoform). The object is to protect the socket while it heals by granulation from the base outwards and also to prevent mechanical or thermal stimulation of the nerve fibres which are already hyperalgesic. It also keeps food from collecting and decomposing in the socket. Alternatively a pack of zinc oxide–eugenol cement incorporating some whisps of cotton wool can be placed in the socket, but this is not as good as the first suggestion. Analgesics such as aspirin may be taken.

**Causalgia**

There is some confusion about this condition so it is considered in an historical and general context. As the name implies, causalgia is a burning pain. It follows traumatic injury, and was first described by Mitchell (1872) who investigated traumatic injuries of the limbs during the American Civil War.

In modern times Noordenbos (1959) similarly described it as a severe, continuous burning pain, arising spontaneously and aggravated by stimuli, local, general and emotional.'The patient is most unwilling to have the part examined, resents even the slightest touch or movement, and often protects the affected limb in damp towels. Vasomotor and sudomotor phenomena are prominent, though varying in type and degree; there may be abnormal vasoconstriction with profuse sweating; the limb then looks cyanosed and feels cold and clammy; in other cases it may be warm and dry. Trophic changes are present: the skin becomes smooth and presents a glossy appearance, the nails may be long, curved and brittle.' A further diagnostic criterion is that the condition is temporarily relieved by sympathetic block (Bonica, 1954).

The author has not seen such a condition in the trigeminal system, and questioning ten consultant dental and oral surgeons working in the Liverpool Hospitals revealed that they had not either. Moreover, Mitchell himself wrote (1872) that he had made many attempts to bring about trophic changes in the face by irritating or partially wounding the sympathetic fibres, but without success. This suggests that causalgia as described above does not occur in the trigeminal system.

However, it is clearly possible for there to be injuries of the main branches of the trigeminal nerve and such an injury may be associated with constant burning pain; though not the classical causalgia described above this might still be described as minor causalgia. Such a condition could arise, for example, as a result of extracting teeth with roots near the inferior dental nerve. In the bony canals there would be opportunity for interaction between the somatic fibres and those of the sympathetic system (Gregg, 1974).

Not to be confused with causalgia is burning pain which affects the oral mucosa. This has a different, possibly unknown aetiology and should not be called causalgia but simply burning pain; such cases will be described in Chapter 15.

One explanation of causalgia is that damage to the nerve disrupts the myelin sheath thus producing an 'artificial synapse'. This is said to permit neural impulses to cross from an active nerve fibre to adjacent fibres which would otherwise have remained inactive. This 'cross-talk' thereby amplifies the effect of peripheral stimuli. Moreover, a nerve fibre stimulated in this way would not simply conduct impulses towards the central nervous system; it would also conduct them towards the periphery (antidromically). Here, it has been postulated (Lewis, 1942), there could be liberation of pain producing substances which would aggravate the condition.

Another explanation which is, perhaps, more acceptable is that nerve injury disrupts the larger nerve fibres, leaving the smaller C fibres active. Normally, the activity in the larger nerve fibres modulates the input along the C fibres (gate control theory, Chapter 4). In the damaged state the modulating activity is lost and a constant burning pain remains. This may last for many years, as in cases of anaesthesia dolorosa following trigeminal nerve section, and it has been suggested that anaesthesia dolorosa is really causalgia of the face (Mumford and Miles, 1977).

Since sympathetic block gives temporary relief of pain it may be supposed that at least part of the input to the central nervous system is by way of visceral afferent fibres. Another possibility is that the sympathetic fibres normally modulate C fibre terminals.

*Treatment*

This is very difficult and, in most cases, it is just a matter of waiting for nerve fibres to recover, usually for months but maybe for years. Meanwhile the patient is encouraged and reassured. There must be no suggestion that the pain is imaginary. Sympathetic nerve block may help. (See also Chapter 16 under Anaesthesia dolorosa.)

## Phantom teeth

Amputees nearly always have a basic phantom limb which tends to fade with time, and about 10 per cent of persistent phantom limbs are painful for at least part of the time (Inman, 1967). It therefore seems reasonable to postulate phantom teeth, and these 'phantoms' might be responsible for cases of pain. Many patients complain of toothache after all the teeth have been extracted and some patients complain of pain in the place formerly occupied by an individual tooth. These cases are ascribed to various factors such as residual infection, spicules of bone, bony eminences, previous painful treatment, etc. These diagnoses might well be correct, but why not phantom teeth?

One objection is that a phantom hand can have its 'position' accurately described. Similarly, a missing tooth should seem as though it is still present as well as being a source of pain. The mouth is certainly capable of giving a clear perception of geometric shape (Gibson, 1967), and Marbach (1978) suggests that cases occur, but the author has seen no convincing case of a phantom tooth after trying to find a case for several years. Whenever the possibility is mentioned the patient or dentist is unable to say that the crown seems present in the dental arch.

## NEOPLASIA

The tumours of odontogenic origin do not usually give rise to pain unless they become infected, but pain does arise from neoplasia. This may be due to expansion of the growth causing pressure on a nerve, or it may be due to infiltration of malignant cells into the nerve trunk. Secondary infection is also an important cause of pain

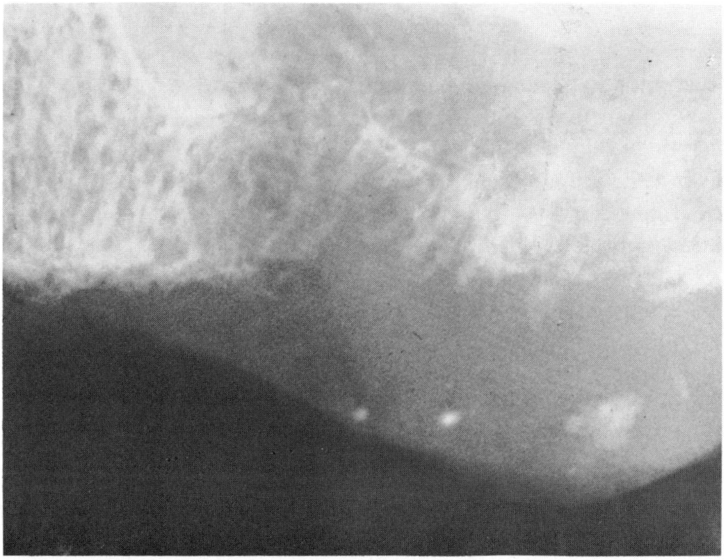

**Fig. 13.17.** Chondrosarcoma of the maxilla causing destruction of the alveolar bone. There is enlargement of the soft tissues in which the radio-opaque areas are presumably cartilage. (Courtesy of Mr P. D. Bird.)

in oral malignancies and, of course, lymph nodes are likely to be involved. In addition to pain, nerve involvement may result in paraesthesia and ultimately anaesthesia. These facial sensory changes are just as important as pain in cases of underlying malignant neoplasms (Boles, 1977).

The radiographic appearance depends upon the type of neoplasm, the stage of development and the site affected. Radiolucence, radiopacity, bone erosion and bone expansion may be present and the teeth subject to drifting. A chondrosarcoma of the maxilla is shown in Fig. 13.17.

When carcinoma involves the maxillary sinus there is frequently pain and, from a survey of 420 cases, Sakai, Shigematzu and Fuchihata (1972) gave the following percentage incidence; pain (39), toothache (29), headache (21), ocular pain (16). Paraesthesia occurred buccally (83) and in the teeth (53). Nasal obstruction and nasal discharge were frequent (68), and they considered the condition to be difficult to differentiate from purulent maxillary sinusitis. However, they stressed two important features; exophthalmos or the slightest degree of continuous bloody discharge must arouse suspicion. From their paper, one might add to this the presence of swelling in the hard palate.

Secondary tumours may occur and cause pain, due to metastasis of primary neoplasms developing elsewhere in the body.

*Treatment*

Great care is needed in handling neoplastic conditions and good cooperation is required between surgeons, radiotherapists and everybody involved. The surgery, radiation and chemotherapy are beyond the scope of this book but appropriate analgesic therapy is now more clearly understood. A primary objective is to keep the patient completely pain free. By giving analgesics at suitable intervals pain is not allowed to return, so the patient ceases to fear it. Though given by the clock the dosage must be adjusted to the individual patient (Twycross, 1978). If the non-narcotic analgesics fail to give adequate pain relief the narcotic analgesics are used. These also give a sense of euphoria which is usually desirable (Houde, 1979). Houde advises doses of 650 mg aspirin; or a weak narcotic analgesic such as 30 mg codeine or 30 mg pentazocine, along with 650 mg aspirin or 650 mg paracetamol. He gives tables of equianalgesic doses which the interested reader should consult, and points out the improvements to be obtained from radiation therapy, steroids and chemotherapy.

If the patient is depressed tricyclic antidepressants e.g. amitryptaline are prescribed; anxiolytics e.g. diazapam, and tranquillisers e.g. chlorpromazine are also considered; diversion therapy is usually indicated (Twycross, 1979).

Nerve blocking with neurolysis may be necessary in some cases (Bonica and Madrid, 1979), and cutting nerve roots in others (Pagni, 1979).

**Osteitis deformans (Paget's disease)**

This slowly progressing bone enlargement may involve the jaws, possibly before affecting other bones. However, the jaws are less likely to be involved than the pelvis or calvarium (Gorlin and Goldman, 1970). The bones show both radiopaque and radiolucent areas producing the so-called 'cotton wool' appearance (Figs. 13.18, 13.19). Enlargement of skull bones produces narrowing of foramina which may transmit nerves and this causes facial pain. Headache, visual disorders and deafness may be present, and advanced cases have the simian appearance of enlarged head, curved back, bowed legs and long arms.

Apart from the neuralgia-like pain which may result from compression of nerves there is often also a dull background 'bone pain'.

*Treatment*

Clinical regression of this disease, and relief of pain, results from administration of calcitonin (calcitare), the daily dose being 160 international units, given subcutaneously or intramuscularly, and is related to the severity of the disease. Alternatively it can be given

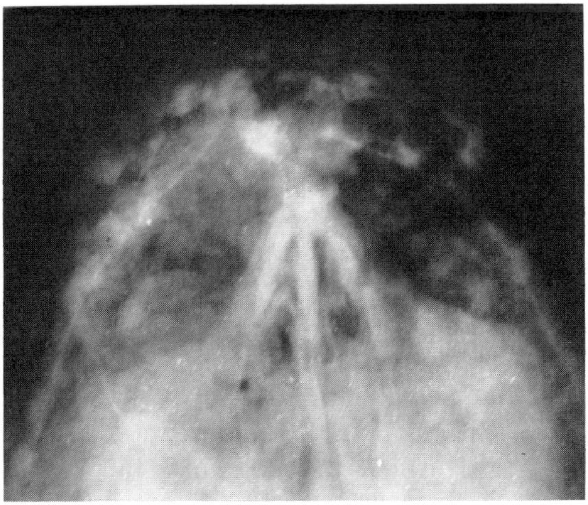

**Fig. 13.18.** Osteitis deformans (Paget's disease). (Courtesy of Dr W. R. Tyldesley.)

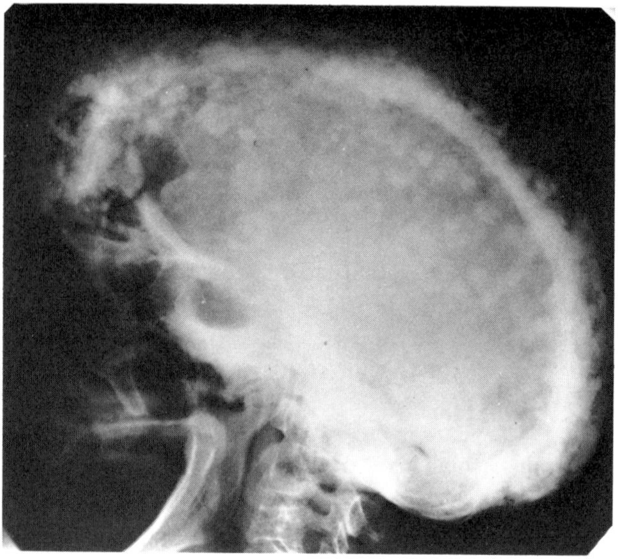

**Fig. 13.19**. Osteitis deformans. Same case as Fig. 13.18. (Courtesy of Dr W. R. Tyldesley.)

as a divided dose, morning and night. The course of the disease and the effect of therapy are monitored by frequent determinations of serum alkaline phosphatase and urinary hydroxyproline, excretion of which begins to show a fall towards normal after 1–2 months of treatment (Tyldesley, 1981).

## Acromegaly

In the early stages of this disease there may be pain which is difficult to diagnose and the case may be placed in the category of atypical facial pain; this is an ill-defined group of conditions which are mainly thought of as being due to psychological illness, so the patient may be placed on a seemingly appropriate drug such as an antidepressant (but see Chapter 19).

Later, the bone changes affect the jaws, especially the lower jaw, and there is spacing of the teeth. Malocclusion develops and abnormal stress causes pain, dentures become too small and no longer fit, causing pressure on the oral mucosa which is painful. Further pain may occur from muscular imbalance, and there can be headache, usually experienced in the middle of the forehead. There is thickening of the facial tissues with bags under the eyes, large jaws, supraorbital and superciliary ridges, enlarged hands and feet, slowed general metabolism and diminished sexual activity. A lateral skull radiograph may reveal enlargement of the sella turcica caused by the pituitary tumour.

*Treatment*

This is directed to the primary cause, with surgery and/or radiation. Pain is treated by appropriate drugs, occlusal adjustment if needed, occlusal splints, or new dentures in controlled cases, or the dentures may be simply left out.

## REFERENCES

Axelsson, A. and Chidekel, N. (1972) Symptomatology and bacteriology correlated to radiological findings in acute maxillary sinusitis. *Acta Otolaryngol.*, **74**, 118–122.

Birch, R. H. (1980) Personal communication.

Birn, H. (1972) Kinines and pain in dry socket. *Int. J. oral Surg.*, **1**, 34–42.

Boles, R. (1977) Paranasal sinuses and facial pain. In *Facial Pain*, 2nd edition, ed. Alling, C. C. and Mahan, P. E. pp. 115–133. Philadelphia: Lea and Febiger.

Bonica, J. J. (1954) *The Management of Pain*. Philadelphia: Lea and Febiger.

Bonica, J. J. and Madrid, J. L. (1979) Cancer pain in the head and neck; role of nerve blocks. In *Adv. Pain Res. Therap.*, ed. Bonica, J. J. and Ventafridda, V. Vol. 2, pp.. 537–542. New York: Raven Press.

Gibson, J. J. (1967) The mouth as an organ for laying hold on the environment. In *Symposium on Oral Sensation and Perception*, ed. Bosma. J. F. pp. 111–136. Springfield, Ill: Thomas.

Gorlin, R. J. and Goldman, H. M. (1970) *Thoma's Oral Pathology*, 6th edition. St Louis: Mosby.

Gregg, J. M. (1974) Neurological disorders of the maxillo-facial region. In *Textbook of Oral Surgery*, ed Kruger, G. O., pp. 620–660. Saint Louis: Mosby.

Houde, R. W. (1979) Systemic analgesics and related drugs: narcotic analgesics. In *Adv. Pain Res. Therap.*, ed. Bonica, J. J. and Ventafridda, V., Vol. 2, pp. 263–273. New York: Raven Press.

Inman, V. T. (1967) Clinical pathologic consideration of pain mechanisms. In *New Concepts in Pain and its Clinical Management*, ed. Way, E. L., pp. 49–53. Philadelphia: Davis.

Lewis, T. (1942) *Pain*. Macmillan, New York.

Marbach, J. J. (1978) Phantom tooth pain. *J. Endo.*, **4**, 362–372.

McGowan, D. A., Murphy, K. J. and Sheiham, A. (1977) Metranidazole in the treatment of severe acute pericoronitis. *Brit. dent. J.*, **142**, 221–223.

Mitchell, S. W. (1872) *Injuries of Nerves and their Consequences*. Lippincott, Philadelphia. Reprinted from the original in 1965 by Dover Publications, New York.

Mumford, J. M. and Miles, J. B. (1977) Thermography and orofacial pain. *Acta Thermographica*, **2**, 155–161.

Noordenbos, W. 1959. *Pain*. Amsterdam: Elsevier.

Pagni, C. A. (1979) Cancer pain in the head and neck: role of neurosurgery. In *Adv. Pain Res. Therap.*, eds Bonica, J. J. and Ventafridda, V., Vol. 2, pp. 543–552. New York: Raven Press.

Sakai, S., Shigematzu, Y. and Fuchihata, H. (1972) Diagnosis and TNM classification of maxillary sinus carcinoma. *Acta Otolaryngol.*, **74**, 123–129.

Seward, M. H. (1969) The effectiveness of a teething solution in infants. *Brit. dent. J.*, **127**, 457–461.

Taverner, D. (1959) Facial pain. *Brit. dent. J.*, **106**, 165–171.
Twycross, R. G. (1978) Relief of pain in advanced cancer. *Prescriber's J.*,Oct., 117–124.
Twycross, R. G. (1979) The Brompton Cocktail. In *Adv. Pain Res. Therap.*, ed Bonica, J. J. and Ventafridda, V., Vol. 2, 291–300. New York: Raven Press.
Tyldesley, W. B. (1981) *Oral Medicine*, Oxford: Oxford University Press.
Wolff, H. G. (1963) *Headache and Other Head Pains*, 2nd edition. New York: Oxford Univ. Press.

# 14

# Pain due to disturbance of the masticatory system

An important source of orofacial pain is the masticatory dysfunction syndrome. Since this is largely caused by stress the incidence of the condition is likely to increase, so it is necessary to have a clear understanding of its nature. Though medical practitioners must be aware of it, treatment of this syndrome falls within the dentist's province and he is well equipped to deal with it in a manner which is frequently gratifying to himself as well as to his patient. Naturally this does not preclude consultation should this be deemed desirable. It is also necessary for neurologists and neurosurgeons to be more aware of it since flashes of pain are sometimes a feature of the condition which might thus simulate idiopathic trigeminal neuralgia.

## MASTICATORY DYSFUNCTION SYNDROME

The patient's chief complaint is of constant aching pain in the side of the face. It may continue all day and be present for weeks or months but its intensity varies. Frequently it is most severe on waking and/or in the evening. The former is due to over-activity of the masticatory muscles associated with either grinding the teeth (bruxism) or clenching the teeth during the night and is accompanied by stiffness of the jaws on waking and some reduced opening of the mouth (trismus). The greater evening intensity is due to general tiredness at the end of the day as well as fatigue of the masticatory muscles. The lower intensity during the main part of the day is partly because of other activities which divert attention.

There is frequently a second pain which occurs on movement of the mandible especially in certain positions, and this can be reproduced by some patients. It is a brief sharp pain of considerable intensity and the patient tries to avoid it by limiting mandibular movement. In a few cases there is a third pain of a shooting or flashing character which simulates idiopathic trigeminal neuralgia. The distribution of pain will be considered later.

There may also be clicking of the temporomandibular joint and abnormal deviation of the mandible on opening.

## Incidence

### *Sex*

Approximately 80 per cent of patients are female (Schwartz and Cobin, 1957; Schwartz, 1968; Thomson, 1971; Butler, Folke and Bandt, 1975; Nally and Moore, 1975; Zarb and Thompson, 1975). However, surveys of people in a general population have revealed that the numbers of males and females affected were more even than this, suggesting that the preponderance of females seeking treatment is due to other social and/or psychological factors (Agerberg and Carlsson, 1972; Helkimo, 1974).

### *Age*

The condition can affect all ages but the peak period is approximately 25–45 years of age (Agerberg and Carlsson, 1972; Helkimo, 1974; Nally and Moore, 1975; Zarb and Thompson, 1975; Butler, Folke and Bandt, 1975).

### *Side*

The condition is unilateral in 90 per cent of cases (Kydd, 1959; Thomson, 1959).

## Aetiology

The mouth frequently reveals spaces due to missing teeth, and irregularities in the occlusion due to tilting, drifting and over-eruption of the remaining teeth, so it is not surprising that such occlusal abnormalities have been blamed for the painful condition and clicking joint. However, these occlusal abnormalities are a common feature of the mouths of numerous people, and in the majority of people do not cause pain, so it would be wrong to jump to conclusions regarding their aetiological significance in these cases. Moreover, many patients who complain of pain due to dysfunction of the masticatory system have good dentitions — indeed, in some cases the dentitions can only be described as excellent (Fig. 14.1). The patient featured in Fig. 14.1 also had normal temporomandibular joints (Fig. 14.2), and she drew the graph in Fig. 14.3. Furthermore, there can be marked changes in the condylar head and the articular tubercle without any symptoms

(Schwartz, 1968). A survey of cases by Thomson (1959), complete with a control group of patients, showed no correlation between occlusal irregularities and the incidence of joint symptoms. However, one form of occlusal irregularity could be a more important predisposing factor than others; that is unilateral mutilation of a dentition causing the patient to masticate only on one side (Franks, 1965).

The essential aetiological feature appears to be psychological stress, one feature of which is bruxism or toothgrinding, especially during sleep. Grinding of teeth is not always noticed by the patient but may be brought to her attention by her husband or other member of the family. It is this activity which causes the teeth to be worn with well defined facets, and which also causes the muscles and jaws to feel tired and aching when the patient awakes. This view is supported by the investigation of Christensen (1967) who caused experimental subjects to perform intensive right-sided bruxism for 20 minutes. Pain was later experienced in

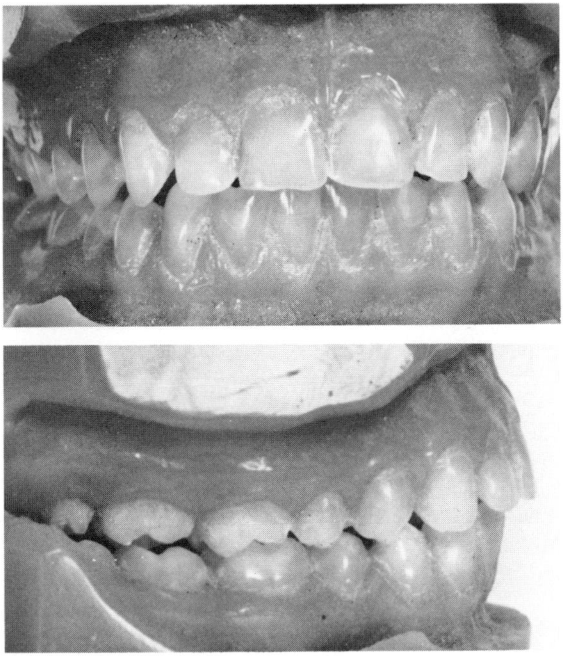

**Fig. 14.1**. Excellent dentition of a patient suffering the pain dysfunction syndrome. The right joint was stiff in the morning, improving during the day, and stiffening again towards the end of the day. On moving the jaw there was a sharp pain.

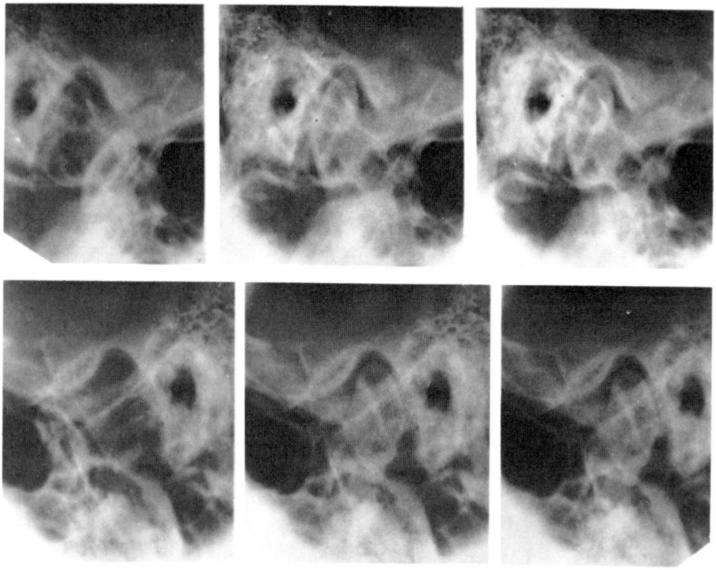

**Fig. 14.2**. Temporomandibular joint radiographs of the patient whose dentition is shown in Fig. 14.1. Above, Right side with the mouth open, in occlusion and at rest. Below, Left side with the mouth open, in occlusion and at rest.

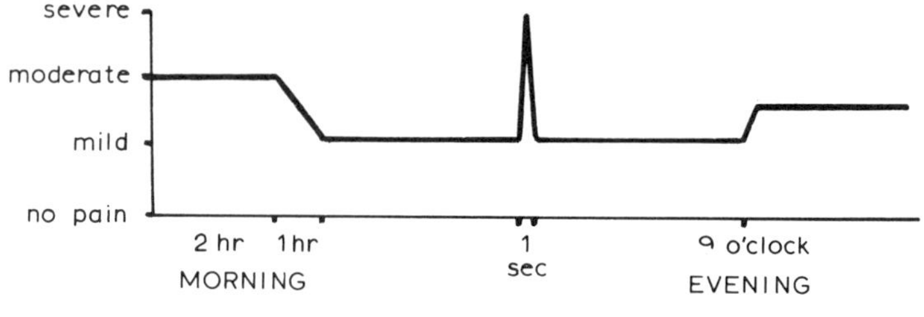


**Fig. 14.3**. The patient (the same as in Figs. 14.1, 14.2) illustrated her pain as above. Chewing caused a severe sharp pain with a duration of approximately 1 second. Pain sometimes became worse in the evening but never as bad as in the morning.

the temporomandibular joints and supra-orbitally, usually after 2–3 hours, but in one case after 30 hours. It was deep, lasted for hours, and tended to radiate to the ear, the zygomatic arch and the frontal region. In further experiments Christensen (1976) splinted the lower teeth, applied a load and had the experimental subjects perform work by actively lowering the load. Pain developed in 8 out of 10 subjects starting from 5 minutes to 24 hours later, and in 4 subjects there was shooting pain. The significance of muscle activity is also supported by work of Trenouth (1979) who applied steel bands to opposing incisors and wired them to a recorder. Patients with the masticatory dysfunction syndrome and bruxism made four times as many contacts during the night as did a control group; they also had contacts of greater duration.

Pain is at least partly due to muscle contraction associated with ischaemia, and raised intramuscular pressure in the temporal and masseter muscles has been demonstrated during exercise by Møller, Rasmusson and Bonde-Petersen (1979). The average intramuscular pressure was below the arterial blood pressure but relative ischaemia during biting was indicated by a marked post-exercise hyperaemia.

Clinical observation suggests that clenching the teeth occurs as frequently as grinding but is less noticeable because it causes neither abrasive facets nor makes a noise; it may be even more damaging than grinding because the latter implies a masticatory force that is not too large to prevent lateral excursions of the mandible with the teeth in contact (Newton, 1981).

It is not always easy to get at the cause of psychological stress and the patient needs to be carefully questioned. She may feel a sense of guilt and be unable to talk freely in front of an audience — even the dental surgery attendant might have to leave the surgery for a while. For example, a lady with an excellent dentition (Fig. 14.1) had been spending a holiday with her husband's family and did not like to admit that this made her feel tense.

Sometimes the reason may be a socially acceptable one, such as a male patient who announced, half proudly, half with annoyance, that he had just driven his family more than 2500 miles on holiday. It is not difficult to imagine his masseters clenching towards the end of a long run as he determined to make the distance. In this case the patient was able to understand the cause and only needed reassurance together with the suggestion that he should (at least for a while) have a quiet alcoholic drink at the end of the day's work.

The masseters are amongst the first muscles to contract in persons who are in a state of tension, determination or desperation, and a moment's thought reveals that this is really common knowledge. In fact it is sometimes possible to produce a deep groove in the masseters by determined effort, such as lifting a heavy weight. Electromyographic examination reveals increased electrical activity

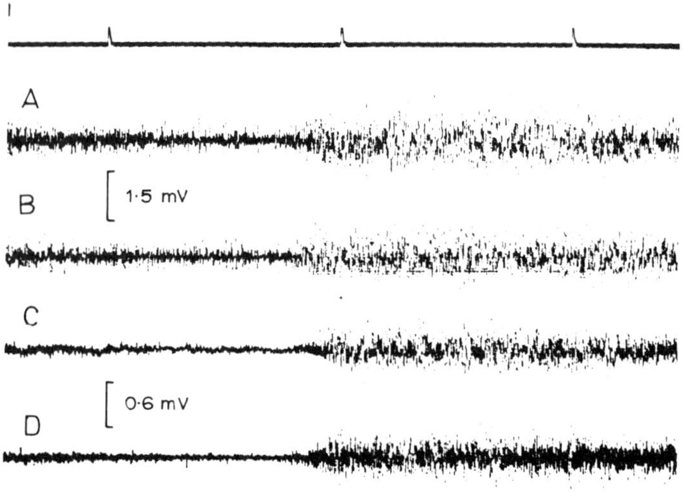


**Fig. 14.4**. Increase in the electrical activity of muscles made to do extra work. A, right temporal; B, left temporal; C, right masseter; D, left masseter. (Courtesy of Mr T. O. Tweedie.)

from masseter and temporal muscles made to do extra work (Fig. 14.4), and this increases when people are subjected to psychological stress (Yemm, 1969, 1971). The time sequence of activity has been investigated and the masseter was always the first muscle to contract, followed by the anterior, then posterior part of the temporal muscle (Steiner, Michman and Litman, 1974). This was true with both hard food (carrots) and soft food (bread). If pain occurs it does so approximately one second after the onset of electrical activity in the masseter and temporalis muscles (MacDougall and Andrew, 1953), and is due to compression of the blood vessels causing a diminished blood supply (Kawamura, 1968). The pain that sometimes occurs in associated neck muscles is probably due to these being recruited to assist the tired muscles of mastication (Krogh-Poulsen and Olssen, 1968).

Sometimes tension is due to local factors, as in a female patient who complained of very severe pain including tightness and soreness of her jaws and masseters when she woke in the morning. Eventually it was discovered that there were exposed pulps in two of her molar teeth. This case illustrates an important point, for the dysfunction was due to pathological processes outside of the muscles and joints — in other words she was suffering from a secondary muscle spasm whereas the muscle spasm is usually primary.

It should be remembered that tension can be self-generated and need not be logical; problems can be magnified or even invented. Indeed, one difficulty in these cases is that once tension is established it becomes self-generating — a state of positive feedback develops; in other words, tension creates the condition which increases tension which aggravates the condition and so on (Newton, 1969). The vicious circle (positive feedback) must be broken and the first step is that the dentist must show confidence in his ability to deal with the problem and be able to give firm reassurance. There should neither be frightening discussion of the diagnosis, nor extensive treatment which would only increase the existing tension. In fact, dental treatment is sometimes an important contributory factor. This may be due to extensive changes in the occlusion brought on in a rapid manner such as by selective grinding, or the placement of a large number of restorations or of new prosthetic appliances. 'Finals cases' are worth a mention; in laudable efforts to present superb examples of their work to the external examiners, students may subject their patients to prolonged periods of having their mouths wide open with resulting strain on the masticatory system and subsequent painful dysfunction; teachers of operative dentistry should look out for these situations and try to prevent such strain occurring.

**Examination**

When examining these patients the jaw movements are tested, with and without restraining pressure from the dentist's hand. Opening, closing, protrusion, retrusion, and lateral excursions are tested, any clicking, pain or deviations being noted. Sometimes deviation from normal opening can be corrected by the dentist's guiding hand and this may prevent the clicks from occurring in the temporomandibular joint, though possibly inducing a sharp pain in the masseter. As mentioned earlier, one can suppose that the mandibular deviation occurs in order to avoid the pain, though it unfortunately leads to the joint clicking.

The masticatory muscles are examined for tenderness, not just by palpating the skin area but also by having a finger in the mouth at the same time, possibly using bimanual palpation. Auscultation of the joint may also reveal clicking or crepitus. The maximum mouth opening that can be achieved is measured, and Schwartz (1968) recommends estimating the strength of the bite as well as checking on the state of the facial nerve by examining activity of the facial muscles.

In general, the distribution of pain in cases seen by the author may be represented by the composite diagram in Fig. 14.5, and some individual cases are presented in Fig. 14.6.

Examination of Figs. 14.5 and 14.6 shows that headache may be complained of in the temporal region, along the temporal ridge, frontally, coronally and in the occipital region. These headaches could just as well be described as muscle contraction headaches (see Chapter 17).

The figures also show that pain can extend into the neck adjacent to the angle of the mandible and also near the sternomastoid muscle. Since pain in muscles tends to lead to nearby muscles becoming involved pain may spread even further into the neck, and this is usually called the myofascial pain-dysfunction syndrome. It

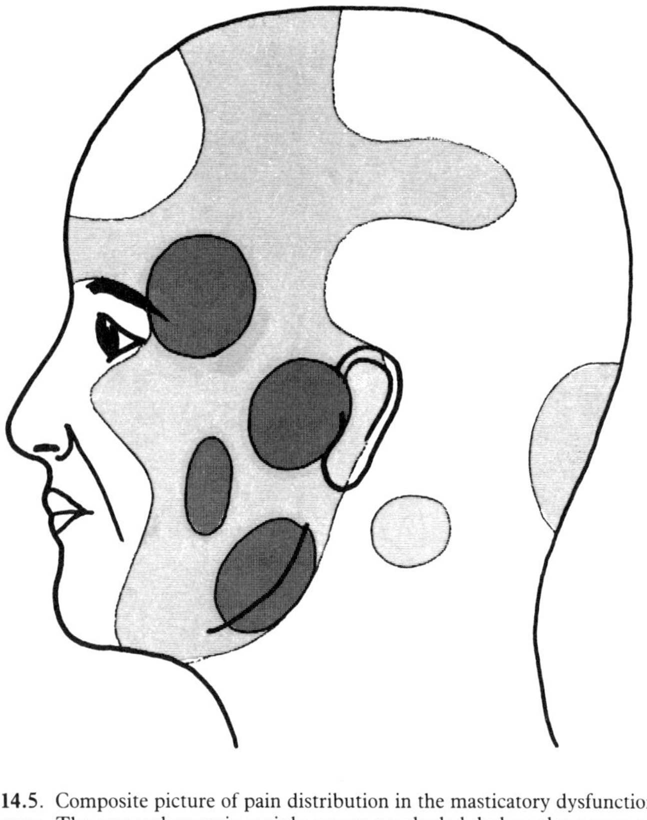

**Fig. 14.5.** Composite picture of pain distribution in the masticatory dysfunction syndrome. The areas where pain mainly occurs are shaded darker; these areas are often tender on pressure and pain is more severe than in the lightly shaded zones. The latter are usually indicated by the patient in an ill-defined manner with a sweep of the hand, whereas the darker zones are likely to be more definitely indicated, often with one finger.

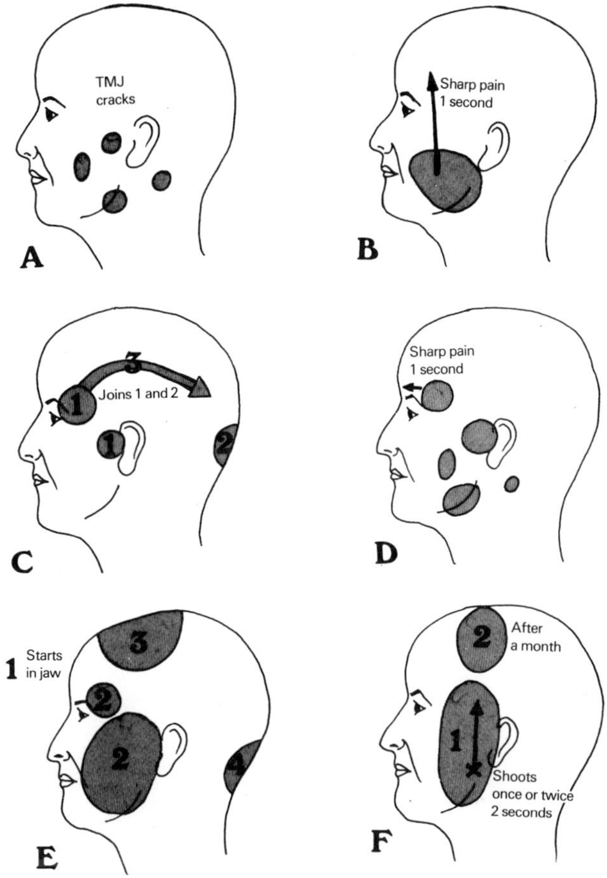


**Fig. 14.6.** Each face represents an individual patient but all are facing one way for comparison.

A. Female, 38 years. A premature sliding contact was ground and pain was largely relieved even before the occlusal splint was fitted.

B. Female, 75 years, wearing the same full upper and lower dentures for 20 years. There was loss of occlusal height, so an occlusal splint was made and pain ceased.

C. Female, 45 years, Many missing teeth. Pain occurred first as shown (1). Then also occipitally (2). The pain seemed to join 1 and 2 (3). Partial dentures were fitted and pain ceased.

D. Male, 55 years. Impacted lower premolar with apex close to inferior dental nerve. Pain, including the shooting pain in the forehead, ceased on surgical removal, (see also Fig. 16.7.)

E. Female, 23 years, married with young child, going out to work, living with parents, house hunting and about to move. Pain started in the jaw. Then was felt in the usual areas (2). Then also at 3 and finally occipitally (4). She said it was severe and she was crying.

F. Female, 42 years, with 3 children but separated from her husband. Four new crowns and had to keep mouth open a long time, but no lower partial denture and loss of occlusal height. Pain started in the usual area (1). Then also at 2. There was also a shooting pain as indicated.

is therefore easy to understand the use of various synonyms for the masticatory dysfunction syndrome which might be regarded as a regional manifestation of a more general syndrome, complicated by the activity of the temporomandibular joints and the various problems which occur within the oral cavity.

The painful muscles frequently have localised areas which are more painful on palpation than elsewhere; these have been described as 'trigger points' and pressure on them is said to cause not only the local pain but also referred pain if this has already been present (Travell, 1976). However, the present author prefers to say that pressure provokes pain, reserving the words trigger and trigger point for the original concept where *light touch* causes the flashing pain in idiopathic trigeminal neuralgia (Chapter 16). Also, when the area of pain extends, apparently involving adjacent structures one should hesitate to say referred to these structures unless one is sure about the patient's ability to localise accurately,

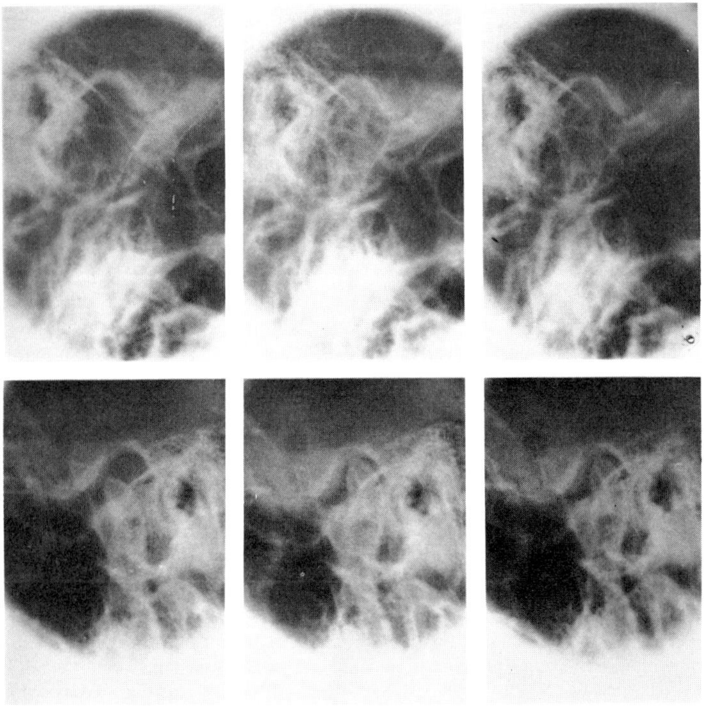

**Fig. 14.7.** Radiographs of the temporomandibular joints in the open, closed and rest positions. The condyl on the affected side (Lower left picture) moves less on opening than does that on the normal side (upper left picture).

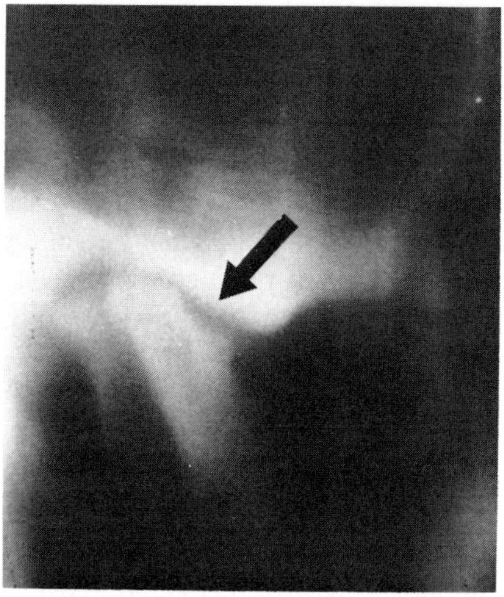

**Fig. 14.8.** Tomograph of temporomandibular joint showing notch in condyle.

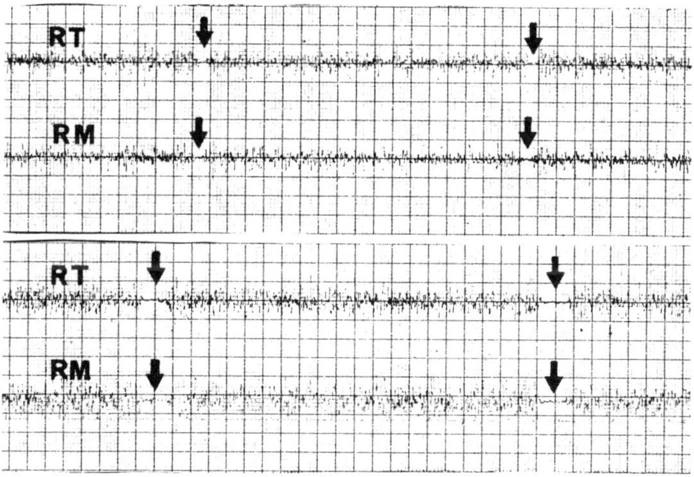


**Fig. 14.9.** Electromyograms of the temporal and masseter muscles in a normal case (above) and one with masticatory dysfunction (below). The silent period is longer in the patient with masticatory dysfunction (Mr T. O. Tweedie's case).

and also sure that the other muscle has not developed its own abnormal painful state (Chapter 18).

Krogh-Poulsen and Olssen (1968) suggested that pain over the eyes originates from the frontalis muscles; pain or headache in the temples from the anterior fibres of the temporalis muscles; pain in front of the ear from the deep masseteric fibres; in the middle of the cheek from the superficial masseteric fibres; pain in the ear may be from the external pterygoid muscle; pain behind the ear from the posterior fibres of the temporalis; pain under the jaw from the medial pterygoid muscle; and pain in the side of the neck from the posterior belly of the digastric muscle.

Radiological examination must include an orthopantomograph to scan the whole of the jaws, and this may reveal dental caries, apical pathology, unerupted teeth, retained roots, etc., which could be causing, or contributing to the condition. It might also give a satisfactory view of the temporomandibular joints, but it is better to take radiographs with the joints at rest and in the closed and open positions. The latter may show that on opening the mouth the condyl on the affected side moves less than that on the other side (Fig. 14.7). The condylar head is usually a smooth curve but it can appear flattened or even notched, although this can also happen in normal cases (Worth, 1974). Moreover, a recognisable structural change need not be associated with the masticatory dysfunction syndrome, eg. the joint shown in Fig. 14.8 had caused the patient a great deal of pain which failed to respond to various treatments such as hydrocortisone injections into both joints, occlusal splinting, and acupuncture; eventually success was achieved by bilateral high condylectomies.

Electromyographic analysis may be made, the pick-up electrodes being placed over the masseter and temporalis muscles on both sides. One feature which might prove to be of diagnostic value is the silent period. When a stimulus such as a tap on the chin is applied to the jaws the electrical recording is affected as shown in Fig. 14.9. The duration of the silent period tends to be longer in patients with masticatory dysfunction than in normal people so this is of diagnostic value, but there is some overlap between the two groups (Tweedie, 1981).

This condition has also been investigated by means of thermography which is thought to have shown that in most cases the skin overlying a tender area of the masseter muscle was hotter than the corresponding area on the opposite side of the face (Berry and Yemm, 1974). This was presumed to be because of inflammation but simple increased vascularity would be sufficient explanation. The method is still in the experimental stage.

## Occlusal abnormalities

In the previous section prime attention has been paid to psychological tension and the muscles of mastication, and it was said that pain was not primarily due to occlusal abnormalities. Nevertheless, the occlusion is important and should be treated on its merits. It is amazing how so many people manage apparently very well with deranged occlusions, but the effect of loss of teeth is insidious. Even the loss of one tooth causes a disturbance of the contact point pressure and teeth start to move within a couple of days. Loss of more teeth allows tilting and drift of adjacent teeth and over-eruption of the opposing teeth, so that adverse occlusal relationships arise which can cause pain. To a considerable extent the masticatory system accommodates to the changed conditions but not always and periods of psychological stress have a bearing on pain production.

Examination of the mouth reveals facets on certain teeth which may also be more mobile than normal. If the dentist places a finger along the buccal side of the arch it is usually possible to detect which tooth is especially subjected to excessive strain.

**Treatment of the masticatory dysfunction syndrome**

Having made a complete examination it is possible to reassure the patient about the condition and the prognosis. In particular, the patient may have been worried about cancer, a brain tumour or arthritis, and reassurance must be firm. The nature of any stressful situation is analysed so that the patient becomes clearly aware of it and is then better able to deal with it even if the situation itself cannot be resolved. It has been suggested that there is need to interpret the symptoms in a way that is credible to the patient — that it must be culturally and psychologically acceptable (Marbach and Lipton, 1978). For example, attributing the problem to psychological factors may upset some people thereby increasing stress, so it would be better to make more of the mechanical factors involved.

Reassurance is the first step in breaking the vicious circle, and tension can be further reduced by prescribing a tranquilliser eg. 5 mg diazepam morning and evening, but only for one week in the first instance. Many people might prefer to have a quiet alcoholic drink on the way home from work or on arriving home. It is appropriate to advise the patient's medical practitioner, partly as a courtesy, but also because he may be able to help regarding the patient's life situation. Some thought should also be given to the amount of caffeine taken by the patient because some people drink more coffee and tea than is good for them; it can often be reduced to a half. Stress relieving activities such as sport, jogging, showers, a weekly hairdressing appointment, and a short sleep after lunch should be encouraged. If the patient becomes aware of muscle ache she should try massaging it away with the jaw hanging loose.

Any natural teeth which are subjected to undue masticatory pressures should be relieved but only a limited reduction is indicated for it is no longer acceptable to make the extensive reductions that were practised some years ago. This aspect of treatment applies especially to any teeth which have been recently restored. Experimentally it is possible to produce functional disturbance and/or pain by simply fitting a raised gold inlay (Randow et al, 1976). A raised gold inlay or an overpacked amalgam filling will eventually wear itself in but porcelain restorations will not. For example, a patient complained of pain in both masseters at the anterior borders, saying that since three porcelain jacket crowns had been placed on her upper incisors she could not close her back teeth together. In attempting to occlude her cheek teeth she was retruding her mandible beyond the normal position, subjecting her masticatory muscles to abnormal effort and causing pain. Examination revealed that the incisal edge of her lower incisors had been ground flat rather than on a slope. Using articulating paper as an aid a minute amount of enamel was removed from the labial edge of the incisal plane of each lower incisor. This was sufficient to restore her occlusion and she cried with relief, having suffered badly for two weeks.

In edentulous cases the full upper and lower artificial dentures may have been in the mouth for many years and have been reduced by wear, as well as being associated with remodelling of alveolar bone. This results in overclosure of the mandible which can be corrected by adding a layer of self-curing resin to the occlusal surface of one of the dentures. If this cures the condition then new dentures are made taking care to establish the correct vertical dimension, or the existing dentures are relined. The opposite condition may also be responsible — if the vertical dimension is too great the lower denture should not be worn for a while. If the condition resolves new dentures are made to the correct vertical dimension.

An important line of treatment is the provision of an occlusal splint (bite raising appliance, etc). This is made to fit over the occlusal surfaces of the arch, either upper or lower — it is not yet known if one is better than the other. The object of fitting the appliance is to eliminate any interfering occlusal contacts and to produce a gentle passive stretch to the elevator muscles of the mandible, thus altering the sensory input and breaking the vicious circle already described. However, if the appliance is badly made it can cause additional pain as well as further stress. It is therefore desirable to make special trays to take a second pair of accurate impressions and even then some adjustment is needed when fitting the appliance. It must cover all of the teeth in the arch so that there are no uncovered teeth which might over-erupt, and it also includes areas where there are missing teeth. It is worn at night or during the evening for about three hours, during several weeks, but many cases resolve in a week or two, and sometimes even in a day or two. Such quick results are probably a result of reducing anxiety, and one patient reported himself cured before the appliance could even be fitted. The psychological influence has also been demonstrated by experiments in which the pain ceased after fake occlusal equilibration, grinding surfaces which had no occlusal relationship (Goodman, Greene and Laskin, 1976).

Electromyographic feedback may be used, the electrical activity being monitored by the patient, possibly via earphones (Dohrmann and Laskin, 1978). By reducing the frequency of noise the patient learns to relax and thus reduce muscle activity. It is probably only an expensive way of helping the patient to relax.

Other adjuncts to treatment include the injection of a local anaesthetic into the painful muscle, spraying the painful area with a refrigerant material, acupuncture, transcutaneous neural stimulation and analgesics.

Cessation of pain is confirmatory evidence of the correct diagnosis, and this adds to the patient's confidence, but she should wear the splint a while longer, perhaps several weeks. It is then placed in a sealed polythene bag together with a little water to prevent it drying out and distorting, so the patient may use it again if necessary. The knowledge that it is available helps to reduce tension. If there are many missing teeth arrangements are made to provide partial dentures and these may have to include onlay portions to establish the best occlusal relationship. Fewer missing teeth may be replaced by bridgework.

### Novice pipe smokers

It is worth noticing that men who have recently taken to smoking a pipe sometimes complain of a dull ache in the jaws and masseter muscles. Rather than encouraging them to get used to holding the pipe in a more relaxed manner it is probably better to persuade them to give up smoking altogether before the habit takes a firmer hold.

**Costen's syndrome**

It was said that because of disturbed function of the temporomandibular joint there was dull pain in the area including within the ears, intermittent or continuously impaired hearing, stiffness in the joints marked about meal times, tinnitus and sometimes snapping in the joint (Costen, 1934, 1937). It was said to be due to over-closure of the mandible causing compression of nerve fibres of either the auriculo-temporal nerve or the chorda tympani, and that over-closure might also cause some deafness as well as producing a defect in the tympanic plate. Though Costen performed a useful function in drawing attention to it the syndrome is no longer accepted, at least in the original form. It seems to be partly a description of the masticatory dysfunction syndrome, and the anatomical part is not tenable. The tympanic plate can have a developmental defect in it and the auriculo-temporal nerve is situated behind the neck of the condyle rather than behind the condyle itself, whilst the chorda tympani nerve is located in the petrotympanic fissure where it is presumably well protected against encroachment by the condyle. Sicher gave a clear account of the unsoundness of this syndrome as early as 1948. Schwartz and Chayes (1968) suggested that the term Costen's syndrome should be abandoned, and it now seems to be less frequently mentioned.

## ACUTE TRAUMATIC ARTHRITIS

Following trauma there is pain and tenderness together with secondary spasm of the masticatory muscles which are treated symptomatically and with rest for several days. Pain and tenderness are located immediately over the joint, and also on palpation via the external auditory meatus. On opening the mouth it deviates to the same side. If there is dislocation of the head of the condyle this is reduced by downward pressure in the molar area together with lift and backward pressure in the anterior region. The patient is advised against opening the mouth too wide in yawning or during dental treatment. Radiographic investigation is essential for there may be a fracture of the condylar head. This is associated with pain in the temporomandibular joint and tenderness over it, oedema in the area being likely to prevent the patient from fully closing his teeth together on the affected side. This subject is properly within the province of the maxillo-facial surgeon.

## RHEUMATOID ARTHRITIS

Also known as proliferative arthritis, in this systemic disease granulation tissue from the synovial membrane proliferates on to the articular surface; being vascularised and innervated, pressure provokes inflammatory symptoms with consequent pain.

The percentage of patients suffering rheumatoid arthritis in whom the temporomandibular joint is affected is probably about 5 per cent compared with 90 per cent in whom the hands are affected (Brod, 1968), but up to 51 per cent has been suggested (Grokoest and Chayes, 1968). The fusiform swellings of the proximal finger joints are an obvious diagnostic factor and the treatment of this condition is a problem for the patient's physician.

## OSTEOARTHRITIS

This is essentially a disease of older people affecting various joints, and the temporomandibular joints may be included. There is degenerative change of the articular surfaces due to wear and tear (old age), trauma and damage due to occlusal dysharmony. Limitation of movement can occur and there may be tenderness not only of the joint and its capsule but also of the masseter and temporalis muscles. However, there is usually no pain even though crepitus is present. The paths of opening and closing may be irregular, although many otherwise normal cases also have irregular paths.

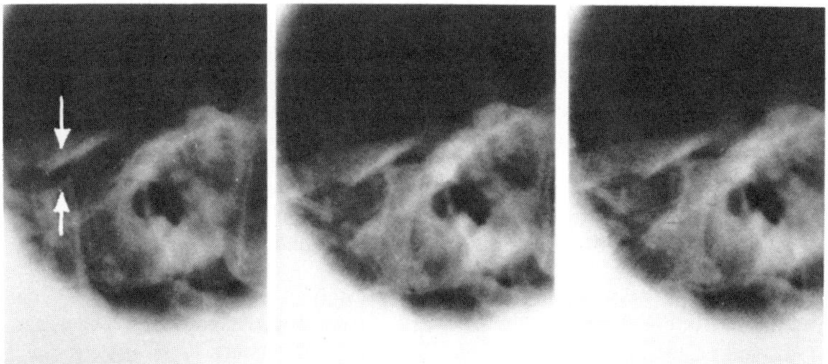

**Fig. 14.10**. Osteoarthritis of the temporomandibular joint in a patient who was 74 years old. Notice the flattened articular surfaces, and compare with the normal joints shown in Fig. 14.2. (Dr W. R. Tyldesley's case.)

Radiographic examination is important (Fig. 14.10) and there are degenerative changes in other joints.

If pain develops the condition becomes, in effect, a masticatory dysfunction syndrome and is treated accordingly (Bell, 1977).

## REFERENCES


Agerberg, G. and Carlsson, G. E. (1972) Functional disorders of the masticatory system: I Distribution of symptoms according to age and sex as judged from investigation by questionnaire. *Acta odont. Scand.*, **30**, 597–613.

Bell, W. E. (1973) *Orofacial Pains — Differential Diagnosis*. Dallas: Denedco.

Berry, D. C. and Yemm, R. (1974) A further study of facial temperature in patients with mandibular dysfunction. *J. oral Rehabilitation*, **1**, 255–264.

Brod, M. S. (1968) Differential diagnosis. In *Facial Pain and Mandibular Dysfunction*, ed. Schwartz, L. and Chayes, C. H., pp. 220–235. Philadelphia: Saunders.

Butler, J. H., Folke, L. E. A. and Bandt, C. L. (1978) A descriptive survey of signs and symptoms associated with the myofascial pain-dysfunction syndrome. *J. Amer. dent. Ass.*, **90**, 635–639.

Christensen, L. V. (1967) Eksperimentelt provokerede ansigtssmerter fra kaebernes bevaegesystem ved bruksisme. *Saetryk af Tandlaegebladet*, **71**, 1171–1181. (English summary.)

Christensen, L. V. (1976) Facial pain in negative and positive work of human jaw muscles. *Scand. J. dent. Res.*, **84**, 327–332.

Costen, J. B. (1934) Syndrome of ear and sinus symptoms dependent upon disturbed function of the temporomandibular joint. *Ann. Otol. Rhin. & Laryng.*, **43**, 1–15. Quoted by Costen, below.

Costen, J. B. (1937) Some features of the mandibular articulation as it pertains to medical diagnosis, especially in otorhinolaryngology. *J. Amer. dent. Ass.*, **24**, 1507–1511.

Dohrmann, R. J. and Laskin, D. M. (1978) An evaluation of electromyographic biofeedback in the treatment of myofascial pain-dysfunction syndrome. *J. Amer. dent. Ass.*, **96**, 656–662.

Franks, A. S. T. (1965) Conservative treatment of temporomandibular joint dysfunction: a comparative study. *Dent. Practit. dent. Rec.*, **15**, 205–210.

Goodman, P., Greene, C. S. and Laskin, D. M. (1976) Response of patients with myofascial pain-dysfunction syndrome to mock equilibration. *J. Amer. med. Ass.*, **92**, 755–758.

Grokoest, A. W. and Chayes, C. M. (1968) Rheumatic diseases. In *Facial Pain and Mandibular Dysfunction*, ed. Schwartz, L. and Chayes, C. M., pp. 110–115. Philadelphia: Saunders.

Helkimo, M. (1974) Studies on function and dysfunction of the masticatory system. IV Age and sex distribution of symptoms of dysfunction of the masticatory system in Lapps in the north of Finland. *Acta odont. Scand.*, **32**, 255–267.

Kawamura, Y. (1968) Mandibular movement, normal anatomy and physiology and clinical dysfunction. In *Facial Pain and Mandibular Dysfunction*, ed. Schwartz, L. and Chayes, C. M., pp. 37–82. Philadelphia: Saunders.

Krogh-Poulsen, W. G. and Olssen, A. (1968) Management of the occlusion of the teeth. In *Facial Pain and Mandibular Dysfunction*, ed. Schwartz, L. and Chayes, C.M., pp. 236–280. Philadelphia: Saunders.

Kydd, W. L. (1959) Psychosomatic aspects of temporomandibular joint dysfunction. *J. Amer. dent. Ass.*, **59**, 31–44.

MacDougall, J. D. B. and Andrew, B. L. (1953) An electromyographic study of the temporalis and masseter muscles. *J. Anat.*, **87**, 37–45.
Marbach, J. J. and Lipton, J. A. (1978) Aspects of illness behaviour in patients with facial pain. *J. Amer. dent. Ass.*, **96**, 630–638.
Møller, E., Rasmussen, O. C. and Bonde-Petersen, F. (1979) Mechanism of ischemic pain in human muscles of mastication: intramuscular pressure, EMG, force and blood flow of the temporal and masseter muscles during biting. In *Advances in Pain Research and Therapy*, Vol. 3, ed. Bonica, J. J., Liebeskind, J. C. and Albe-Fessard, D. G., pp. 271–281. New York: Raven Press.
Nally, F. F. and Moore, D. S. (1975) Psychogenic, diagnostic and therapeutic aspects of temporomandibular joint pain: an analysis of 232 patients with discussion. *J. Canad. dent. Ass.*, **41**, 403–406.
Newton, A. V. (1969) Predisposing causes for temporomandibular joint dysfunction. *J. pros. Dent.*, **22**, 647–651.
Newton, A. V. (1981) Personal communication.
Randow, K., Carlsson, K., Edlund, J. and Öberg, T. (1976) The effect of an occlusal interference on the masticatory system. An experimental investigation. *Odont. Revy*, **27**, 245–256.
Schwartz, L. (1968) The pain-dysfunction syndrome. In *Facial Pain and Mandibular Dysfunction*, ed. Schwartz, L. and Chayes, C. M., pp. 140–155. Philadelphia: Saunders.
Schwartz, L. and Chayes, C. M. (1968) *Facial Pain and Mandibular Dysfunction*. Philadelphia: Saunders.
Schwartz, L. and Cobin, H. P. (1957) Symptoms associated with the temporomandibular joint. *Oral Surg.*, **10**, 339–34.
Sicher, H. (1948) Some aspects of the anatomy and pathology of the temporomandibular articulation. *New York State dent. J.*, **14**, 451–469.
Steiner, J. E., Michman, J. and Litman, A. (1974) Time sequence of the activity of the temporal and masseter muscles in healthy young human adults during habitual chewing of different foods. *Archs. oral Biol.*, **19**, 29–34.
Taverner, D. (1959) Facial pain. *Brit. dent. J.*, **106**, 65–71.
Thomson, H. (1959) Mandibular joint pain. *Brit. dent. J.*, **107**, 243–251.
Thomson, H. (1971) Mandibular dysfunction syndrome. *Brit. dent. J.*, **130**, 187–193.
Travell, J. (1976) Myofascial trigger points: clinical view. In *Advances in Pain Research and Therapy, Vol. 1*, ed. Bonica, J. J. and Albe-Fessard, D. G., pp. 919–926. New York: Raven Press.
Tweedie, T. O. (1981) Personal communication.
Worth, H. M. (1974) The role of radiological interpretation in disease of the temporomandibular joint. In *Temporomandibular Joint — Function and Dysfunction, II*, ed. Melcher, A. H. and Zarb, G. A. *Oral Sciences Reviews*, **6**, 3–51. Copenhagen: Munksgaard.
Yemm, R. (1969) Variations in the electrical activity of the human masseter muscle occurring with emotional stress. *Archs. oral Biol.*, **14**, 873–878.
Yemm, R. (1971) A comparison of the electrical activity of masseter and temporal muscles of human subjects during experimental stress. *Archs. oral Biol.*, **16**, 269–273.
Zarb, G. A. and Thompson, G. W. (1975) The treatment of patients with temporomandibular joint pain dysfunction syndrome. *J. Canad. dent. Ass.*, **41**, 410–417.

15

# Pain due to soft tissue lesions

Both local and systemic conditions may leave the soft tissues of the mouth more susceptible to trauma including that caused by hard substances in food such as bones. Though chronic gingivitis is not usually painful lateral periodontal abscesses occur (Chapter 12) and there can also be local abrasions and small gingival abscesses which cause a small amount of pain for a few hours.

## ULCERATION

### Acute ulcerative gingivitis

This disease might be expected to cause more pain than it does, but only occasionally is pain severe, and most patients complain of soreness rather than pain. More usual complaints are of bleeding gums, bad taste in the mouth and halitosis, the latter being so bad that diagnosis can sometimes be made upon the patient entering the surgery. However, all cases are not straightforward and there may well be pain on percussion which could conceivably give a false idea of periapical abscess, but electric pulp testing reveals a vital pulp.

Pain is more likely to be a feature when acute ulcerative gingivitis affects the erupting lower third molars, and any patient with the disease may experience pain on eating.

*Treatment*

Metranidazole (Flagyl) is prescribed as 200 mg tablets, taken with water, 3 times a day for 3 days. Oral hygiene instruction and care are essential.

### Traumatic ulcers

Small ulcers can be caused by a foreign body or bone in food (Fig. 15.1). They can also be caused by the patient's finger nail and, occasionally, this is done deliberately by the patient who is trying to attract attention, and the psychological background of such a case must be considered. It is worth noting that low grade trauma may cause a level of pain which some people find pleasurable (in the metaesthetic range). Many people have noted this with the application of matrix bands or copper rings to teeth, and also with some lip biting. The latter can lead to traumatic ulcers usually during the time that the lower lip is anaesthetised following an inferior dental injection, though pain is not experienced until the anaesthesia wears off. The position of such an ulcer is related to the incisal edges of the teeth. Similar ulcers can be caused by a blow to the mouth (Fig. 15.2).

An unusual case is illustrated in Fig. 15.3 which shows the emergence from the lower lip of part of the crown of an upper incisor fractured a year earlier and buried in the tissues.

Traumatic ulcers are also produced by dentures, and pain due to dentures will be considered later in this chapter.

**Chemical burns**

The oral mucosa can be damaged by phenols or other chemicals injudiciously applied or which leak during treatment (Fig. 15.4). Patients may apply chemicals such as aspirin and cause similar damage.

**Aphthous ulcers**

Although they are usually small, aphthous ulcers cause patients considerable discomfort and may interfere with eating. The first

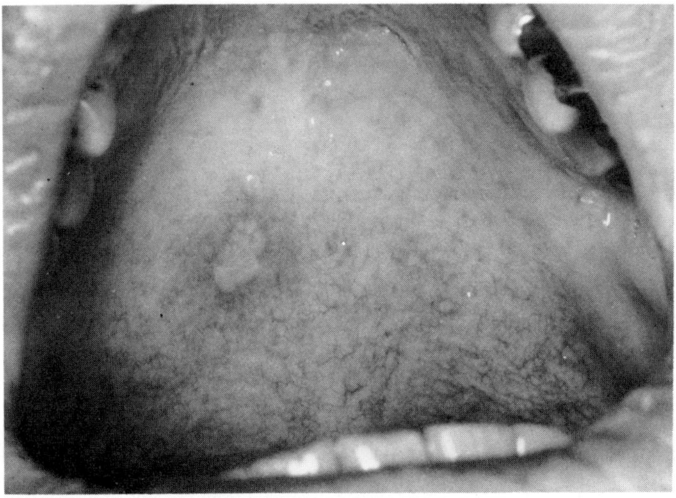

**Fig. 15.1.** Traumatic ulcer in the palate caused by a bone in food.

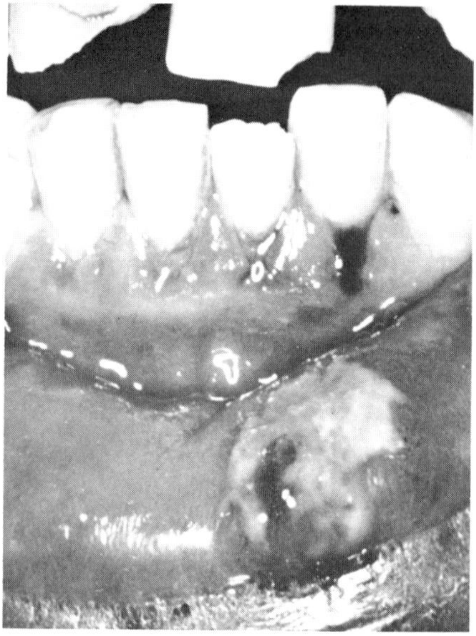

**Fig. 15.2**. Traumatic ulcer of the lower lip caused by a blow to the mouth. Notice also the fractured teeth and the damaged gingival margin.

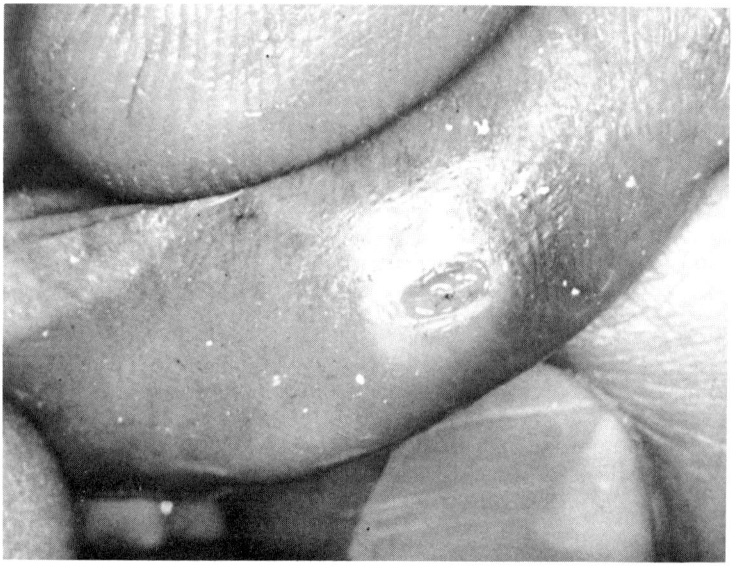

**Fig. 15.3**. Part of an upper central incisor emerging from the lower lip. It was fractured a year earlier, buried in the lip and forgotten.

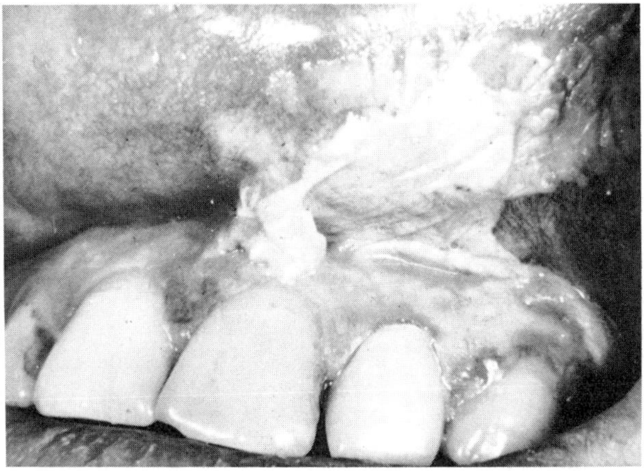

**Fig. 15.4**. Chemical burn.

sign is a prickly or burning sensation in the mucosa which becomes reddened. and an ulcer forms within 24 hours. Most ulcers are small, 2–3 mm diameter, oval shaped, yellowish craters, each one surrounded by a red base which is slightly raised (Fig. 15.5). They are not really painful until subjected to stimulation by food when they 'smart'.

The lesion heals of its own accord in a few days without scarring, but outbreaks of aphthous ulcers occur at intervals for no obvious reason, though stress is a factor, possibly by its effect on autoimmune activity.

Major aphthous ulcers also occur. These are more severe variants of the same condition (Lehner, 1968) and may be as large as 2 cm diameter. They last longer and cause considerable discomfort (Fig. 15.6). They gradually increase in size, unlike herpetiform lesions which enlarge by coalescence of a number of smaller ulcers. Many different foods cause pain, for example, salty foods which should be avoided.

The considerable pain and discomfort experienced by some patients may become serious, leading to anorexia, loss of weight, anaemia, depression and even suicidal tendency (Walker, 1973). They heal with the formation of scars which might even distort the soft palate (Tyldesley, 1973b).

*Treatment*

The aetiology of aphthous ulceration is poorly understood, so they are treated symptomatically. A 0·2 per cent mouthwash of chlorhe-

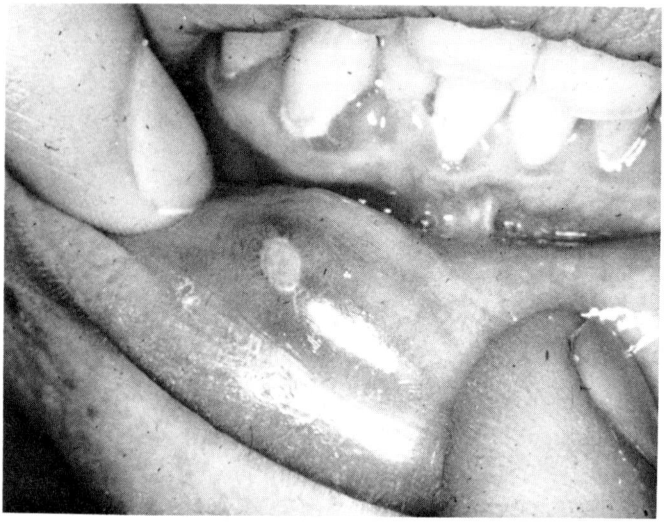

**Fig. 15.5.** Small aphthous ulcer on the lip showing the crater of the ulcer and the surrounding inflamed mucosa. (Professor E. D. Farmer's case.)

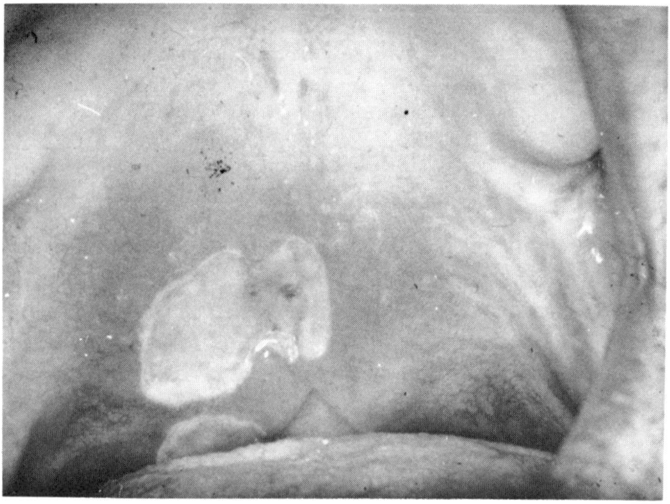

**Fig. 15.6.** Two major aphthous ulcers on the soft palate, one almost hidden. The unpleasantness of this can be understood. (Professor E. D. Farmer's case.)

xidine gluconate (hibitane) is used in 10 ml quantities for a minute twice a day, and this reduces discomfort. The ulcers can be covered by a protective layer which adheres long enough for the patient to eat a good meal, such as carboxymethylcellulose gelatin paste (Orabase). This material may have a steroid added which is anti-inflammatory and thus reduces pain. Steroids may also be used locally as pellets (Corlan) 2·5 mg dissolved in the mouth in contact with the ulcer 4 times a day for children as well as adults. In very severe cases it might be justified to use steroids systemically but such treatment should be avoided because of the risk of adrenal suppression (Tyldesley, 1981).

There are also a number of proprietary gels available with various compositions and these are massaged onto the ulcers several times a day, usually before meals or before going to bed.

**Herpes**

The primary infection with herpes is acute herpetic stomatitis which occurs early in life, possibly being mistaken for teething trouble (Cawson, 1974). There is malaise with raised temperature and submandibular lymphadenitis, this area being tender. Groups of vesicles occur in the oral mucosa and break down to form ulcers. During this period the mouth is sore but the condition resolves in about 10 days (Tyldesley, 1973a).

Alternatively the primary infection may be almost subclinical, but in both cases the infection remains in the tissues for life and any debilitation of the patient can lead to outbreaks of herpes or cold sores. These occur on or near the lips but can be farther afield. The first sign is a slight burning sensation or irritation of the affected area. By next day vesicles form; these break down and become crusted over as the typical cold sore (Fig. 15.7). This is

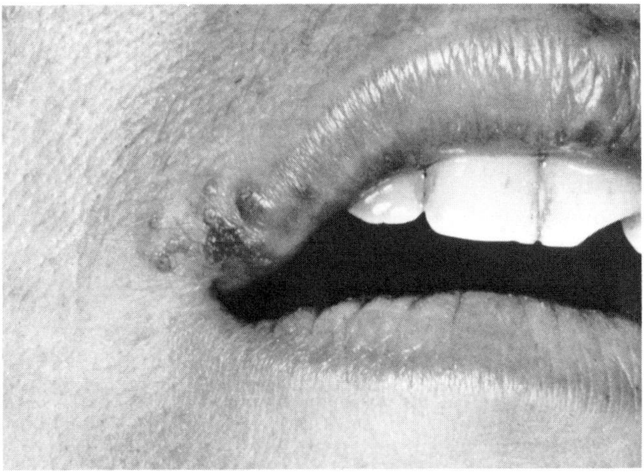

**Fig. 15.7.** Herpetic lesion at the corner of the mouth involving the skin and vermilion border.

uncomfortable rather than painful and, though the surface heals, it tends to break down again because of the mobility of the lips, and this allows secondary infection. The submandibular lymph nodes become enlarged and tender on pressure.

When herpetic lesions spread farther afield and there is considerable pain it is important to consider the differential diagnosis of herpes zoster (Chapter 16).

### Herpetiform ulcers

Numerous tiny vesicles occur on the oral mucosa, especially the lateral borders of the tongue. They are grey, without a red border, and are difficult to see. They soon break down to form ulcers which may coalesce, at which stage they are very painful, sufficiently so to justify treating them with a 2 per cent tetracycline mouthwash, despite objections to using antibiotics in this way (Tyldesley, 1973b).

*Treatment*

A 2 per cent tetracycline mouthwash decreases pain by reducing secondary infection. It also reduces the number of new ulcers occurring (Denman and Schiff, 1979). However, there are objections to using antibiotics in this way especially for recurrent conditions so the method should be used only in emergency; use of hydrocortisone cream is also controversial (Tyldesley, 1981).

For skin lesions the early application of 5 per cent idoxuridine several times a day relieves irritation.

There are a number of proprietary ointments and gels which can also be used in the treatment of oral ulceration, stomatitis, cheilitis and denture irritations. (Also, see Angular cheilitis later in this chapter).

### Neoplastic ulcer

A squamous celled carcinoma can occur in any part of the oral mucosa and may ulcerate, such as that occurring on the side of the tongue (Fig. 15.8). Pain occurs because nerve endings are no longer protected by the lost surface tissue, because there may be nerve involvement and because of infection of the damaged tissue. Movement of the tongue makes the pain worse so chewing, swallowing and speech are all more difficult. The pain is a mixture including a burning sensation, and there may also be pain referred to the ear. An additional problem is halitosis.

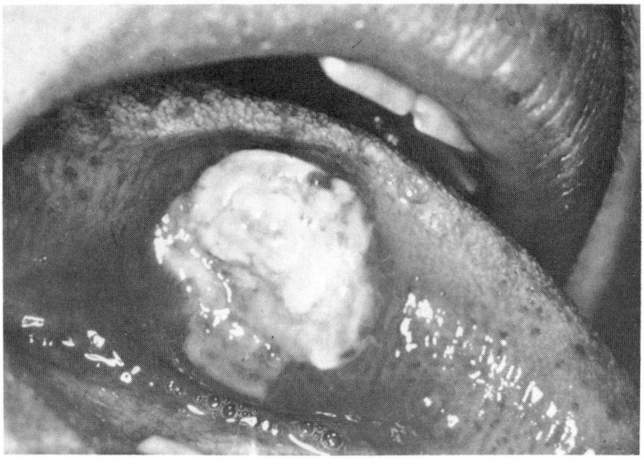

**Fig. 15.8.** Carcinoma of the tongue (Dr W. R. Tyldesley's case).

*Treatment*

This is complex, requiring the attention of many different health professionals (Chapter 13).

## GLOSSODYNIA

Glossodynia is often thought of as being pain in the tongue without obvious cause and, if the condition remains idiopathic, it is possible to adduce evidence for emotional conflict, sexual maladjustment and cancerphobia (Ziskin and Moulton, 1946). However, before doing so it is necessary to consider other conditions including those which occur frequently.

The tongue is frequently subjected to trauma, especially by the patient biting his tongue as a result of momentary incoordination during chewing. The pain is immediate and the patient stops chewing forthwith while he assesses the situation. He then goes back to chewing rather more carefully, at least for a while. Such cases are so common that, as a rule, the patient does not even present himself for treatment. Pain, though it can be momentarily severe, rapidly subsides to a mild level which causes only slight inconvenience. It ceases in a few hours to two days, unless biting is repeated. Related to the above was the case of a 70 years' old lady who complained, not of pain, but of intense soreness. The tongue took up too much room, especially when she was not busy. It appeared normal but the lingual enamel of her lower incisors was worn to a sharp edge.

Trauma during dental operations also causes pain in the tongue and care is naturally taken to avoid this by proper techniques and by using guards where necessary. The patient's attention should not be drawn to his tongue because he then moves it about unnecessarily.

Trauma from ill-fitting dentures, bridges, crowns and other restorations can also cause pain in the tongue, as can sharp edges of enamel associated with caries or fractures. The patient is often able to indicate the cause himself but, occasionally, careful examination is needed.

Pain in the side of the tongue may be of a constant burning character and related to galvanism (see later). However, some patients complaining of a sore tongue may only be doing so as an indirect way of saying that they do not like their new dentures.

When an ulcer occurs on the side of the tongue and has lasted for some time in any age group but especially in an older person, a squamous celled carcinoma must be considered (Fig. 15.8).

When there is deficiency of vitamin B12, folic acid or iron an early sign can be pain or a burning sensation in the tongue, the tip and margins of which become smooth and red. Disturbance of taste may also occur. These are not constant findings, however, and there may be no soreness of the mouth even in advanced anaemias (Jones, 1973). This author also suggested that a burning sensation might arise in association with diabetes because of the poor reaction to infection in such patients.

Rarely, pain in the tongue may be due to glossopharyngeal neuralgia (Chapter 16). In the first instance pain is likely to be attributed to some other factor such as a lower denture (Franks, 1970) and only when easing this fails might the true condition be diagnosed.

Pain in the tongue may occur in trigeminal neuralgia (Chapter 16), and Cohen (1959) stated that it is almost invariably a feature or trigeminal neuralgia affecting the mandibular division.

*Treatment*

Biting of the tongue and cheek is controlled by the patient but it is helpful to palpate the teeth to detect and then remove sharp cusps and sharp edges. Only small amounts of tissue need be ground away to restore comfort. The same procedure is used for crowns, bridges and partial dentures. Denture clasps also need consideration and the patient is likely to indicate what is wrong.

Ulceration is treated as suggested earlier, and neuralgic pains are included in the overall treatment of idiopathic trigeminal neuralgia (Chapter 16), provided that any denture overextension has been eliminated as a possible cause.

Possible nutritional deficiency should be investigated and faults rectified, giving Vitamins where indicated. Iron deficiency is treated with 200 mg ferrous sulphate twice daily, folic acid deficiency with 5 mg folic acid once a day, or both materials given if needed. Burning sensations are considered later.

It is frequently appropriate to reassure the patient that the tongue symptoms do not indicate cancer.

## PAIN AND SALIVATION

Increased flow of saliva may be provoked by noxious stimulation of the oral tissues, and a jet of saliva is sometimes seen spurting from the orifice of the sublingual duct. Similarly, tears may appear brimming over the lower eyelids when a hypodermic needle is inserted near the upper anterior teeth, often to the patient's embarrassment. Stimulation of the anterior part of the oral cavity has a greater effect in provoking salivary flow than stimulating other orofacial areas, and painful stimulation provokes more saliva than does gustatory stimulation (Kawamura and Yamamoto, 1977).

When patients experience pain on the thought of eating, salivary gland disease must be suspected, although it may be necessary to actually start eating before pain occurs. The salivary glands are firmly encapsulated which means that pressure rises if saliva cannot escape into the mouth. The result is that the patient feels the area to be tense. Pain in the upper part of the parotid gland may be confused with a temporomandibular joint problem. In some cases there is a purulent salivary discharge from the orifice of the duct, the orifice being possibly inflamed.

Mumps is a virus disease which causes enlargement of the parotid gland, usually followed by the contralateral gland within a few days. There is pyrexia, malaise, trismus, pain and tenderness in the area, and flushing of the overlying skin. Swelling is variable but reaches a peak in 2 days, after which it subsides during a week or two.

### Calculus in the duct

The effect of a calculus in the submandibular salivary duct depends on its size, the duct being blocked to a greater or lesser extend, so that as saliva forms it cannot escape, the gland swells, pressure rises and there is pain. Gradually the saliva escapes, the swelling subsides and pain decreases. A lateral radiograph sometimes shows the calculus in the duct, but an occlusal radiograph might reveal it better (Fig. 15.9), and sialography might show the blockage (Fig. 15.10). The patient whose calculus is shown in the above figures illustrated the pain as in Fig. 15.11.

It is interesting that the above patient did not have the calculus removed and returned 3 years later. By this time the condition had become more chronic and the calculus had grown in size, so that it was readily palpated. (The operator places one hand under the submandibular region, supporting it while he uses his other forefinger to palpate in the mouth). Although the pain was chronic there were acute exacerbations during which time 'life became difficult'. At this stage he illustrated the pain by drawing a rather different graph (Fig. 15.12). At this time pain developed more slowly, taking about 2 minutes to reach a mild intensity which it never exceeded, and fading away over a period of about 10 minutes

When a calculus is left untreated it is possible that pieces may occasionally be shed, and that there will be some fibrosis within the gland together with a reduction of secretory activity. The gland

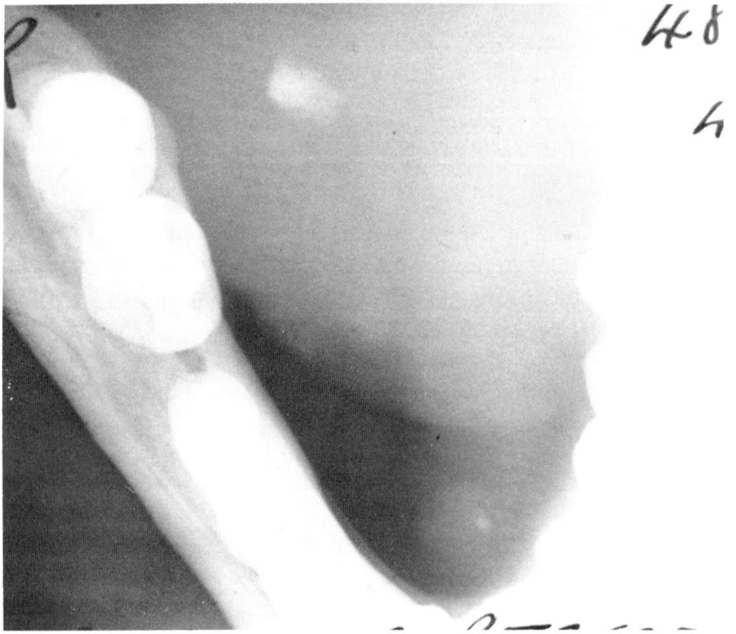

**Fig. 15.9.** Calculus in the submandibular duct (occlusal view).

may atrophy, or it might become hypertrophic with the result that the area over it looks swollen as seen from the neck.

Experimentally, back pressure has been applied to the submandibular gland of a human subject via a small polyethylene tube inserted into the duct (Kawamura and Funakoshi, 1964). When the back pressure approached 60 mm mercury the subject experienced

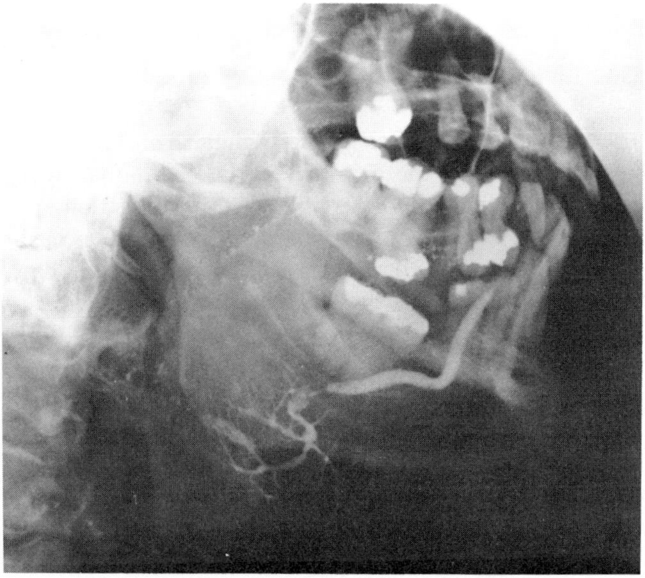

**Fig. 15.10**. Submandibular sialogram, showing dilatation of the main duct on both sides of the calculus. Same case as Fig. 15.9.

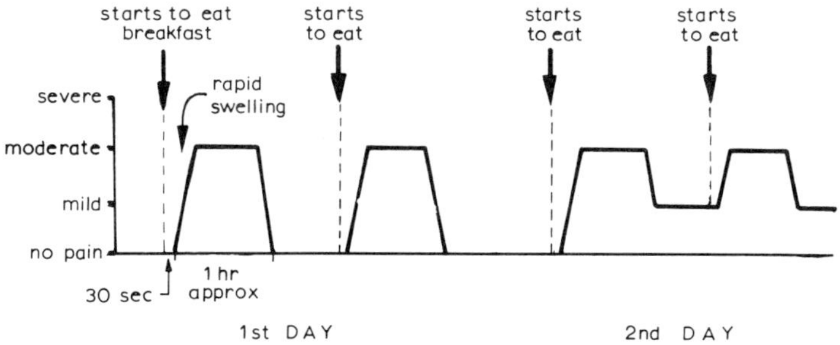


**Fig. 15.11**. Pain due to a calculus blocking the submandibular gland. The patient suffered several bouts during 2 days. About half a minute after starting to eat there was rapid swelling of the gland which was painful for about 1 hour. On the first day he was completely free of pain between bouts, but on the second day pain never ceased completely.

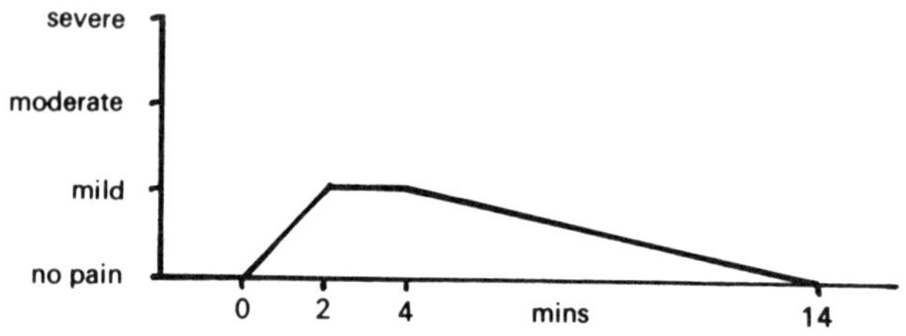


**Fig. 15.12.** Same patient as Fig. 15.11 but 3 years later. Pain is only mild. It rises over about 2 minutes, stays at its peak for about 2 minutes and subsides over about 10 minutes. The patient cannot really tell if the pain has ceased.

a diffuse swelling sensation along the sublingual area of the floor of the mouth, and when the pressure reached 90 mm mercury the sensation became painful. Extending their investigations to dogs Kawamura and Funakoshi found that the nerve impulses mediating pain were carried in the chorda tympani nerve. Also on dogs, they showed that increasing the back pressure to 104 mm mercury induced only a slight dilation of the ductal system.

*Treatment*

Mumps is treated by analgesic antipyretics e.g. soluble aspirin. Severe inflammation requires antibiotic treatment.

Calculus sometimes comes away in fragments but surgical treatment is usually required.

## PAIN DUE TO DENTURES

### New dentures

When dentures are inserted, especially the first dentures to be worn, the patient may suffer a great deal of pain. How much pain depends on various factors, not least being the amount of planning beforehand and the care taken in all stages of construction. For these reasons 'immediate' dentures, placed after extraction and surgical adjustment of the tissues, usually cause less pain and discomfort than do 'temporary' dentures made and inserted during the early post-extraction period (Anderson and Storer, 1973).

Pain due to new dentures may occur from the time they are first inserted but proper adjustment at the fitting stage at least partly alleviates this. Generalised discomfort may arise from movement of the dentures on the mucosa, faulty occlusal relationships and incorrect occlusal height.

More troublesome pain takes a little longer to develop, and may be due to over-extension of the periphery of the denture causing ulceration. Ulceration and pain are also likely to occur whenever there is a bony protuberance, especially in the area of the canine eminence (Fig. 15.13). In such situations the mucosa is subjected to excessive pressure and abrasion from the denture. On the lingual side of the denture pain may arise from pressure on a thin mylohyoid ridge. Also in this area, over-extension of the denture flange may cause a 'sore throat'.

Patients may complain of pain in a well defined area, occurring on eating but not on talking. This pain is often severe with a burning quality, and can also radiate. For example, a patient complained of pain shooting towards the eyes from the regions where the upper canine teeth had been, and it was found that the mucosa over both canine eminences had been severely abraded. This is a good example of how pain from dentures can be bilateral, a possibly helpful point in diagnosing.

At other times the patient is unable to localise the pain to any particular place or places. This makes the dentist's task very difficult for if he 'eases' the denture he may spoil the final fit and retention, and this may also prolong discomfort. On the other hand there may be places on the denture which could be trimmed only slightly to give considerable relief of pain, if only the places could be detected!

In diagnosing these cases it may be helpful to use pressure relief cream. The fitting surface of the denture is dried and the cream is

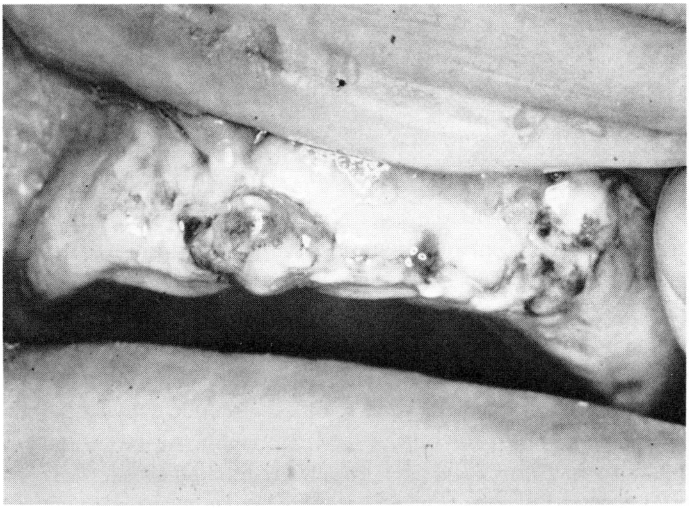

**Fig. 15.13.** An edentulous patient with a traumatic ulcer over the left canine eminence (indicated by the finger tip). (Mr A. V. Newton's case.)

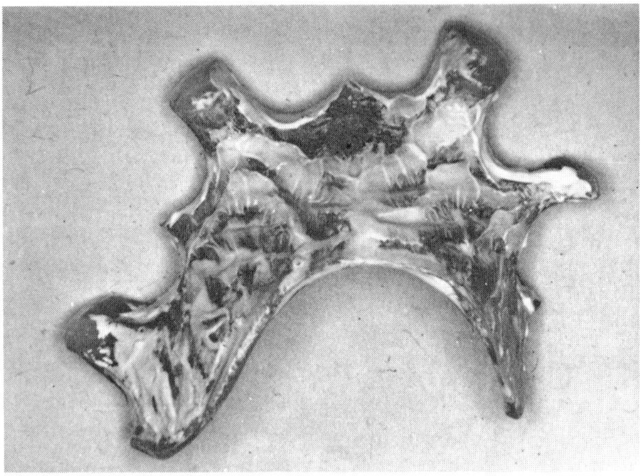

**Fig. 15.14.** Fitting surface of partial denture covered with pressure relief cream which is missing where pressure is greatest, behind the upper central incisors.

applied evenly to the entire surface. The oral tissues are kept moist with saliva. The denture is seated in the mouth using pressure which simulates biting; this has a slight backward component in the lower jaw and a forward component in the upper jaw. On removing the denture the area of undue pressure is indicated by an area denuded of cream (Fig. 15.14). The denture is reduced in this zone, cream re-applied, and the procedure repeated until pressure becomes evenly distributed.

In cases such as that illustrated it is fortunate that this method of diagnosis is available because they can be confusing. In addition to pressure on the gingiva there is a tendency to 'strip' the gingiva away from the tooth thus leaving exposed cervical dentine which may be sensitive to hot, cold and sweet foods. Pain may have been occurring for months and may last for hours. Even if the correct adjustments are made damaged tissues do not stop hurting for some time, so the entire situation is difficult for both patient and dentist. It is not surprising that, in some cases, the dentist only pretends to trim the denture and, provided a thorough examination is made of the mouth and denture, this is sound psychological treatment, for at least the patient knows that the dentist has examined him and nothing serious is amiss. Included in the examination will be a search for buried teeth, fragments of tooth and bone sequestra which might be pressing on the mucosa from below. Pain is likely to be greater when there is thinner mucosa as in older people, occlusal forces being less well distributed. Also when the underlying alveolar ridge is irregular and sharp.

*Treatment*

It is usually possible to evaluate overextended dentures by careful observation and manipulation of the tissues. Such dentures are appropriately reduced and the roughened surface polished again. In some cases pressure relief cream is used as described above. Other dentures may be improved by the use of soft linings, but it may be necessary to start afresh with new dentures, perhaps with a different material, a different design or a more carefully estimated occlusal height. Since this approach is extravagant an attempt is first made in most cases to encourage the patient and reassure him about the successful outcome.

In treating such cases the dentist must call on all his understanding of people to try to assess not simply the physical condition, but also the patient's psychological state and attitude to pain, both real and anticipated. Some patients who are very co-operative and try hard to adjust to their dentures actually persevere too long with the result that damage becomes greater than it should be allowed to do, and pain persists for a correspondingly longer time. Patients should be re-examined a day or two after the dentures have been inserted.

**Pressure on the mental nerve**

One special case worth mentioning is that in which the lower dentures presses directly on to the mental nerve. This situation arises following extensive physiological resorption and remodelling of the alveolar bone, with the result that the mental foramen comes to lie much nearer to the upper border of the mandible. Pain may be localised near the mental foramen or it may spread backwards along the line of the mandible, and paraesthesia of the lower lip and chin might even occur. Such a case may be confused with a true trigeminal neuralgia.

*Treatment*

The area of the mental foramen has less pressure applied to it by having the denture (or a new one) relieved in the area.

**Pain due to sliding movements**

The pain and discomfort experienced early in the life of a denture may wear off and the denture appear to be satisfactory, but after a time pain may occur due to faulty occlusion.

For example, a patient with complete upper and lower dentures complained of pain in the midline on the lingual aspect of the lower alveolar ridge. No obvious fault was found on examination of the mouth, with and without the dentures in place, but when the up-

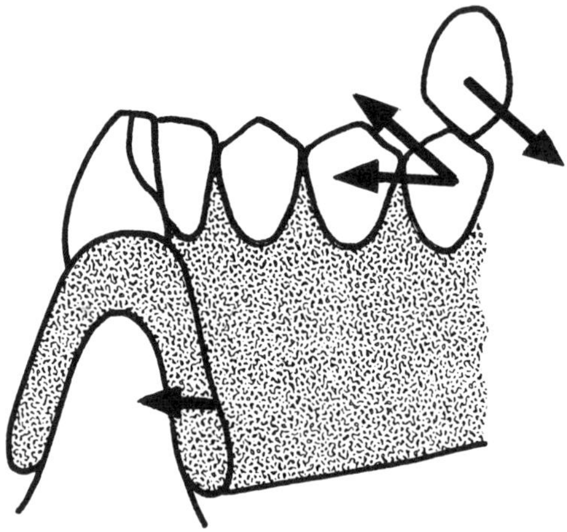

**Fig. 15.15.** Sliding contact in the premolar area produced a resolved component of force which pushed the lower denture forwards, causing pain on the lingual aspect of the alveolar ridge in the anterior region.

per and lower teeth occluded there was an obvious displacement of the lower denture which precipitated the pain (Fig. 15.15).

*Treatment*
Suitable grinding of the cusps eliminates the forward displacement and pain ceases.

**Angular cheilitis**
If the patient's dentures allow overclosure of the mouth the skin at the corners of the lips may crack and allow infection to occur with candida albicans and other micro-organisms. Sometimes the submandibular lymph glands are affected and tender. The condition is uncomfortable with small increases in pain as the partially healed lesion cracks again.

Angular cheilitis may also occur in a number of conditions (such as anaemias) when the general health of the patient is poor. But it is worth noting that the general health may not appear to be poor, so, if no obvious denture fault exists e.g. occlusal height, investigations for nutritional deficiency must be considered.

*Treatment*
New dentures are made, taking special care to obtain the correct occlusal height.

**Denture sore mouth**

The mucosal area underlying an upper denture frequently becomes affected by this condition, although under lower dentures the mucosa is less often affected. The cause is denture trauma followed by secondary invasion by candida. Small areas of inflammation develop first around the orifices of the ducts of the palatal mucous glands, and spread to produce a generalised hyperaemia of the entire denture bearing area (Newton, 1962). Denture sore mouth may take years to develop and, despite inclusion of the word 'sore' in the name, the condition is not usually painful and may never be noticed by the patient.

## BURNING PAIN

Systemic causes of burning sensation in the mouth include menopause, diabetes and nutritional deficiencies, including vitamin B12, folic acid or iron. Local causes include sharp edges and cusps on teeth due to dental caries and wear, especially lower incisors, and also due to incorrectly packed and contoured fillings. Dentures are important in a number of ways including a rough fitting surface especially if there is undue movement of the denture. Lack of freeway space means that excessive pressure may be applied to the alveolar ridge. Overextension of the periphery, badly designed and positioned clasps, and inadequate space for the tongue are also factors. Excessive residual monomer may be present, or the denture may be inadequately cleaned. These problems are made worse if the tongue is active, and the tongue is probably the most frequent site of burning sensation in the mouth. The palate and alveolar ridge are also affected. Any cancerphobia can make sensations seem more sinister as well as more intense, and this fear is also likely to be associated with the condition of geographic tongue.

In addition to the problems mentioned dentures also interfere with the normal sensory input, the texture of food being not so well appreciated. In other words there is presumably decreased activity in nerves mediating the sense of touch, so there is diminished modulation of activity in the smaller nerve fibres (Chapter 4) and this partly explains the burning pain.

Burning sometimes seems to be associated with galvanism, i.e. electrolytic activity between metallic restorations with different electrode potentials (Chapter 9). There is no doubt that electric currents occur and these may be sufficient to cause pain but the electric cell polarises rapidly and the current decreases with the result that pain ceases to occur. However, small currents might still be able to produce the burning sensation which some people complain of.

Misuse of mouthwashes, toothpaste or other drugs must be considered, and drug idiosyncrasy, whether systemic or by direct contact, is sometimes responsible for burning sensations. Sometimes patients complain of painful areas of the oral mucosa which are sufficient to prevent them from eating but which appear normal to the dentist. It is conceivable that some of these are postherpetic but it is not easy to tell. In such cases a local anaesthetic test can be used. The usual method of infiltration or regional injection is not advised because, although the mucous membrane will be anaesthetised, so will the deep structures, and this will not allow accurate definition of the suspected area. For this reason the local anaesthetic should be applied as a surface agent whenever it is suspected that the pain is of mucosal origin. If considered desirable the patient can be shown how to apply the surface anaesthetic himself, and relief of pain allows him to have a good meal, which is morale-raising in itself. Although the cause is not necessarily known the patient can usually be reassured.

Occasionally patients complain that the gums and mucous membrane are hurt by certain foods. One lady said that when she ate tomatoes they hurt her mouth and seemed as though they were 'taking the skin off'. Regrettably, the only helpful suggestion was that she should stop eating tomatoes.

Similarly, cheese eaten in considerable quantities can leave some mouths sore, presumably by an osmotic effect. A really hot curry, though pleasurable to some people, may be not just distasteful but actually painful to others; Keele (1971) has explained that the stimulation produced is in the metaesthetic range for the former groups, but in the algaesthetic range for the latter (Chapter 5).

Certain toothpastes, perhaps used in excessive amounts, can 'sting' when first applied or can leave the oral mucosa feeling 'tight', presumably by its astringent action.

*Incidence*

In a survey of 392 patients attending general dental practice it was found that 5 per cent of patients had experienced a prolong burning sensation at some time, half of whom had it at the time of questioning (Basker, Sturdee and Davenport, 1978). These authors also found that 20 per cent of 114 women attending a menopause clinic had burning sensations in the mouth. They found that 10 per cent of 110 patients being treated for diabetes had burning sensations in the mouth or strange tastes. These results seem high, but they were responses promoted by questionnaire and it might be thought preferable to obtain results from a survey of patients whose complaints were unprompted.

*Treatment*

In most cases it is appropriate to deal with the local factors first. Sharp edges of cusps and other dental faults are corrected. If galvanism seems a likely cause restorations made of different metals are to be avoided, and replacement with composite restorations may be helpful even though they are not really strong enough for routine use. Dentures are adjusted or even new dentures made if necessary, perhaps to a different design, with different materials, with minimum coverage of tissue, accurate fit and correct occlusal height. Sliding pressures are avoided and clasps placed even more carefully than usual to avoid 'inviting' the tongue to play with them; they may even be avoided altogether. The patient must not wear them at night and perhaps not even in the day for the misery of a constant burning pain may exceed the patient's natural wish to look nice.

Systemic factors are dealt with by making good dietary deficiencies of vitamins and iron, by diabetic control or by appropriate hormonal treatment.

Food such as cheese or tomatoes or anything else the patient notices can be avoided, but intractable cases will need the attention of a specialist in allergy problems.

The patient should try different toothpastes and not use excessive amounts unnecessarily often.

Reassurance is given that the burning pain does not indicate a cancer to patients with anxiety about it.

Psychological problems are considered and stressful situations avoided or reduced. Since excessive tea or coffee drinking provides too much caffeine the amount may have to be reduced.

Regrettably some cases still persist but the patients need to know that they can still bring their problems to the clinician. Fortunately, when everything has been tried and apparently failed the burning pain sometimes ceases so one should not give up trying.

**Post-incisional pain**

Post-incisional pain is said to occur most often after thoracotomy, herniorrhaphy and lateral cervical incisions (Maroon and Janetta, 1973); the onset of pain may begin immediately after operation or may start 'explosively' some weeks or months later. Sometimes this seems to happen in the mouth following a Caldwell Luc operation for the investigation and treatment of the maxillary sinus, but there are also cases following apicectomy operations. The patient complains of pain in the area and the pain may be burning. He may have been seen by several different specialists and there may also be suggestions that the pain is psychological. Sometimes the patient points to the scar or near it. In both cases it may be found that the apicectomy has been imperfectly performed.

*Treatment*

Occasionally, removal of the scar stops the pain but it may not do so. However, this is a simple operation to do, using electrocautery or cryosurgery, and should be tried.

Alternatively, a repeat apicectomy is done if there is even a small suggestion of an untreated lateral canal or a spicule of apex left.

However, some cases seem to have psychological features, so the surgeon may be reluctant to repeat an operation.

REFERENCES


Anderson, J. N. and Storer, R. (1973) *Immediate and Replacement Dentures*, 2nd ed. Oxford: Blackwell.

Basker, R. M., Sturdee, D. W. and Davenport, J. C. (1978) Patients with burning mouths. A clinical investigation of causative factors, including the climacteric and diabetes. *Brit. dent. J.*, **145**, 9–16.

Cawson, R. A. (1974) Oral Ulceration. *Prescriber's Journal*, **14**, 13–20.

Cohen, H. (1959) Facial neuralgias. *Brit. dent. J.*, **107**, 9–18.

Denman, A. M. and Schiff, A. A. (1979) Recurrent oral ulceration treated with mysteclin: a controlled study. *Brit. med. J.*, **1**, 1248–1249.

Franks, A. S. T. (1970) Lecture to the Liverpool and District Odontological Society. 16 March 1970.

Jones, J. H. (1973) The oral mucous membrane markers of internal disease. *Brit. dent. J.*, **134**, 81–90.

Kawamura, Y. and Funakoshi, M. (1964) A study of baro-receptive nerve fibres from the submandibular gland of the dog. *Japan. J. Physiol.*, **14**, 528–537.

Kawamura, Y. and Yamamoto, T. (1977) Salivary secretion to noxious stimulation in the trigeminal area. In *Pain in the Trigeminal Region*, ed. Anderson, D. J. and Matthews, B., pp. 395–404. Amsterdam: Elsevier/ North Holland.

Keele, K. D. (1971) A physician looks at pain. *J. Roy. Coll. Surg. (Edin).*, **16**, 15–23.

Lehner, T. (1968) Autoimmunity in oral diseases, with special reference to recurrent oral ulceration. *Proc. Roy. Soc. Med.*, **61**, 515–524.

Maroon, J. C. and Janetta, P. J. (1973) Pain following peripheral nerve injuries. In *The Neurosurgical Approach to the Relief of Pain*, pp. 20–32. Chicago: Year Book Medical Publishers.

Newton, A. V. (1962) Denture sore mouth; a possible aetiology. *Brit. dent. J.*, **112**, 357–360.

Tyldesley, W. R. (1969) *Oral Diagnosis*. Oxford: Pergamon.

Tyldesley, W. R. (1973a) Oral medicine for the dental practitioner. 2. Infections of the oral mucosa. *Brit. dent. J.*, **135**, 449–455.

Tyldesley, W. R. (1973b) Oral medicine for the dental practitioner. 4. Recurrent ulcers. *Brit. dent. J.*, **135**, 537–541.
Tyldesley, W. R. (1981) *Oral Medicine*. Oxford: Oxford University Press.
Walker, J. E. G. (1973) Aphthous ulceration and vitamin B12 deficiency. *Brit. J. oral Surg.*, **11**, 165–170.
Ziskin, D. E. and Moulton, R. (1946) Glossodynia: a study of idiopathic oral pain. *J. Amer. dent. Ass.*, **33**, 1422–1432.

# 16

# Neuralgia

Neuralgia is a word frequently used in a loose and inaccurate way to mean a dull constant pain, especially in the face, such wrong usage being not confined to lay people. The word is also used to mean pain along the course of a nerve, the area affected corresponding with the anatomical distribution of the nerve. This is alright up to a point but in many cases pain cannot be said to be along the nerve (Fig. 16.1). It is better to think of neuralgia as indicating pain due to something wrong with the nerve itself and/ or its central connections (primary neuralgia) as opposed to other diseases which involve the nerve or encroach on it in some way (secondary or symptomatic neuralgia). In other words, neuralgia is

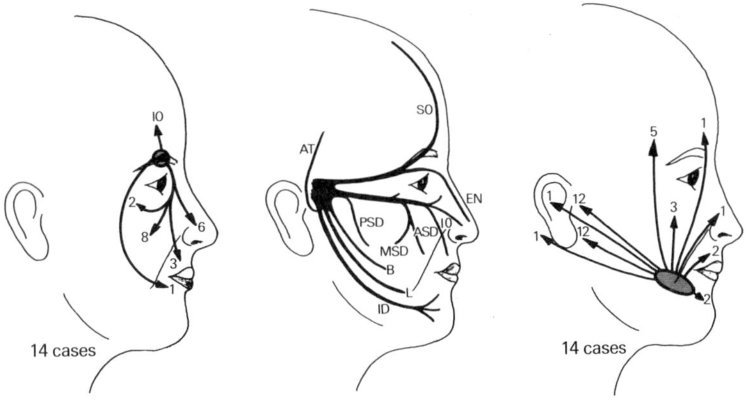


**Fig. 16.1** The main branches of the trigeminal nerve are represented in the middle drawing. The results of Rasmussen (1965) are re-drawn at each side.

On the left are 14 cases with a trigger point in the eyebrow showing the directions of the shooting pains reported. The 10 upwards are along the course of a nerve, and so are the 6 along the nose, but the 2, 8, 3 and 1 are *not* along the course of a nerve.

On the right are 14 cases with a trigger point in the lower lip area. The 26 to the ear are along the course of a nerve, and also 2 to the lower lip. The upward directed 2, 1 and 3 are not. Still less the 5 to the temple and 1 to the supraorbital area.

The same argument applies to the 51 cases represented in Fig. 16.2.

what it says — nerve pain, and its main feature is usually a severe shooting pain of sudden onset and brief duration with little or no stimulation needed to produce it, and occurring intermittently. Whatever it is that is wrong with the nerve is not fully understood so the condition is idiopathic.

## IDIOPATHIC TRIGEMINAL NEURALGIA

In severe cases pain can occur spontaneously but in most cases there is a recognisable stimulus which is most likely to be touch, eating, talking, washing, shaving, or cold winds and draughts. These activities stimulate an area of skin or oral mucosa called a trigger zone (see later) causing a severe, unilateral, paroxysmal, shooting pain which seems to be superficial in most cases. There may be only one jab of pain or several in quick succession, each lasting about a second or less. The person appears transfixed, hardly daring to move until the attack ceases, this occurring either abruptly or more gradually. Afterwards, there is a pain-free period until the next attack. So severe is the pain in some cases that the patient lives in fear of it and avoids activity that might provoke it. For example, the skin may not be washed or shaved, the teeth and gums not cleaned or the hair not brushed. The patient may wear a scarf to protect the face against cold air or he may walk backwards into the wind.

In such a classical or typical case diagnosis is straightforward, but many cases are non-classical or atypical and present difficulties. Also, there is no simple division into typical and atypical cases; rather is there a continuum from one to another. Moreover, there are other orofacial conditions which cause comparable severe shooting pain and these have not always been recognised. Add to this some semantic confusion and it is not surprising that precise description varies from one author to another.

The duration of an attack may be only seconds (Kerr, 1970) but although the jabs of severe pain are thought to last only seconds, the effective duration of the attack is also described as one or two minutes (Kugelberg and Lindblom, 1959; Rasmussen, 1965), and Fothergill's early description (1776) of a quarter to half a minute still sounds good. After recognising the jab as being only about a second the patient may say that she has to wait 5–10 minutes while the pain dies.

The intensity of an attack and its duration can vary from day to day or even hour to hour, so the case may seem different at different examinations (Kugelberg and Lindblom, 1959). There may be transient contractions at the angle of the mouth or of the eyelids, coincident with the attack, and these give the disease one of its names — tic douloureux. There may also be increased lacrimation and associated rhinorrhoea, but this is not peculiar to idiopathic trigeminal neuralgia for it occurs with other pain in the anterior part of the mouth and face (Kawamura and Yamamoto, 1977) (Chapter 15).

There is then an interval before the next attack and this is very variable, possibly lasting for weeks, days, hours, or maybe only minutes in which case the patient may describe the pain as being almost continuous in an on and off manner.

Remission periods of months or years sometimes supervene, during which attacks do not occur.

There are no abnormal neurological findings such as loss of corneal reflexes, anaesthesia, paraesthesia, muscular atrophy or muscle weakness. If such features are present it is not a case of idiopathic trigeminal neuralgia but a secondary neuralgia, symptomatic of some other condition.

**Incidence**

In a series of 286 patients suffering from facial neuralgia Cohen (1959) found that 270 had trigeminal neuralgia compared with only 12 who had glossopharyngeal neuralgia, 2 with geniculate neuralgia and 2 with great auricular neuralgia.

*Sex*

The condition is more common in women, as recognised by Fothergill (1776) and Patrick (1914), the latter recording 96 males and 104 females, but Peet and Schneider (1952) give a proportion of 3 males to 4 females.

*Age*

Cases have been reported in the first and second decades of life and the number of cases increases in each decade to peak in the 5th and 6th decade before falling off (Patrick, 1914; Peet and Schneider, 1952; Rowbotham, 1954; Onofrio, 1975).

*Side*

The condition is unilateral except in 3 per cent of 689 cases (Peet and Schneider, 1952), 413 cases (Petr, 1970) and 526 cases (Rothman and Wepsic, 1974). Approximately two thirds of cases affect the right side (Patrick, 1914; Peet and Schneider, 1952; Rowbotham, 1954; Rasmussen, 1965; Rothman and Wepsic,

1974), although this is not related to the patient's dominant handed ness or any other factor yet identified. White and Sweet (1969) compiled 16 reports with a total of 6719 patients and found a right side to left side ratio of 1.7:1.

*Division*

The trigeminal nerve divisions involved are given in Table 16.1 from which it can be seen that the ophthalmic division is affected in approximately 30 per cent of cases, the maxillary division in approximately 75 per cent of cases and the mandibular division in approximately 60 per cent of cases. According to Cohen (1959) trigeminal neuralgia affecting the mandibular division is almost invariably accompanied by pain in the tongue.

Lesser parts of the trigeminal system have been described as giving rise to neuralgias, including sphenopalatine neuralgia, auriculotemporal neuralgia and neuralgia of the nerve of the pterygoid canal, but there is some doubt about these being separate entities.

**Table 16.1** Incidence of trigeminal neuralgia (expressed as a percentage of cases with some approximations by JMM)

| Division involved | Peet and Schneider (1952) 689 cases | Rasmussen (1965) 284 cases * | | Petr (1970) 413 cases |
|---|---|---|---|---|
| | | Typical | Atypical | |
| 1st | 3 | 5 | 6 | 7 |
| 1st and 2nd | 14 | 23 | 15 | 12 |
| 2nd | 17 | 16 | 18 | 22 |
| 2nd and 3rd | 37 | 25 | 33 | 34 |
| 3rd | 16 | 19 | 19 | 13 |
| 1st and 3rd | 0.1 | 1 | 2 | 9 |
| 1st, 2nd and 3rd | 12 | 11 | 7 | |
| Bilateral | 3 | | | 3 |

*number in each column not specified

## Trigger zones

Trigger zones are an important feature of trigeminal neuralgia and can be located almost anywhere in the trigeminal receptive area (Table 16.2) but they are most common in the nasolabial fold, on the upper lip, the angle of the mouth and the lateral part of the lower lip (Fig. 16.2). Together, these places account for between 53 and 84 per cent of trigger zones (Table 16.2). Kugelberg and Lindblom sometimes found two trigger zones, and sometimes a zone shift from one place to another during the course of the dis-

**Table 16.2** Distribution of trigger zones (expressed as a percentage of the total with some approximations by JMM)

| Trigger zone | Peet and Schneider (1952) 689 cases | Kugelberg and Lindblom (1959) 30 cases | Rasmussen (1965) * Typical | Rasmussen (1965) * Atypical |
|---|---|---|---|---|
| Nasolabial fold and wing of the nose | 33 | 38 | 32 | 25 |
| Upper lip | 26 | 10 | 19 | 15 |
| Lower lip | 10 | 7 | 14 | 19 |
| Angle of mouth | 15 | | 5 | 4 |
| Eyebrow and upper eyelid | | 3 | 9 | 7 |
| Malar eminence | 9 | | | |
| Diffusely over an area | | 21 | 9 | 22 |
| Skin at lower border of side of chin | | 7 | | |
| Oral cavity | | 14 | 12 | 8 |
| Lower jaw | 7 | | | |

*Based on a study of 284 cases.

ease; sometimes the trigger zone was large and diffuse but in most cases it was small and well defined, as little as 1 or 2 square millimetres. This is in accordance with the small area of receptor fields in the region. Darian-Smith (1970) has suggested that the preponderance of mechanoreceptor fields in the perioral region could account for the high incidence of trigger points in this area.

Onset of pain may be triggered by sneezing or blowing the nose, talking or yawning, swallowing or laughing, washing or shaving, but touch is the effective stimulus rather than stronger stimuli and a tickling sensation is even more effective. As Patrick (1914) stated, 'the peripheral stimulus may be wondrously light', and it is interesting that he actually mentions trigger teeth (though this is not generally accepted).

In addition to the light stimulus it seems essential that the trigger zone and the underlying tissues must be apparently normal, so use of the expression trigger point in other situations is undesirable. For example, when there is a periapical abscess, pressing the finger tip over the apex of the tooth, either on the mucous membrane or on the skin, causes pain, but this is simply tenderness; it is not a trigger point. This can also happen occasionally if the tongue is pressed on the palate overlying an abscessed tooth. In an edentulous area pressure on the alveolar ridge overlying a retained root or irregular bone can also cause a pain which may be quite sharp, but this does not indicate a trigger point. Myofascial pain can often be provoked by pressure over certain areas which are sometimes described as trigger zones; this needs heavy pressure whereas a trigger zone needs only a light touch or tickle. The term should be reserved for situations where a tiny stimulus gives a big effect somewhat as a light touch on a rifle trigger leads to a big energy output.

*Refractory period*
In many cases the attack is followed by a period when triggering does not occur, so touching the trigger zone does not provoke an attack. Occasionally the patient will finger around the area 'searching' for the trigger if the clinician asks. Patients report that they can eat alright or talk in this phase. These are the fortunate ones but others are scared to eat and some sufferers lose a great deal of weight.

*Direction of the shooting pain*
With careful questioning the patient is usually able to indicate the direction taken by the shooting pain and Rasmussen (1965) has taken great trouble over this, analysing his results with respect to the various trigger zones and also whether the cases were regarded

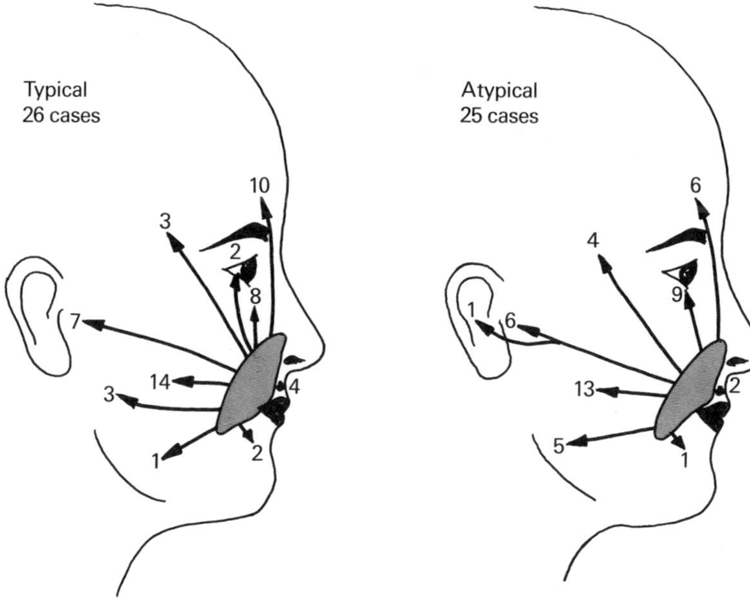


**Fig 16.2.** These cases of idiopathic trigeminal neuralgia are from Rasmussen (1965) but have been redrawn. Rasmussen presented the cases as typical or atypical and it is interesting that the shooting pains reported by his patients are so similar in the two groups.

as typical or atypical. The interested reader should consult this work but two groups are presented in Fig. 16.2, both based on trigger zones in the nasolabial fold and adjacent lips. Though Rasmussen has carefully divided the cases into typical and atypical ones, the shooting pains, taken as two collections, seem almost identical. From this same trigger zone 83 per cent of shooting pains were described as superficial whereas 17 per cent went deep. In comparison, when the trigger zone was in the upper gingiva 53 per cent of shooting pains were described as superficial whereas 47 per cent went deep.

Considerable questioning is needed in some cases to elicit the information and it should not be forgotten that the patient may be very anxious, fatigued and upset, so care is needed. In one case a patient had told me of the shooting pain and I asked, 'Where does it shoot to?' She fixed me with a withering look and replied, 'I

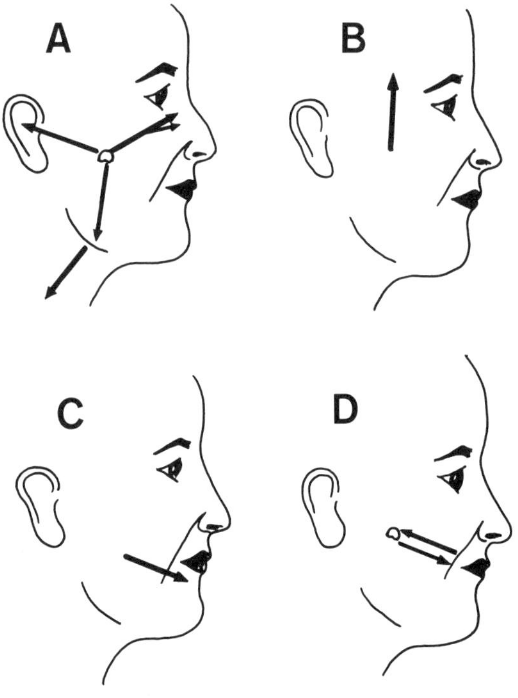


**Fig. 16.3**. Examples of shooting pains proved by successful treatment to be from dental disease. In these examples the sites and directions seem somewhat different from comparable ones in idiopathic trigeminal neuralgia.
A. Acute pulpitis of upper second molar and second premolar.
B. Deep caries of upper canine, and sinus near lateral incisor.
C. Dry socket after extraction of lower second molar.
D. Shooting from upper molar and back to it. Acute pulpitis.

am in no mood for sarcastic questions'. Nevertheless, the information elicited may prove valuable since patients report shooting pains in many other conditions besides idiopathic trigeminal neuralgia. These include herpetic neuralgia, masticatory dysfunction syndrome, malignancy, acute pulpitis, dry socket, pressure on the mental foramen from a denture or residual cyst, and even (rarely) an abrasion cavity or a leaking filling. Such shooting pains may only occur once or a few times, as distinct from the frequent occurrence in idiopathic trigeminal neuralgia. Also, at least in some cases, they start from different sites and move in different directions (Fig. 16.3).

**Aetiology**

The circum-oral skin is richly innervated with thermoreceptors, nociceptors and mechanoreceptors, the latter including hair cells, touch receptors and pressure receptors. The lips in particular have great tactile sensitivity and a delicate touch or tickle at the edge of the vermilion border can be quite unpleasant even in normal circumstances. It is not suggested that there is anything wrong with the skin in idiopathic trigeminal neuralgia but sensory input is essential and this is along nerves with large myelinated axons; without it there is no pain however important more central factors may be in the aetiology of this condition. Similarly, the trigeminal nerve peripheral to the ganglion is not held to be responsible.

However, the condition of the trigeminal ganglion and the immediate postganglionic portion of the root are considered to be of great importance. This part of the trigeminal system has a built-in point of compression where it crosses the petrous ridge of the temporal bone and this causes a considerable bend in the mandibular and maxillary division, though there is much less of a direction change for the fibres of the ophthalmic division (possibly a factor in why this division is less affected?). If, for any reason associated with ageing, the brain should tend to sink further into the posterior fossa the extra compression at the petrous ridge might produce a lesion in the nerve fibres, but this effect is not generally accepted. It seems that ordinary Wallerian degeneration need not occur; instead there can be retention of the axon with loss of myelin (Kerr and Miller, 1966; Moses, 1967). Since the axons thus come to lie closer together, there is opportunity for ionic movements between adjacent fibres so that an impulse in one fibre could be communicated to another — cross talk (Granit, Leksell and Skoglund, 1944). The effect of this could be that neural impulses starting from mechanoreceptors in the skin and travelling in A fibres could set up impulses in the smaller 'pain fibres' thereby increasing the total number of impulses to the level of a barrage which might be the basis of the shooting pain. Kerr (1967) has demonstrated disorganisation of the myelin, and Calvin, Howe and Loeser (1977) agree with him that this is the primary microanatomical pathology of idiopathic trigeminal neuralgia.

Such a demyelinated site might give rise to backward propagation of neural impulses (Howe, Calvin and Loeser, 1976; Calvin, Loeser and Howe, 1977). On reaching the skin these antidromic impulses might set up additional orthodromic impulses thus increasing the total number of impulses. There might be a reverberatory effect if there were not just one reflection site but two, and this would further increase the number of neural impulses. Goldstein and Rall (1974) have suggested a mechanism for this, and Kerr (1967) has pointed out that there is no myelin in the initial glomerulus of Cajal (the part of the limb of the T-junction next to the cell body).

The petrous ridge has therefore received considerable attention. Its height has been measured radiographically in controls as well as in cases of idiopathic trigeminal neuralgia (Gardner, Todd and Pinto, 1956) and it was found that the disease occurred three times as often on the side of the higher petrous ridge than on the lower. Bjerrum and Thornval (1959) obtained a similar result but an investigation of 526 cases by Rothman and Wepsic (1974) found that the height of the petrous ridge could only be a weak factor at the most. Nevertheless the angle of the petrous ridge is very variable (Smith and Mumford, 1980) and this might be a factor independently of its height; though the mean angle in 18 dried skulls was approximately 77° the range was 37–116°. Any influence of the petrous ridge is compatible with the view of Kerr at that time (1970b), that the lesion is located in the immediate post ganglionic portion of the root where fibres of the three divisions are still somewhat separated. Although a strict somatotopic distribution has not been demonstrated in the ganglion there is a tendency for nerve fibres from the perioral area to be more ventrally placed (Kerr, 1970a) and there is some separation of the divisions even in the medulla, so this could be a factor in the greater incidence of pain in the maxillary and mandibular divisions.

In this region the vascular system may have an important influence. The superficial petrosal sinus runs along the petrous ridge between the cavernous and lateral venous sinuses but it may lie above the nerve roots, or between them and the bone (when it might act as padding), or even in a bony canal (Smith and Mumford, 1980). Pressure changes in the sinus might be a factor (Lee, 1937). The internal carotid artery lies inferior to the ganglion, close to it, sometimes intimitely so, and pulsation might be a factor sensitizing the ganglion cells (Kerr, 1979). However, the main vascular factor is thought by others to be pressure from a branch of the superior cerebellar artery (Jannetta, 1967, 1968); he found that 9 out of 11 successful cases (13 attempted) were due to arterial compression. Later, Jannetta (1976) said that the superior cerebellar artery was responsible in cases affecting the maxillary and mandibular divisions whereas the opthalmic division was affected by the anterior inferior cerebellar artery. In this series 6 per cent of cases were due to multiple sclerosis, 6 per cent to tumour or angioma and 88 per cent to vascular compression. However, it should be understood that many procedures in this zone can stop the disease, at least temporarily, and these include

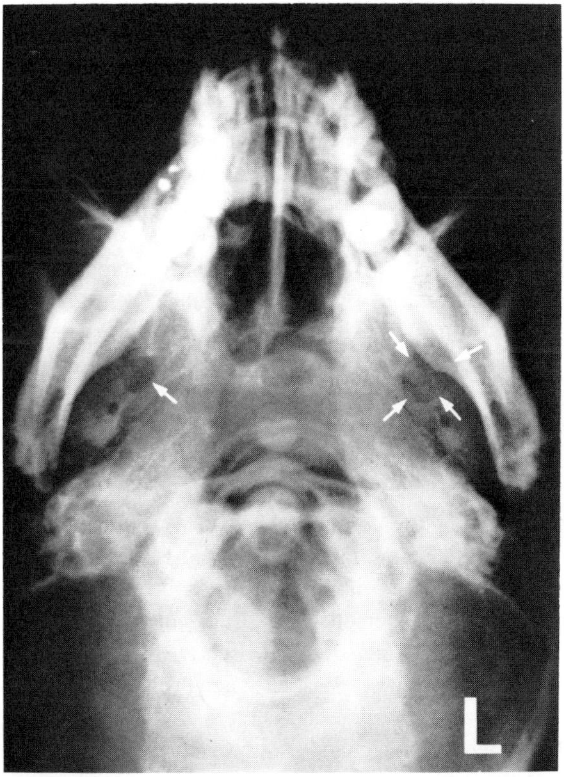


**Fig. 16.4.** Submento-bregmatic radiograph of skull showing expansion of the left foramen ovale by a tumour (Mr John Miles' case).

various forms of small decompressive procedures (Taarnhøj, 1952; Malis, 1967). At present Haines, Jannetta and Zorab (1980) only suggest an association between the condition and arterial compression.

An important cause of compression is that brought about by tumours in the area. Diagnosis of these is aided by the other symptoms and signs that they produce, e.g. an acoustic neuroma causes progressive deafness as well, or there might be radiologically visible changes (Fig. 16.4). At this stage it may be noted that once the cause is found the condition is no longer idiopathic, though the mechanism is not fully explained. The various causative factors also partly account for the atypical forms of trigeminal neuralgia (Yonas and Jannetta, 1980).

Considering next the central connections of the trigeminal nerve, an interesting point may be made about the effect of tooth extraction. Idiopathic trigeminal neuralgia can occur whether the teeth are present or absent, and the teeth are not considered to be a factor in themselves. However, they have a rich nerve supply so extraction is associated with considerable deafferentation in terms of both pulpal and periodontal nerve fibres. It might be expected that degeneration of the nerve fibres would be confined to the parts peripheral to the trigeminal ganglion but degeneration proximal to the ganglion also occurs — transganglionic degeneration — and involves restricted areas of the spinal nucleus (Westrum, Canfield and Black 1976a, b). In cats there is spontaneous neural hyperactivity (Black, 1974) and the cats also demonstrated altered behaviour in so far as they avoided contacts with the affected side of the face (which, of course, is what human patients often do). If deafferentation from loss of teeth were proved to be an important factor it would partly explain the preponderance of the disease in the maxillary and mandibular divisions as opposed to the ophthalmic division.

An important factor could be the failure of inhibition (Denny-Brown, Kirk and Yanagisawa, 1973). Since gamma-aminobutyric acid (GABA) is the commonest inhibitory transmitter in the central nervous system (Iversen, 1979) it is conceivable that deficiency of this could be a factor. The effectiveness of the neurotransmitter at the receptor sites is enhanced by diazepam and other drugs of the benzodiazepine class (Iversen, 1979), so one can wonder if this is why clonazepam is successful in treating some cases. Also it has been suggested that there might be such extensive presynaptic inhibition of small fibres that the threshold of excitation was actually exceeded leading to both orthodromic and antidromic transmission (Calvin, Howe and Loeser, 1977; Calvin, 1979). Calvin also suggested that carbamazapine might work by decreasing presynaptic inhibition.

Other features of importance include summation, both temporal and spacial. In younger patients who have paraesthesia and numbness of the face multiple sclerosis must be considered. With this disease 3 per cent of cases get trigeminal neuralgia (Kerr, 1970 b). Conversely 4 per cent of cases of trigeminal neuralgia were found to have multiple sclerosis (Moses, 1967). The more the case deviates from the classical condition the more necessary does it become to make further investigations including radiography of the skull, angiography and computerised axial tomography.

*The shooting pain*

It is conceivable that cross-talk near the petrous ridge could permit neural impulses in adjacent nerve fibres, one after another, with impulses going to the brain and being interpreted as coming from the periphery, one place after another, so the pain shoots along in a certain direction. But it is also possible to think a barrage of impulses is experienced which, in fewer numbers, would have been interpreted as causing pain from one peripheral site and the patient only interprets them as a shooting effect. If the former explanation were to be correct the shooting effect should presumably be in more than one direction at a time, but this seldom seems to happen. No definite views on this have been found in the literature.

## TREATMENT

The treatment of idiopathic trigeminal neuralgia is either medical or surgical and both approaches may be associated with unfortunate side effects so, before embarking on long term drug therapy or neurosurgical procedures, it is essential to be quite certain that there is not a more peripheral cause of the pain. For this reason it is desirable that a meticulous examination should be made by a dentist.

### Dental

The dentist should preferably be a person who is interested in this subject because the large majority of cases will truly be medical or surgical problems and the tediousness of the dental examination will usually be fruitless and disheartening. Moreover dentists tend to be, quite rightly, conservative; for example, when working on

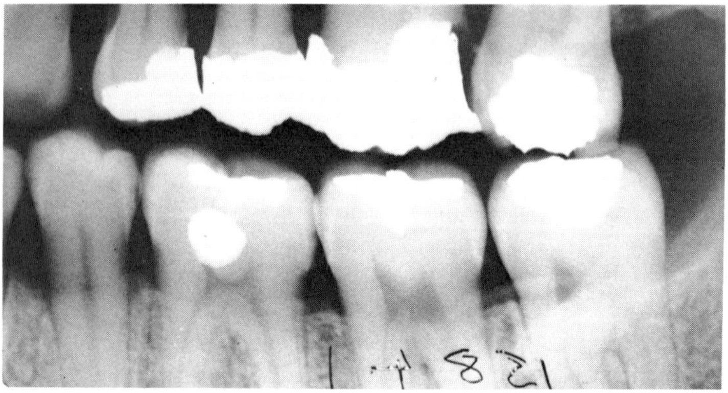

**Fig. 16.5.** After examination by a dentist further radiographs were taken, including computerised axial tomography, and all unnecessary. In a difficult case the deep and badly made filling in the upper molar should have been removed without hesitation. The pulp was found to be exposed and the tooth extracted.

deep dental cavities the dentist probes gently to avoid exposing the pulp, but in cases with pain of unknown origin the probe should be applied strongly so that it can penetrate a thin layer of dentine when the underlying pulp may be diseased. Fillings that might otherwise be left may be better removed (Fig. 16.5). It is hoped that teeth will not be uselessly extracted causing unnecessary mutilation but pulps can be extirpated and the teeth restored after endodontic procedures. In a few cases the dentist's contribution to the problem meets with success and these may involve dentinal faults, pulp disease, retained roots, cysts, impacted teeth, faulty dentures and masticatory dysfunction (Mumford, 1978). Pathological lesions within the bone itself may also be found (Grundt, 1937; Rothen et al, 1974; Ratner et al, 1979; Roberts and Parson, 1979). This means, of course, that the condition was not idiopathic trigeminal neuralgia but some cases are presented which are more surprising.

A female patient, aged 36 years, had a generalised discomfort of the right side of her face, which never completely ceased, with severe attacks of shooting pain. When the pain shot to the ear it always left a sense of deafness and tenderness of the ear. For both the latter reasons she took to holding the telephone against her other ear. Examination revealed that she was somewhat deaf and the neurosurgeon considered the possibility of an acoustic neuroma. Fortunately, a bite wing radiograph revealed deep dental caries in two teeth. Removal of the fillings and caries revealed that both dental pulps were exposed. Both teeth were extracted and histological examination showed acute inflammation of the pulp in each case. Pain ceased, and it transpired that deafness was coincidental.

An edentulous patient was diagnosed as having idiopathic trigeminal neuralgia affecting the third division but radiographic examination revealed a residual cyst close to the mental foramen (Fig. 16.6). This was removed and pain ceased.

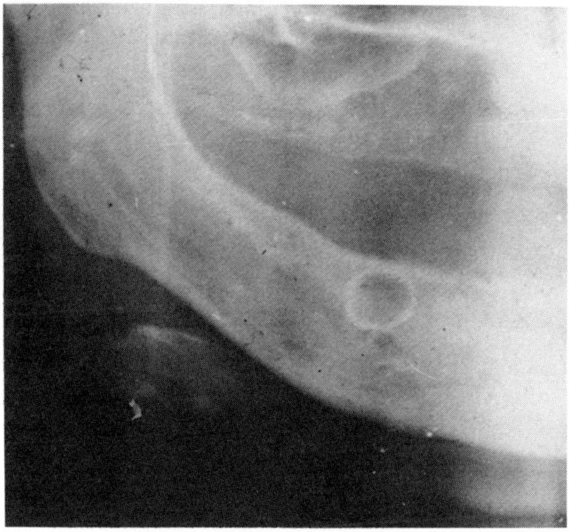

**Fig. 16.6**. After diagnosing idiopathic trigeminal neuralgia of the third division an orthopantomograph revealed a retained cyst. This was dissected out, taking care to avoid the mental nerve, and pain ceased.

Another edentulous patient did have idiopathic trigeminal neuralgia but radiographic examination revealed an additional problem — an unerupted wisdom tooth. This was removed and, remarkably, he recovered 30 pounds in weight that he had previously lost. He looked better and felt much happier and became a much fitter subject for further treatment of the idiopathic trigeminal neuralgia.

Another patient diagnosed as having idiopathic trigeminal neuralgia had a shooting pain just above his left eyebrow. Radiographic examination of this middle-aged man revealed an unexpected impacted lower left second premolar (Fig. 16.7). This was removed with even more care than usual since levering it might have compressed the inferior dental nerve. Pain ceased.

Even when the dentist's efforts have no such dramatic result it is still important to attend to the patient's oral hygiene. Unfortunately this is often overlooked; yet the patient may be frightened

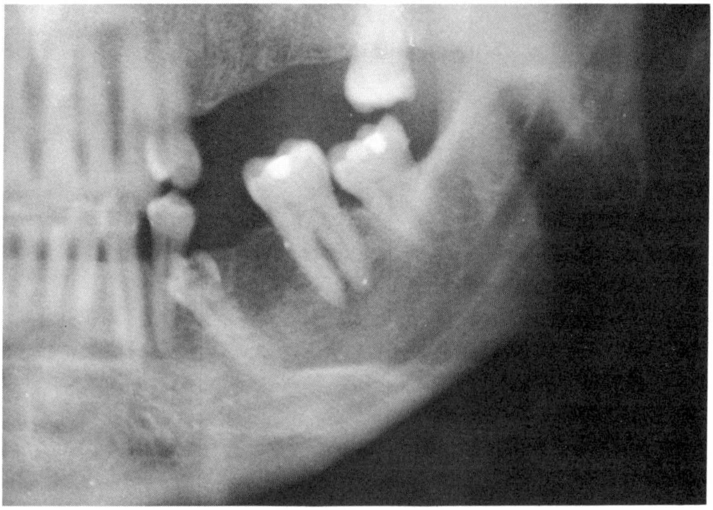

**Fig. 16.7.** With a shooting pain in the forehead this patient was suspected of having idiopathic trigeminal neuralgia of the first division, but there were also aching muscles that made masticatory dysfunction a likely diagnosis (see also Fig. 14.6D). The routine orthopantomograph revealed an impacted second premolar which was removed, taking care to avoid levering it against the inferior dental nerve, and pain ceased right away.

to clean his or her teeth leaving the breath foul and the gums diseased. Proper oral hygiene is needed and the help of a dental hygienist is valuable. It may also be desirable to prescribe a regular mouthwash of 0.2 per cent w/v aqueous solution of chlorhexidine, suitably flavoured.

Summarising the dental requirements, every case should:

1. Be seen by a dentist with more than average understanding of the problem.
2. Have an orthopantomograph of the jaws.
3. Have proper oral hygiene instituted and maintained.

**Medical**

Carbamazapine (Tegretol) is the drug most commonly used. There are two ways of giving it, the most usual being to start with a small dose of 100 mg twice a day and building up to the dose required to control the pain. Alternatively, a larger dose of 600 mg a day may be given and this is likely to work within a couple of days thereby confirming the diagnosis, controlling the pain and raising the patient's morale enormously. Moreover, such a patient can then start to experiment with a progressively smaller dose. However, even larger doses may be needed in some cases, up to

1600 mg a day in four divided doses; this relieves the pain in 75 per cent of cases (Loeser, 1973).

Unfortunately, there are side effects such as nausea, dizziness, drowsiness and even aplastic anaemia so control is needed including blood examination. Tolerance also develops so that this treatment may only be a means of delaying neurosurgery. Nevertheless, it may help the patient to reach a better frame of mind and helps the surgeon to plan the timing and type of surgery (Miles, 1980).

If carbamazapine is not completely successful in relieving pain it may be supplemented with analgesics, or phenytoin (Epanutin) in an equivalent dose may be tried (Hayward, 1977). This should start at 300–400 mg per day and be increased until there is pain relief or toxicity (Loeser, 1977).

**Surgical**

Before any surgical procedure it may be desirable to give an ordinary local anaesthetic nerve block so that the patient gets a reasonable idea of the area and sense of 'deadness'. Some might prefer the pain.

Neurolytic injections may be tried, using either absolute alcohol or phenol, applied either to branches or divisions or even into the ganglion, and these are effective for variable periods usually from months to about two years.

Branches such as the infraorbital or mental nerves may be avulsed, or coagulated using a cryosurgical probe (Gregg et al, 1978; Barnard, Lloyd and Glynn, 1978). These methods are usually successful for a time.

The method of choice for many years has been open operation to cut the sensory root, approaching the root via either the middle cranial fossa or the posterior cranial fossa, the choice depending partly on technical factors and partly on any suspected abnormality in either fossa. The sensory root can be completely divided, taking care to preserve the motor root, or partly divided so as to retain the fibres of the ophthalmic division, this being of great importance to maintain the corneal reflex functioning properly. Introduction of the operating microscope has greatly improved the safety of the posterior fossa approach (Miles, 1980). This can also be used when the intention is to mobilise the posterior superior cerebellar artery (Jannetta, 1976).

Nowadays the method of choice seems to be radiofrequency coagulation of the sensory root. A cannula is directed through the foramen ovale under or through the ganglion to the sensory root in the trigeminal (Meckel's) cave. The end of the cannular is uninsulated and subjected to a radiofrequency current so that it becomes hot and part of the sensory root is coagulated.

When other surgical procedures have been tried and failed the neurosurgeon can resort to cutting the spinal tract of the trigeminal system (trigeminal tractotomy). It should rarely be the initial procedure (Loeser, 1977).

## Anaesthesia dolorosa

Following major operations dividing the trigeminal nerve there are occasional fatalities or various other complications including keratitis following corneal insensitivity. Amongst these is anaesthesia dolorosa which occurs in about 3 per cent of cases (Olivecrona, 1947; Petr, 1970) and, as its name implies, is a painful area in a part that is anaesthetic. However, *analgesia* dolorosa also occurs, some touch sensation being preserved (Sweet, 1976). There may be nothing to see but, after many years, the sufferer may contemplate suicide.

A possible method of investigation is by thermography which shows that the temperature in the area is raised by about 1°C (Fig. 16.8). This does not help treatment but it does help the patient who likes to think the doctor knows that there is objective evidence and the pain is not just imagined (Mumford and Miles, 1977). It may also prove of value in attempting to understand the cause of the pain. One possibility, from animal experiments, is

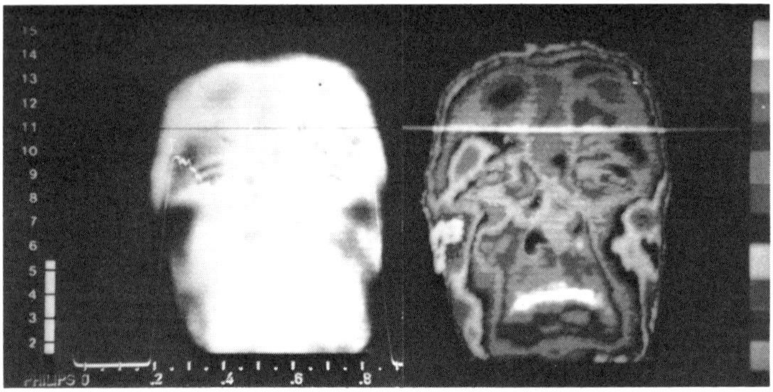

**Fig. 16.8**. Thermographs of a patient with anaesthesia dolorosa affecting the left forehead and orbital area.

*Left*. Black and white thermograph with temperature trace (white) along a selected line (black) across the forehead. White trace shows a temperature 1·2°C higher in the painful area.

*Right*. Original taken in colour with a colour scale of temperature to the right of illustration. This also showed a temperature 1·2°C higher in the painful area.

that the unpleasant sensation is due to activity in the cut and sprouting nerve fibres (Wall, Scadding and Tomkiewicz, 1979). Some cases which seem to be closely related are seen quite often in dental practice after the inferior dental nerve has been damaged in various operative procedures. These patients complain of a burning, tingling sensation in the lower lip which can be so unpleasant as to interfere with eating and cause loss of weight. This condition usually resolves in several months but may take 2 or 3 years.

*Treatment*

Anaesthesia dolorosa is difficult to treat but combinations of analgesics and psychotrophic drugs may be tried, clonazepam being most favoured at the moment (Miles, 1981).

## IDIOPATHIC GLOSSOPHARYNGEAL NEURALGIA

The pain of glossopharyngeal neuralgia is similar to that of trigeminal neuralgia and the paroxysm is similarly triggered by swallowing, chewing, talking, yawning, coughing or sneezing. The timing of the pain is similar to that of trigeminal neuralgia. The trigger zones and the pain are in the tonsils, the pharyngeal wall, the base of the tongue and the ears (Fig. 16.9). As might be expected, eating is an ordeal so there is likely to be loss of weight. The clinician's finger on the tonsil provokes the pain, and the only case who came directly to the author actually lost consciousness on one occasion — according to the patient and his wife. The ex-

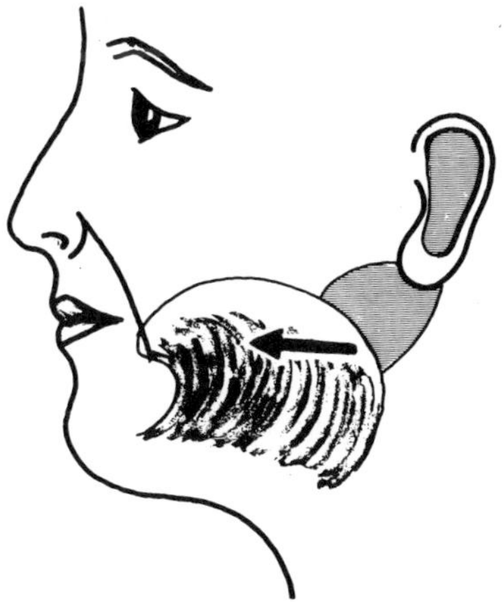

**Fig. 16.9.** Idiopathic glossopharyngeal neuralgia. The shooting pain in the tongue did not reach the anterior part of the tongue. Pain in the ear was like earache, and pain in the tonsillar area was like tonsillitis.

planation of this is said to be that neural impulses from the tonsillar trigger point proceed centrally and are interpreted as coming from the carotid sinus, also innervated by the glossopharyngeal nerve, and the heart slows reflexly. Riley et al (1942) cite two similar cases.

*Incidence*

As stated earlier, Cohen (1959) found 12 cases of glossopharyngeal neuralgia compared with 270 cases of trigeminal neuralgia. The two conditions may be present simultaneously according to Petr (1970) who found 5 such combined cases in a series of 480 cases of trigeminal neuralgia (1 per cent); the pain of both ceased after transection of the sensory root of the trigeminal nerve. Kerr (1967) stated that idiopathic trigeminal neuralgia was 100 times more common than idiopathic glossopharyngeal neuralgia and this proportion seems acceptable.

Even neurosurgeons will see these cases only rarely and a dentist may never see one. However, he will have to consider the problem occasionally when a patient complains of a pain near the tonsil or the posterior part of the lower alveolar ridge and mylohyoid ridge. The likely cause of this is from an over-extended flange of a lower denture which could be stimulating the lingual nerve. Such a denture has the flange reduced and repolished and pain should cease. Also the denture can be left out for a while. Such a case is possible when a patient has worn the same denture for many years and the alveolar ridge has been resorbed, thus allowing the denture to settle lower in the mouth.

*Aetiology*

The aetiology is similar to that of idiopathic trigeminal neuralgia. Ishii (1976) investigated 7 cases and found that 5 had myelin degeneration, especially in the large myelinated fibres. Kerr (1979) reported myelin degeneration in 7 out of 8 cases.

*Treatment*

Carbamazepine is given as for trigeminal neuralgia. If this fails the glossopharyngeal nerve is cut, approaching via the posterior cranial fossa or via the neck.

**Geniculate neuralgia**

This is the analagous condition affecting the seventh cranial nerve and is also known as intermediate neuralgia, the intermediate nerve being the sensory root of the facial nerve. Pain is usually felt deep in the ear, the trigger zone being near the eardrum on the postero-superior wall of the external auditory meatus (Cohen, 1959). The condition is rare.

**Great auricular neuralgia**

There is pain behind the ear and it may be felt at the angle of the jaw (Cohen, 1959), though Kerr (1967) said that idiopathic neuralgia did not occur in the first, second and third cervical nerves.

## HERPETIC NEURALGIA

Herpes zoster (shingles) is a painful affliction caused by latent varicellar-zoster virus infection of a nerve, mainly the ganglion. It frequently affects the trigeminal nerve and, when reactivated, causes intense pain in the distribution area of the affected division, most often the ophthalmic.

In the pre-eruptive phase there is malaise and paraesthesia followed several days later by the eruption of numerous vesicles on both the skin and mucous membrane, the oral lesions being similar to those of herpetic stomatitis but unilateral. Pain occurs spontaneously or may be precipitated by touching some part of the mouth such as the angle of the lips, in which case the patient tends to hold his face immobile. There may also be flushing of the face or upper neck. Pain is described as sharp and lasting approximately one second, or burning (perhaps red hot) and lasting about a minute. The latter may be preceded by a tingling sensation for about a minute. Attacks of pain occur for several days, a week or even two weeks, but it is several weeks before the rash gradually disappears, the face meanwhile being somewhat blotchy in appearance.

As stated above, one of the chief sites affected by herpes zoster is the ophthalmic division of the trigeminal nerve. This is unfortunate for the lesions might involve the cornea where secondary infection, which is always a risk, could lead to scar tissue formation at the site of ulcers. This might endanger vision so it is very important in such a case to institute early antibiotic therapy to control secondary infection. Swelling of the eyelids in such cases may cause the eyes to be temporarily closed. There may also be a second pain — a constant dull ache behind the eye, lasting for several days.

Herpes may involve the facial or glossopharyngeal nerves causing a burning aching pain and redness of the ear, possibly spreading along the upper jaw, and also affecting the tonsil. As with all herpes there may be slight or moderate palsy. The combination of facial paralysis and auricular herpes, with or without tinnitus and vertigo is called the Ramsay Hunt Syndrome.

**Post herpetic neuralgia**

By far the greater number of cases of herpes zoster heal completely and remain pain free (Noordenbos, 1959). Unfortunately, in about 20 per cent of cases (Hope-Simpson, 1975) pain persists as post-herpetic neuralgia, perhaps for months, and may even last for years. Pain is burning or itching in character or may be described as a dull ache. It occurs spontaneously but is made worse by contact, with the result that the patient may withdraw from the clinician's examining hand, i.e. there is hyperalgesia. There may also be a stabbing pain, as well as paraesthesia and some weakness of the masseter and pterygoid muscles on the affected side.

In this disease there is a loss of the larger diameter nerve fibres via which an inhibitory effect is usually exerted over the smaller diameter fibres which are important in the mediation of pain (Chapter 4). Since the larger diameter fibres are lost and they can no longer exert this influence there is less presynaptic inhibition and the area becomes painful.

*Treatment*

At the earliest opportunity, preferable within 2 days of the rash appearing, 0.5 per cent idoxuridine in dimethyl sulphoxide is prescribed and the patient paints this on the lesions and their erythematous bases 4 times a day for 4 days. It penetrates to the deeper layers where the virus is replicating and stops it doing so. The result is a reduction in the period of vesiculation and the duration of pain. Application of stronger solutions, or more frequently gives no advantage (Dawber, 1974; Simpson, 1975).

The reason for early treatment is that once the post herpetic neuralgia starts it has a tendency to become intractable. Various treatments for this have been tried, including acupuncture, transcutaneous neural stimulation, and nerve blocks, but a more hopeful approach is the use of 0.1–0.2 mg buprenorphine taken sublingually. The dose is varied both in quantity and frequency to meet the needs of the case, and side effects must be considered but the sharp, shooting pains and the itch are relieved whilst the tingling, burning sensations and hyperaesthesia are reduced (Brown, 1979).

## Auriculo-temporal syndrome

Also called Von Frey's syndrome, this condition is due to damage of the auriculo-temporal nerve causing a paradoxical gustatory reflex. There are paroxysms of unilateral burning pain in the temple and/or temporomandibular joint area, associated with flushing and sweating when the patient eats. Between the attacks the skin may be hyperaesthetic.

REFERENCES

Barnard, J. D. W., Lloyd, J. W. and Glynn, C. J. (1979) Cryosurgery in the management of intractable facial pain. *Brit. J. oral Surg.*, **16**, 135–142.

Bjerrum, J. and Thornval, G. (1959) Roentgenography in trigeminal neuralgia. *Acta Radiol. (Stockholm)*, **51**, 289–296.

Black, R. G. (1974) A laboratory model for trigeminal neuralgia. In *Advances* in Neurology, Vol. 4, ed Bonica, J. J., pp. 651–658. New York: Raven Press.

Brown, D. (1979) Sub-lingual buprenorphine in post-herpetic neuralgia. *Proc. Intractable Pain Soc. of U.K.*, held in Dublin (unpaged).

Calvin, W. H. (1979) Some design features of axons and how neuralgias may defeat them. In *Advances in Pain Research and Therapy*, Vol. 3, ed. Bonica, J. J., Liebeskind, J. C. and Albe-Fessard, D. G., pp. 207–309. New York: Raven Press.

Calvin, W. H., Howe, J. F. and Loeser, J. D. (1977) Ectopic repetitive firing in focally demyelinated axons and some implications for trigeminal neuralgia. In *Pain in the Trigeminal Region*, ed. Anderson, D. J. and Matthews, B. pp. 125–136, Amsterdam: Elsevier North Holland.

Calvin, W. H., Loeser, J. D. and Howe, J. F. (1977) A neurophysiological theory for the pain of tic douloureux. *Pain*, **3**, 147–154.

Cohen, H. (1959) Facial neuralgias. *Brit. dent. J.*, **107**, 9–18.

Darian-Smith, I. (1966) Neural mechanisms of facial sensation. *Int. Rev. Neurobiol.*, **9**, 301–395.

Dawber, R. (1974) Idoxuridine in herpes zoster: further evaluation of intermittent topical therapy. *Brit. med. J.*, **2**, 526–527.

Denny-Brown, D. Kirk, E. J. and Yanagisawa, N. (1973) The tract of Lissauer in relation to sensory transmission in the dorsal horn of spinal cord in the Macaque monkey. *J. comp. Neurol.*, **151**, 175–200.

Fothergill, J. (1776) Of a painful affection of the face. *Med. Obsv. and Inquiries*, **5**, 129–142.

Gardner, W. J., Todd, E. M. and Pinto, J. P. (1956) Roentgenographic findings in trigeminal neuralgia. *Amer. J. Roentgenol.*, **76**, 346–350.

Goldstein, S. and Rall, W. (1974) Changes of action potential shape and velocity for changing core conductor shape and geometry. *Biophys. J.*, **14**, 731–757.

Granit, R., Leksell, L. and Skoglund, C. R. (1944) Fibre interaction in injured or compressed region of nerve. *Brain*, **67**, 125–140.

Gregg, J. M., Banerjee, T., Ghia, J. N. and Campbell, R. (1978) Radiofrequency thermoneurolysis of peripheral nerves for control of trigeminal neuralgia. *Pain*, **5**, 231–243.

Grunt, B. (1937) Über die Behandlung der Trigeminusneuralgie peripher natur. *Acta Psychiat. Neurol. Scand.*, **12**, 585–595.

Haines, S. J., Jannetta, P. J. and Zorub, D. S. (1980) Microvascular relations of the trigeminal nerve. An Anatomical study with clinical correlation. *J. Neurosurg.*, **52**, 381–386.

Hayward, M. (1977) Headache and pain in the head and neck. In *Persistent Pain: Modern Methods of Treatment,* Vol. 1, ed. Lipton, S., pp. 35–60. London: Academic Press.

Hope-Simpson, R. E. (1975) Postherpetic neuralgia. *J. Roy. Coll. Gen. Pract.*, **25**, 571–575.

Howe, J. F., Calvin, W. H. and Loeser, J. D., (1976) Impulses reflected from dorsal root ganglia and from focal nerve injuries. *Brain Res.*, **116**, 139–144.

Ishii, T. (1976) Glossopharyngeal neuralgia: surgical treatment and electronmicroscopic findings. *Laryngoscope,* **86**, 577–583.

Iversen, L. L. (1979) The chemistry of the brain. *Scient. Amer.*, **241**, 118–129.

Jannetta, P. J. (1967) Arterial compression of the trigeminal nerve at the pons in patients with trigeminal neuralgia. *J. Neurosurg., Suppl.,* **26,** 159–162.

Jannetta, P. J. (1968) Trigeminal accessory fibres rediscovered. *World Medicine,* Aug. 27th, 13–14.

Jannetta, P. J. (1976) Microsurgical approach to the trigeminal nerve for tic douloureux. *Prog. neurol. Surg.*, **7**, 180–200.

Kawamura, Y. and Yamamoto, T. (1977) Salivary secretion to noxious stimulation in the trigeminal area. In *Pain in the Trigeminal Region,* ed. Anderson, D. J. and Matthews, B., pp. 395–404. Amsterdam: Elsevier/North Holland.

Kerr, F. W. L. (1967a) Pathology of trigeminal neuralgia: light and electron microscopic observations. *J. Neurosurg.*, **26**, 151–156.

Kerr, F. W. L. (1967b) Evidence for a peripheral etiology of trigeminal neuralgia. J. Neurosurg., **26**, 168–174.

Kerr, F. W. L. (1970a) Fine structure and functional characteristics of the primary trigeminal neuron. In *Trigeminal Neuralgia,* ed. Hassler, R. and Walker, A. E., pp. 11–21. Stuttgart: Thieme.

Kerr, F. W. L. (1970b) Peripheral versus central factors in trigeminal neuralgia. In *Trigeminal Neuralgia,* ed. Hassler, R. and Walker, A.E., pp. 180–190. Stuttgart: Thieme.

Kerr, F. W. L. (1979) Craniofacial neuralgias. In *Advances in Pain Research and Therapy,* Vol. 3, ed. Bonica, J. J., Liebeskind, J. C. and Albe-Fessard, D. G., pp. 283–295. New York: Raven Press.

Kerr, F. W. L. and Miller, R. H. (1966) The pathology of trigeminal neuralgia. *Archs. Neurol.*, **15**, 308–319.

Kugelberg, E. and Lindblom, U. (1959) The mechanism of the pain in trigeminal neuralgia. *J. Neurol., Neurosurg., Psychiat.*, **2**, 36–43.

Lee, F. C. (1937) Trigeminal neuralgia. *J. Med. Ass. Georgia,* **26,** 431–436.

Loeser, J. D. (1973) Neuralgia. *Postgrad. Med.*, **53**, 207–210.

Loeser, J. D. (1977) The Management of tic douloureux. *Pain,* **3**, 155–162.

Malis, L. I (1967) Petrous ridge compression and its surgical correction. *J. Neurosurg.*, **26**, 163–167.

Miles, J. (1980) Trigeminal neuralgia. In *Persistent Pain*, Vol. 2. ed Lipton, S., pp. 223–247. London: Academic Press.

Miles, J. (1981) Personal Communication.

Moses, H. L. (1967) Comparative fine structures of the trigeminal ganglia, including human autopsy studies. *J. Neurosurg.*, **26**, 112–126.

Mumford, J. M. (1978) Role of the dentist in trigeminal neuralgia. *Pain,* **5**, 83–92.

Mumford, J. M. and Miles, J. B. (1977) Thermography and orofacial pain. *Acta Thermographica,* **2**, 155–161.

Noordenbos, W. (1959) Pain. Amsterdam: Elsevier.

Olivecrona, H. (1947) La cirugia de dolor. *Arch. Soc. Cirujanes Hosp.*, **17**, 366–372. *Arch. Neurocirg.*, **4**, 1–10.

Onofrio, B. M. (1975) Radiofrequency percutaneous Gasserian ganglion lesions. Results in 140 patients with trigeminal pain. *J. Neurosurg.*, **42**, 132–139.

Patrick, H. T. (1914) The symptomatology of trifacial neuralgia. *J. Amer. med. Ass.*, **62**, 1519–1525.

Peet, M. M. and Schneider, R. C. (1952) Trigeminal neuralgia; review of 689 cases with a follow up study on 65 per cent of the group. *J. Neurosurg.*, **9**, 367–377.

Petr, R. (1970) Results of trigeminal rhizotomy. In *Trigeminal Neuralgia*, ed. Hassler, R. and Walker, A. E., pp, 22–25. Stuttgart: Thieme.

Rasmussen, P. (1965) Facial Pain. Copenhagen: Munksgaard.

Ratner, E. J., Person, P., Kleinman, D. J., Shklar, G. and Socransky, S. S. (1979) Jawbone cavities and trigeminal and atypical facial neuralgias. *Oral Surg.*, **48**, 3–20.

Riley, H. A., German, W. J., Wortis, H., Herbert, C., Zahn, D. and Eichna, L. (1942) Glossopharyngeal neuralgia imitating or associated with cardiac arrest. *Trans. Amer. neurol. Soc.*, **68**, 28–29.

Roberts, A. M. and Person, P. (1979) Etiology and treatment of idiopathic and atypical facial neuralgias. *Oral Surg.*, **48**, 298–308.

Rothman, K. J. and Wepsic, J. G. (1974) Side of facial pain in trigeminal neuralgia. *J. Neurosurg.*, **40**, 514–516.

Rothen, F., Dolfi, G., Mumenthaler, M. and Neuner, O. (1974) Zahnärztlîche Aspekte der Gesichtsschmerzen, insbesondere der Trigeminusneuralgie. *Z. Neurol.*, **208**, 39–51.

Rowbotham, G. F., (1954) Trigeminal neuralgia; pathology and treatment. *Lancet, 796–798.*

Simpson, J. R. (1975) Idoxuridine in the treatment of herpes zoster. *The Practitioner*, **215**, 226–229.

Smith, D. G. and Mumford, J. M. (1980) Petrous angle and trigeminal neuralgia. *Pain.*, **8**, 269–277.

Sweet, W. H. (1976) Treatment of facial pain by percutaneous differential thermal trigeminal rhizotomy. *Prog. neurol. Surg.*, **7**, 153–179.

Taarnhøj, P. (1952) Decompression of the trigeminal root and the posterior part of the ganglion as treatment in trigeminal neuralgia. *J. Neurosurg.*, **9**, 288–290.

Wall, P. D., Scadding, J. W. and Tomkiewicz, M. M. (1979) The production and prevention of experimental anesthesia dolorosa. *Pain*, **6**, 175–182.

Westrum, L. E., Canfield, R. C., and Black, R. G. (1976a) Transganglionic degeneration in the spinal trigeminal nucleus following removal of tooth pulps in adult cats. *Brain Res.*, **101**, 137–140.

Westrum, L. E., Canfield, R. C. and Black, R. G. (1976b) Axonal degeneration patterns in the cat brainstem spinal trigeminal nucleus after tooth pulp removal. In *Advances in Pain Therapy*, Vol. 1, ed. Bonica, J. J. and Albe-Fessard, D. G., pp. 161–164. New York: Raven Press.

White, J. C. and Sweet, W. H. (1969) *Pain and the Neurosurgeon*, 2nd ed. Springfield, I11: Thomas.

Yonas, H. and Jannetta, P. J. (1980) Neurinoma of the trigeminal root and atypical trigeminal neuralgia: their commonality. *Neurosurg.*, **6**, 273–277.

# 17

# Pain of vascular origin

Pain in the face and deep to the face is probably associated with vascular changes more often than is usually thought. It may be just a throbbing artery that the patient notices and becomes anxious about, or it may be one of the well known conditions, chief of which is migraine. This word derives from the original description — hemicrania, half the skull — and hence one-sided headache.

## CLASSICAL MIGRAINE

The classical migraine headache is a unilateral headache with a variable intensity which may be severe and throbbing. It is preceded by various premonitory symptoms mainly involving the eyes. These visual disturbances include blurred vision, coloured lights before the eyes, blind spots and photophobia (so the pa-

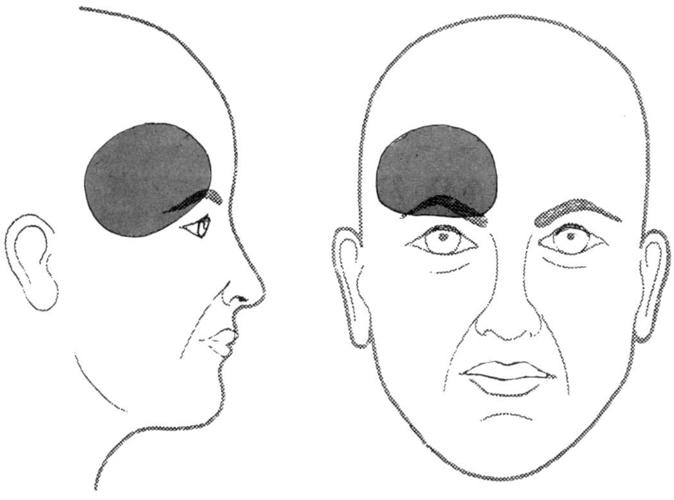

**Fig. 17.1.** Migraine pain is frequently described as temporal or frontal or both.

tient may sit in a darkened room). There may be fortification spectra; i.e. ramparts, turrets, or zig-zags. These premonitory symptoms, which are a valuable warning of impending attack, last for minutes, perhaps half an hour. As they diminish the headache develops and is usually throbbing as well as unilateral. Patients usually indicate the area affected as temporo-frontal (Fig. 17.1), and there is accompanying nausea, dizziness, and probably vomiting.

The intensity and duration of an attack are variable, from several hours to 2 days, and greatly affected by medication and how soon the medication is taken (see below). During this time there may be slurred speech or inability to choose the correct word or phrase, and one patient said that her children laughed when she asked for a 'tup of cea'.

**Mechanism**

The mechanism is vascular, the first phase of the attack, the premonitory symptoms, being due to vasoconstriction of arteries which are branches of the internal carotid artery system. Thus, spasm of the posterior cerebral artery causes ischaemia of the occipital area of the cortex and this produces the visual disturbances already mentioned. If both posterior cerebral arteries are affected simultaneously there may be tunnel vision or even transient blindness (Hayward, 1977). If fainting occurs this is due to the influence of the vertebral-basilar artery system, whereas any confusion of the patient depends upon changes in the carotid system. The vascular effect on the cortex may even prevent the patient from talking properly (as mentioned above) or walking properly — hemiplegic migraine, which may be associated with facial weakness. All of these effects can be frightening.

The second phase of the attack is due to vasodilatation of various branches of the external carotid artery, notably the anterior branch of the superficial temporal artery, but other branches become involved. The arrival of the arterial pulse momentarily increases the blood pressure, increases the number of neural impulses and gives the throbbing quality. At this stage pressure on the artery, which feels full and tender, may reduce the ache.

Although dilatation of the extracranial arteries is so important the skin can be pale, with sweating in severe attacks, and this seems contradictory. However, thermography shows the skin temperature to be approximately 1°C cooler in most cases (Lance and Anthony, 1971; Lance, 1978). This interesting phenomenon supports the view that blood is shunted away from the skin during a migraine attack in spite of the dilatation of the larger arteries, thus leaving the capillary bed under-supplied with blood, so the area is blanched (Saxena, 1978).

**Incidence**

It is estimated that 10 per cent of people suffer from migraine, but only a minority of these have classical migraine. Oleson et al (1979) examined 756 patients with migraine and considered that only 10 per cent were classical cases (which presumably means that only one per cent of the population suffers from classical migraine).

*Sex*

Females represented 75 per cent of cases (Oleson et al, 1979).

*Age*

The first attack of migraine is likely to be in the second decade of life.

*Side*

Although the disease was originally defined as unilateral Oleson (1978) found that no more than 56 per cent of patients had unilateral pain. This seems on the low side but it did derive from a study of 750 cases. However, even when the headache is unilateral there is a tendency for it to spread further afield and become bilateral, and Lance (1978) points out that the definition has widened to include this. Moreover, a headache that was perpetually one-sided without ever affecting the other side would arouse suspicion that there might be an intracranial fault such as an arteriovenous malformation (Miles, 1981).

*Nausea*

This was present in 86 per cent of 750 cases (Oleson, 1978).

*Vomiting*

This was present in 47 per cent of cases (Oleson, 1978).

*Status migrainosus*

This is when the patient wakes each day with the headache.

## COMMON MIGRAINE

In this form of migraine there are no premonitory symptoms, and little or no nausea. It should not be regarded as a separate condition from classical migraine; rather is there a gradient from the most to the least severe, though Lance (1978) distinguishes an intermediate migraine in which the neurological features accompany the headache. At the lesser end of the gradient common migraine shades into ordinary headache. It often seems that patients say they suffer from migraine rather than a headache, because migraine confers a better status (migraineur status) on the patient than does headache, and this should be considered when prescribing treatment.

**Aetiology**

The cause of migraine is not known but many factors have been considered. These include too much sleep, premenstruation, contraceptive hormones, and alcohol, especially red wine. Various foods have been implicated, including cheese, tomatoes, oranges and plain chocolate, and it has been thought that the amino-acid tyramine could be a common factor. Free fatty acids have also been considered, including oleic, palmitic and linoleic acids (Anthony, 1978). Research using the method of dietary exclusion suggests that two thirds of migraineurs are allergic to certain foods (Monro et al, 1980). On the other hand, missing a meal has been implicated. Changes in barometric pressure have been considered, and there may be a familial tendency (Miller, 1965; Bickerstaff, 1967).

The algogenic agents (described in Chapter 10) are thought to be important in migraine, and may accumulate around the dilated arteries. These include histamine (from mast cells) and neurokinin which is related to bradykinin. More than one of these agents might be involved. There is a chronic aggregation of blood platelets associated with a slight rise in serotonin (5HT) at the onset of a migraine attack and the level falls sharply with the onset of headache (Dalessio et al, 1978; Lance, 1978). Sicuteri (1976, 1978) believes that deficiency of cerebral serotonin lowers the pain threshold, and that headache may be of central origin, being genetically determined by deranged metabolism of brainstem monoamines, especially serotonin. He considers as unproven the conventional view that vasodilatation is the chief mechanism in causing pain (1979). Blau (1978) also rejects the conventional view, suggesting that variation in the calibre of vessels in the pia mater can either excite or inhibit the cortex locally, thus producing visual disturbances, etc. This phase is succeeded by a more diffuse alteration in the meningeal blood flow in arteries, capillaries and venous sinuses which affects nociceptive nerve endings in the walls of the venous sinuses especially.

**Treatment**

There is likely to be self treatment in the first instance, and this is appropriate since the trouble might be a simple headache. Simple analgesics such as aspirin or paracetamol are appropriate. If these are not successful a combination of the two, perhaps with codeine is tried.

Once the patient visits his medical practitioner ergotamine can be prescribed in its various forms. Ergotamine tartrate, placed sublingually as 1–2 mg tablets is effective, especially if taken early in an attack before the headache really develops. The dose may be repeated in half an hour (Lance, 1978). Unfortunately, ergotamine tartrate may cause nausea, so use of an ergotamine inhaler may be better, and rapid absorption occurs. The dose is 0.36 mg and can be repeated up to 6 doses at 5 minute intervals, the maximum daily dose being 4 mg. Ergotamine suppositories may be necessary because of nausea and vomiting, or an intramuscular injection of 0·25–0·5 mg. Ergotamine can be given in combination with caffeine, i.e. Cafergot, which consists of 1 mg ergotamine tartrate with 100 mg caffeine. It is taken as 1 or 2 tablets at the onset, maximum 6 daily or 10 in one week. Cafergot suppositories contain 2 mg ergotamine tartrate with 100 mg Caffeine. At onset one is used, with a maximum of 3 daily or 5 in a week. Ergotamine almost certainly acts by direct selective vasoconstriction of the external carotid artery (Lance et al, 1978).

However, the treatment of choice may now be that developed by Wilkinson et al (1978) at the London Migraine Clinic. They give an anti-emetic, such as metaclopramide, 10 mg intramuscularly, along with soluble aspirin 1 g, or paracetamol 1 g. In addition anxious patients are given diazapam, and about 10 per cent are given ergotamine tartrate 1–2 mg orally or 0·25 mg intramuscularly. Over 90 per cent of their patients were either symptom-free or had only a slight residual headache after 4 hours. The earlier the treatment was given the fewer were the headaches experienced in the following 7 days. The better the patients slept whilst in the clinic the better was their recovery when they came to leave, and this was more so with classical migraine than common migraine. A similar approach has been used with similar results in the Copenhagen Acute Headache Clinic (Oleson et al, 1979). These authors also recognised over use of ergotamine in 6 per cent of their series of 756 cases.

Methysergide 1–4 mg daily (Deseril) may be useful as a prophylactic because it antagonises serotonin. So does pizotifen (Sanomigran) the dose of which is 0·5–3·0 mg daily. Monoamineoxidase inhibitors raise blood serotonin levels and may help, according to Anthony and Lance (1969). Clonidine, an antihypertensive agent, may be used in subhypotensive doses, and is thought to stabilise vascular reactivity (Fanchamps, 1975). Drugs blocking the β-adrenergic receptors on the blood vessels may help by diminishing the vasodilator response, such as propranolol (Inderal) (Fanchamps, 1975).

Sleep rationing should be considered. One of the synonyms of migraine is 'weekend headache' which occurs because people are able to stay in bed longer. There seems to be a general assumption that everybody must have 8 hours sleep but this is not the case; still less are 9 hours needed which some patients mention. It is worth trying a reduction of an hour or so, and it is probably a good idea if migraineurs do any reading before they go to bed rather than read in bed because the latter habit keeps them lying down longer. Nevertheless, once migraine has started some people say that sleep is their best treatment, and relaxation was found to be helpful by Oleson et al (1979).

If women taking hormonal contraceptives suffer more frequent or more severe migraine headaches then these contraceptives may have to be stopped altogether, but alternative preparations and doses can be tried first.

Although it is right to start treatment for migraine, before very long it is wise to consider whether special investigation is necessary for possible intracranial pathology, especially in cases of hemiplegic migraine. Now that non-invasive techniques of investigation are so well developed, especially computerised axial tomography, it is desirable in such cases to eliminate potentially lethal disease. Moreover, reassurance is an important part of treatment, especially if the patient is anxious about a possible intracranial tumour, and can only really be given after full investigation; this is also needed for reassurance to be effective. An additional advantage is that successful reassurance reduces the need for tranquillisers or antidepressants.

Once an appropriate line of treatment is established patients learn to deal with the condition expeditiously, taking proper heed of the premonitory symptoms. This is advantageous for two reasons. The first is that the earlier the treatment is commenced the sooner does the pain cease and the less are any after effects (Wilkinson et al, 1978). The second reason is that the accompanying nausea, and possibly vomiting, may make it impossible to take drugs orally, so that suppositories become necessary.

The patient should observe the effects, or rather the after-effects of alcohol and either avoid it, reduce it or choose his or her 'poison' carefully. Similarly, diet should be considered and the patient should observe any possible connection of a particular food with any attack.

Training patients to relax is aided by biofeedback, using various methods such as alpha rythm, electromyograms, muscle relaxation exercises and skin temperature feedback. Diamond and Medina (1978) surveyed 556 patients who had been taught to use biofeedback and obtained 413 replies; 28 per cent had migraine and 69 per cent a combination of migraine and muscle tension headache; 39 per cent believed that biofeedback helped them permanently, and 32 per cent for a limited period. However, it should be remembered that about 36 per cent of patients with many different conditions are helped by the placebo effect. Moreover, an extensive survey of the literature on biofeedback therapy for headache (Jessup et al, 1979) revealed that there were inadequate controls or insufficient cases, that biofeedback is of no more value than relaxation training, and that the application of feedback techniques to migraine is of unproven value.

Other treatments include acupuncture, hypnosis, neck manipulation and transcendental meditation.

## FACIAL MIGRAINE (PERIODIC MIGRAINOUS NEURALGIA)

There is a problem over naming this syndrome, and it is also known as lower half headache or cluster headache, the latter name being given because the attacks come in groups or clusters. However, pain occurs in the face so face ache would be more accurate than headache. The name migrainous neuralgia is inappropriate because the condition is not a neuralgia, being mediated by the perivascular neural plexus (Wyke, 1968), and Lance (1978) also regards the name migrainous neuralgia as a misnomer. The condition used to be known as Horton's Syndrome because Horton (1941) was able to provoke it by injecting histamine which is a vasodilator, but eponymous terms should be avoided whenever possible. The expression facial migraine is intended to convey only the idea that pain has its origin in vascular changes as does migraine, but without necessarily being fundamentally the same condition.

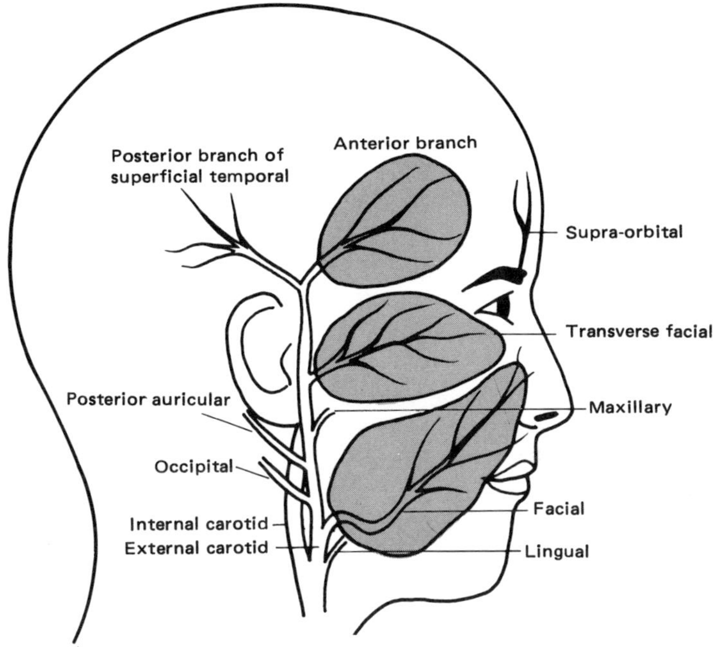


**Fig. 17.2** Superficial arteries of the face. Pain may occur in areas such as the three shaded zones.

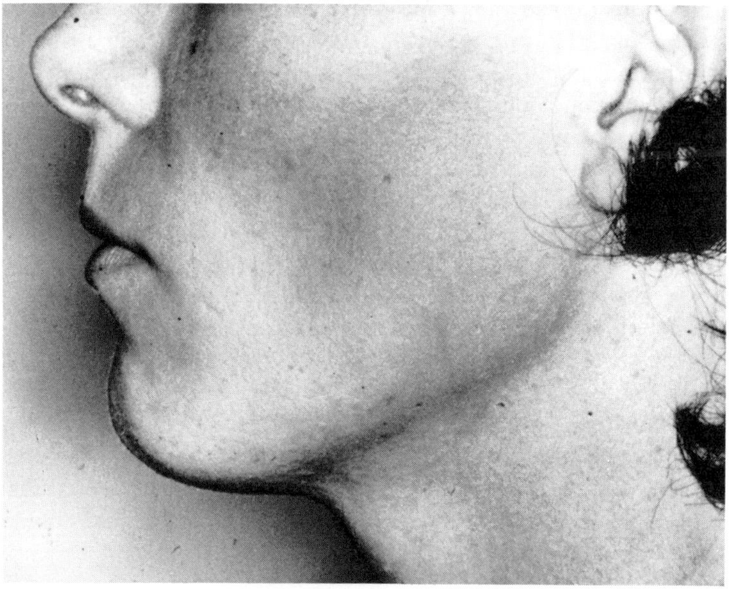

**Fig. 17.3**. Flushing of the cheek and zygomatic area in a case of periodic migrainous neuralgia. This was unilateral and is much more obvious on the subject or in a colour photograph.

The attacks may come day or night, those at night occurring regularly for a short period between midnight and three o'clock and each attack lasts 10 minutes to three hours (Turner, 1959; McArdie, 1970). Since it wakens the patient regularly it has also been called 'alarm clock headache'. After a week to several weeks the 'cluster' of headaches ceases, and there is spontaneous remission for months or years.

Pain occurs unilaterally in the distribution area of one of the facial arteries (Fig. 17.2) which is found to be tender on pressure. More than one artery may be affected and the patient shown in Fig. 17.3 seems to have flushed in the area *between* the facial and transverse facial arteries, as though it were in the capillary area common to these two large vessels. The pain is described as boring or burning, but is only throbbing in 10 per cent of cases (Pearce, 1980). The conjunctival vessels may be involved so the eye is red and watery, which may allow overflow of tears and also a running nostril. Similarly the vessels of the nasal mucosa may be affected. There are no visual disturbances, and no nausea and vomiting, because the cerebral blood vessels are not affected.

Lance (1978) says that the pain can also be experienced in the upper and lower gingiva and in the roof of the mouth. This is not the author's experience but pain cases are very selective in the kind of practitioner they go to or are sent to.

Occasionally during an attack there may be ptosis and a smaller than normal pupil (Horner's syndrome) presumably because carotid vasodilation compresses the enveloping sympathetic nerve plexus, fibres of which reach the pupil via the deep petrosal nerve and the sphenopalatine ganglion.

When the anterior branch of the superficial temporal artery is affected the area involved is similar to that of migraine headache (Fig. 17.1 left, and Fig. 17.2), and also pain due to undue tension in the anterior fibres of the temporalis muscle (Fig. 14.5); these two conditions might go together to some extent. Similarly, involvement of the posterior branch of the superficial temporal artery might be confused with undue muscle tension in the posterior fibres of the temporalis muscle. This area may be supplied by the lesser occipital nerve which could be involved in disease of the upper cervical vertebrae (Fig. 18.8). Ekbom (1974, 1975) considered that cases affecting the orbital and supraorbital area might be mainly due to change distally in the internal carotid system.

### Aetiology

The blood level of histamine is raised during an attack whilst the serotonin level is unchanged (Anthony and Lance, 1971), whereas in migraine the histamine level does not change whilst the plasma serotonin does, suggesting a different biochemical basis of the two conditions (Hayward, 1977).

Thermographic studies have shown that the skin temperature in the affected area was raised by 1–3°C in 3 out of 5 cases (Lance and Anthony, 1971). Also 2 cases had a cold spot over one eye, early in the attack, which suggests decreased blood flow in the internal carotid artery. This can be related to the colder areas in both migraine and icecream headaches (see below).

**Incidence**

In a series of 859 patients Oleseon et al (1979) found only 3 cases of 'cluster headache', and this small percentage would not justify much space in a book this size, but it seems possible that comparable vascular factors, not yet properly understood, account for a greater percentage of cases than this, possibly loosely classified as atypical facial pain.

**Age and sex**

It starts in the second and third decade of life and about 85 per cent of cases are male (Bickerstaff, 1967; Eggleston, 1970; Ekbom, 1974; Lance, 1978; Pearce, 1980). This contrasts with only about 25 per cent of migraine cases being male.

*'Red migraine'*

This is the old name when there is a flushed face, which occurs in 20 per cent of cases (Lance and Anthony, 1971).

**Treatment**

Since there are no premonitory signs it is inappropriate to use oral ergotamine because this is only effective if given before the vessels dilate, but injection of 1–2 mg ergotamine tartrate is effective. However, administration as an inhalent is easier and effective.

The painful area can be treated with a pain relieving spray, such as PR spray (Boots), which is a mixture of trichlorofluoromethane, 85 per cent, and dichlorodifluoromethane, 15 per cent, used straight from the aerosal can. It is essential that the spray does not go into the eyes or nose, so the patient must be suitably draped. The clothing around the neck should also be covered. The spray is applied in slow sweeps from side to side.

During a cluster bout ergotamine suppositories may be used as a prophylactic, or dihydroergotamine is taken, 1–2 mg three times a day. Also methysergide (Deseril) 2 mg orally three times a day. Pizotifen (Sanomigran) 1 mg three times a day may be used as an antihistamine, antiserotonin agent. The drugs are decreased as the end of a bout is anticipated, to avoid giving them unnecessarily.

For the few individuals who fall into a chronic cluster state, suffering attacks almost daily for years, cryosurgery may be necessary on the arterial branch responsible (Graham, 1974).

### Chronic paroxysmal hemicrania

This is a variant of facial migraine which still occurs unilaterally but does not occur in clusters; rather does it occur at night, has shorter duration, and is mainly in females (Sjaastad, 1978).

## OTHER HEADACHES OF VASCULAR ORIGIN

### Temporal arteritis

This is a condition which affects middle-aged and elderly people. There is persistent pain in the temple and forehead sometimes associated with occasional stabs along the course of the temporal artery or its branches (Appenzeller, 1979). The temporal arteries are tortuous and stand out, this being part of more generalised vascular disease. Exercise provokes the pain or makes it worse, the arteries being narrowed. Lying on the affected side may be avoided because the temporal artery is tender. This contrasts with headaches due to vasodilation in which pressure may give some relief.

Patients with temporal arteritis may suffer pain and stiffness on chewing, and this has been called intermittent claudication of the jaw (Appenzeller, 1979). The condition is likely to be accompanied by general malaise, aching muscles, loss of appetite, exhaustion and depression, which make matters worse (McArdie, 1970).

Temporal arteritis is said to affect females more than males in the ratio of 7 to 4 (Lance, 1978).

The importance of diagnosing lies in the possibility that the arteries of the orbit may be affected, with the risk of occlusion of the retinal arteries (Hayward, 1977) or of the arteries to the optic nerve (Spillane, 1975), and consequent possibility of blindness. Examination shows the erythrocyte sedimentation rate to be raised.

### Treatment

Corticosteroids are given, such as prednisolone 60 mg per day, reducing to 20 mg as a maintenance dose.

## Hypertension headache

Though moderate hypertension does not cause headaches, severe hypertension does, possibly associated with papilloedema, and throbbing in character. A severe case may be a medical emergency requiring immediate treatment with hypotensive drugs.

## Ice cream headache

Sometimes when people eat cold ice cream or gulp iced drinks quickly they develop a pain in the head. This is most likely to be in the centre of the forehead (Fig. 17.4), supraorbitally (Fig. 17.5) or below the eyebrows and at the inner canthus. It can also be felt at the side of the forehead and the anterior part of the

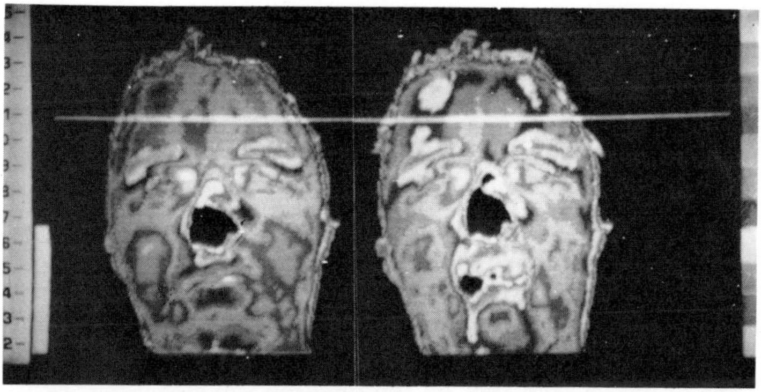

**Fig. 17.4**. Thermographs showing subject before eating ice cream (left) and when the ice cream headache occurred (right). Pain was experienced in the centre of the forehead where the temperature fell by about 1°C (original in colour).

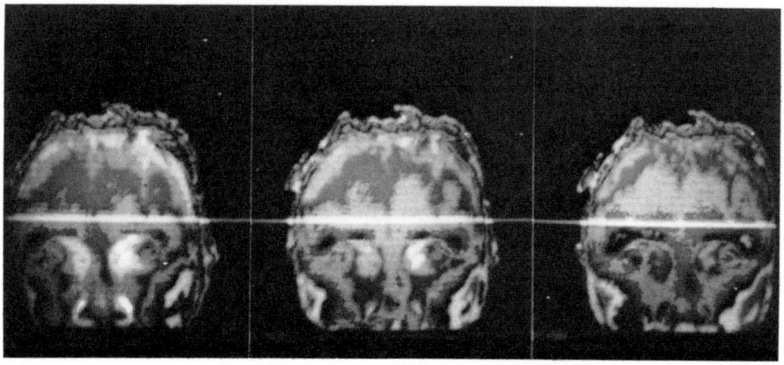

**Fig. 17.5**. Thermographs showing subject before eating ice cream (left) when the ice cream headache occurred (middle) and with the headache still present. Pain was experienced in the supraorbital area on both sides where the temperature fell by about 1°C (original in colour).

temple. Less often it can be experienced behind the eye or deep in the middle of the head. In a survey of 27 people the pain was always described as deep (Mumford, 1979). It is experienced by males and females of all ages, and is most likely to occur on a hot day when the person is hot after exercise.

After starting to imbibe the cold ice cream or liquid there is a latent period of about half a minute before pain develops. For this reason the older explanation that it is a referred pain from the pharynx is considered unlikely; it seems more likely that the mechanism is vascular (Mumford, 1979). The cold mass in the pharynx is separated from the carotid artery system only by a relatively thin layer, and it is supposed that the arteries are subjected to cooling and vasoconstriction. This affects the ophthalmic artery and its branches which supply the nasal sinuses and the skin of the forehead above the eyes. Thermographic investigation revealed a fall in temperature of the skin in the painful areas of approximately 1°C.

Ice cream headache does not matter in the sense that people do not have to eat ice cream or can eat it more slowly, but some people are relieved at the explanation, and it might have a bearing on migraine and other painful conditions. Thus, Raskin (1976) found that only 31 per cent of non-migrainous people had experienced ice cream headache whereas 93 per cent of migraineurs had. Moreover, the ice cream headache was more severe in the migraine group. A cold spot on the forehead can also occur with internal carotid obstruction (Mora et al, 1976; Rocco et al, 1976; Winsor and Winsor, 1976).

**Hangover headache**

People who have drunk alcohol unwisely, frequently awake with a headache which may be throbbing. This is because of the effect of alcohol on blood vessels together with some disturbance of fluid balance. The cause is seldom in doubt and the patient treats himself with analgesics, plain food, fresh air and mild exercise. If he has any sense he learns to drink only the right amount of the right kind of liquor.

**Rebound headache**

Vasoconstriction due to smoking, or caffeine in coffee or tea, may be followed by a rebound dilation which causes a dull headache which goes with more smoking or caffeine.

### Effort headache

Intense exercise can produce a headache similar to a migraine headache but it does not last as long, perhaps an hour or less. It can occur from prolonged exercise, especially in the presence of some additional factor such as high altitude.

### Motorbike or cold wind headache

It is possible to develop a headache in the centre of the forehead at quite low speeds e.g. 40 kph, even if the wind is not particularly cold. The small blood vessels contract whilst the larger ones are still dilated. Lance (1978) suggests that this imbalance causes the pain, but mild anoxia could be the cause.

### Other conditions

Patients, and sometimes people who are not patients, occasionally complain about sensations in the mouth, face, and deep behind the eyes or nose. All too often the condition is rather vague but sometimes a vascular explanation can be given. For example, a throbbing or twitching in the lip can be due to a labial artery, and the patient accepts this. A throbbing deep behind the eye that has gone on intermittently for years with no other obvious symptoms or signs is likely to arise in the maxillary artery or one of its branches. The person complaining often seems depressed and probably more introspective than usual, so the sensations are noticed. This is related to the problem of atypical facial pain (so-called), and possibly the older descriptions, Sluder's sphenopalatine neuralgia, Charlin's nasal nerve neuralgia, Vail's vidian nerve neuralgia and greater superficial temporal neuralgia.

Sometimes when people complain of burning sensations in the lips it seems to be due to small extravasations of blood with release of algogenic agents.

A colleague always had an ache in the region of the anterior branch of the superficial temporal artery, with tenderness on pressure, before he developed herpetic lesions at the corner of the mouth, on the same side.

### Muscle contraction headache

This is not vascular in origin but migraine is frequently associated with muscle contraction headache so it is convenient to include the latter here, especially since it is probably the most common form of headache. Moreover, activity has been shown to increase in the masseter, temporalis and sternomastoid muscle during the peak periods of migraine pain (Møller et al, 1980).

Persistent contraction of the scalp and occipital muscles cause a dull ache which involves a wide area; not so localised as in migraine. Patients may describe the headache as being like a tight band, or a heavy weight pressing on the head. It is essentially due to an inability to relax the muscles and is related to the masticatory dysfunction syndrome (see Chapter 14).

*Treatment*

Most people successfully treat themselves with analgesics but the physician or dentist may be consulted. In this case the patient can be reassured that the ache does not indicate serious disease and that analgesics are appropriate. The area affected can be massaged, usually by the patient himself. Coffee and tea may help to remove the ache but in some people excessive intake of caffeine from coffee and tea may be largely responsible for the patients tension so the number of cups drunk must be reduced.

In persistent cases a stressful situation may have arisen and a sympathetic hearing by the family physician can be helpful. Tranquillisers, eg. diazepam, may be of value but should only be used for a week or so. Moderate amounts of alcohol help by promoting relaxation. When the ache is experienced regularly in the periorbital region it might be due to subconscious attempts to improve vision, so consultation with an ophthalmologist is appropriate since spectacles may be needed.

## REFERENCES


Anthony, M. (1978) Role of individual free fatty acids in migraine. *Res. clin. Stud. Headache*, **6**, 110–116.

Anthony, M. and Lance, J. W. (1969) Monamine oxidase inhibition in the treatment of migraine. *Archs. Neurol.*, **21**, 263–268.

Anthony, M. and Lance, J. W. (1971) Histamine and serotonin in cluster headache. *Archs. Neurol*, **25**, 225–231.

Blau, J. N. (1978) Migraine: a vasomotor instability of the meningeal circulation. *Lancet*, **11**, 1136–1139.

Dalessio. D. J., Otis, S. and Smith, R. (1978) Vasomotor phenomena, platelet antagonism and migraine therapy. *Res. clin. Stud. Headache*, **6**, 34–40.

Diamond, S. and Medina, J. L. (1978) Value of biofeedback in the treatment of chronic headache: the patients' opinion. *Res. clin. Stud. Headache*, **61**, 155–159.

Eggleston, D. J. (1970) Periodic migrainous neuralgia. *Oral Surg.*, **29**, 524–529.

Ekbom, K. (1974) Migraine in patients with cluster headache. *Headache*, **14**, 69–72.

Ekbom, K. (1975) Some observations on pain in cluster headache. *Headache*, **14**, 219–225.

Fanchamps, A. (1975) Pharmacodynamic principles of anti-migraine therapy. *Headache*, **15**, 79–90.

Graham, J. R. (1974) Cluster headache. *Postgrad. Med.*, **56**, 181–185.

Hayward, M. (1977) Headache and pain in the head and neck. In *Persistent pain: Modern Methods of Treatment*, ed. Lipton, S., pp. 35–60. London: Academic.

Horton, B. T., (1941) Histaminic cephalgia; erythromelalgia of the head. *J. Amer. med. Ass.*, **116**, 377–383.
Jessup, B. A., Neufeld, R. W. J. and Merskey, H. (1979) Biofeedback therapy for headache and other pain. *Pain*, 7, 225–270.
Lance, J. W. (1978) *Mechanisms and Management of Headache*. 3rd ed. London: Butterworths.
Lance, J. W. and Anthony, M. (1971) Thermographic studies in vascular headache. *Med. J. Austral.*, **1**, 240–243.
Lance, J. W., Spira, P. J., Mylecharane, E. J., Lord, G. D. A. and Duckworth, J. W. (1978) Evaluation of drugs applicable to treatment of migraine in the cranial circulation of the monkey. *Res. clin. Stud. Headache*, **6**, 13–18.
McArdie, M. J. (1970) Atypical facial neuralgia. In *Trigeminal Neuralgia Pathogenesis and Pathophysiology*, ed. Hassler, R. and Walker, A. E., pp. 35–42. Stuttgart: Thieme.
Miles, J. (1981) Personal Communication.
Miller, H. (1965) The treatment of migraine. *Prescriber's J.*, **5**, 74–77.
Møller, E., Bakke, M., Olesen, J. and Tfelthansen, P. (1980) Action of cranial muscles during provoked attack of "common migraine". *J. dent. Res.*, **59**, Special Issue B, p993, Abstr. 426.
Monro, J., Brostoff, J., Carini, C. and Zilkha, K. (1980) Food allergy in migraine. *Lancet*, July 5th, 1–4.
Mora, L., Morganti, R. and Sharboro, V. (1976) Thermographic follow-up of medical treatment in extracerebral carotid insufficiency. *Acta Thermographica*, **1**, 12–17.
Mumford, J. M. (1979) Thermography and ice cream headache. *Acta Thermographica*, **4**, 33–37.
Oleson , J. (1978) Some clinical features of the acute migraine attack. An analysis of 750 patients. *Headache*, **18**, 268–271.
Oleson, J., Aebelholt, A. and Veilis, B. (1979) The Copenhagen Acute Headache Clinic: Organization, patient material and treatment results. *Headache*, **19**, 223–227.
Pearce, J. M. S. (1980) Chronic migrainous neuralgia: a variant of cluster headache. *Brain*, **103**, 149–159.
Raskin, N. H. (1976) Biologic correlates of migraine. In *Current Reports in Neurology*, p. 8. Rahway, Merck and Co. Quoted by Lance, J. W. (1978). See above.
Rocco, P., Gangemi, M. and Cennamo, G. (1976) Thermography in cerebral vascular pathology. *Acta Thermographica*, **1**, 201–203.
Saxena, P. R. (1978) Arteriovenous shunting and migraine. *Res. Clinic. Stud. Headache*, **6**, 89–102.
Sicuteri, F. (1976) Migraine, a central biochemical dysnociception. *Headache*, **16**, 145–159.
Sicuteri, F. (1978) Endorphines, opiate receptors and migraine headache. *Headache*, **17**, 253–256.
Sicuteri, F. (1979) Headache as the most common disease of the antinociceptive system; analogies with morphine abstinence. In *Advances in Pain Research and Therapy*, Vol. 3, ed. Bonica, J. J., Liebeskind J. C. and Albe-Fessard, D. G. pp. 359–365, New York: Raven Press.
Sjaastad, O. (1978) Pathogenesis of the cluster headache syndrome. *Res. clin. Stud. Headache*, **6**, 53–64.
Spillane, J. D. (1975) *An Atlas of Clinical Neurology*. London: Oxford.
Wilkinson, M., Williams, K. and Leyton, M. (1978) Observations on the treatment of an acute attack of migraine. *Res. clin. Stud. Headache*, **6**, 141–146.
Wyke, B. (1968) The neurology of facial pain. *Brit. J. Hosp. Med.*, Oct., 46–65.
Winsor, T. and Winsor, D. (1976) Disorder of the cardiovascular system. *Acta Thermographica*, **1**, 142–149.

# 18

# Referred pain

If a tooth is diseased and neural impulses pass from it to the central nervous system with the result that pain is felt in that tooth it is misleading to describe it as pain referred to the tooth. The neural impulses are interpreted as originating in the tooth, but the word referred has a specialised significance in pain studies, referred pain being pain experienced in a part of the body not otherwise involved in the causative disease but having common innervation. This seems simple enough but it is not always easy to decide when to speak of referred pain, poorly localised pain or pain which has spread to involve a larger area. Also the primary disease can cause secondary conditions which are painful in themselves. The following remarks may help clarify the matter.

If the diseased tooth is painful and pain extends to adjacent teeth this is not referred pain. If the diseased tooth is a lower premolar and the patient indicates pain as being over the adjacent part of the mandible this is sufficiently close to the diseased tooth to be regarded as pain in the primary site.

If an acute periapical abscess is present on an upper tooth and drains to the submandibular gland causing it to be painful on pressure, this tenderness is not referred pain but a separate focus of disease causing pain in itself. If pain in a molar tooth causes muscle tension so that masticatory muscles become painful this is not referred pain; it is pain in muscle which is temporarily functioning badly, albeit as a result of the primary pain. If a diseased tooth causes pain which is experienced in the tooth and also along the course of the inferior dental nerve it is better to describe such pain as spreading rather than referred.

In cases of acute traumatic periodontitis the patient may suffer pain, not only in a newly restored tooth which shows 'high spots', but also on the opposing tooth, but this is not referred pain. Harmful forces have been equal and opposite on the two teeth and both periodontal membranes are affected.

It should also be remembered that pain in one jaw is not

necessarily referred pain just because an obvious lesion is present in the other jaw; there may also be a hidden lesion at the site of the apparently referred pain. For example, a patient who complained of pain in both upper and lower jaws was found to have an exposed pulp in the lower first premolar. When this was treated pain in the mandible ceased but pain in the maxilla remained. Eventually it was found that the upper lateral incisor also had an exposed pulp, and when this was treated all pain ceased, so this was not a case of referred pain. Another patient with an acute maxillary sinusitis had pain which alternated between the upper lateral incisor and the lower second premolar, and pain in the latter tooth seemed to be referred, but this tooth was found to have exposed pulp. A diagnosis of referred pain should not be made too hastily.

Fig. 18.1 illustrates some examples which are not referred pain whereas cases of referred pain are represented in Fig. 18.2.

## PAIN REFERRED BETWEEN THE JAWS

An excellent example of referred pain is of a dental colleague who complained of pain in a lower premolar but firmly announced that the lower teeth were healthy and that the 'trouble' must be in the upper jaw (Fig. 18.2A). Pain ceased within several minutes of anaesthetising the upper first molar and, following treatment of the molar, pain did not recur. This is a perfect example of how referred pain ceases on applying local anaesthesia to the primary disease focus.

Within the same week a young woman complained of pain in the upper premolars which, on examination, appeared healthy (Fig. 18.2B). One of the lower premolars had obvious deep caries and needed treatment even if it did not prove to be the source of pain, but she was very reluctant to have the lower tooth treated because she naturally regarded relief of pain in the upper tooth as more important. The principle of referred pain was explained and the lower tooth was anaesthetised, whereupon pain in the upper tooth ceased, and the patient was quite impressed though still somewhat mystified. Since this treatment was successful it might be thought that the diseased tooth could have been treated without explanation, but patient education is important, and this might not have been a case of referred pain after all. A further point to note about this patient is that the lower premolar was diseased and needed to be treated even if pain was due to some other fault. It frequently happens that the source of pain cannot be determined and patients have to be treated in an empirical manner, obvious

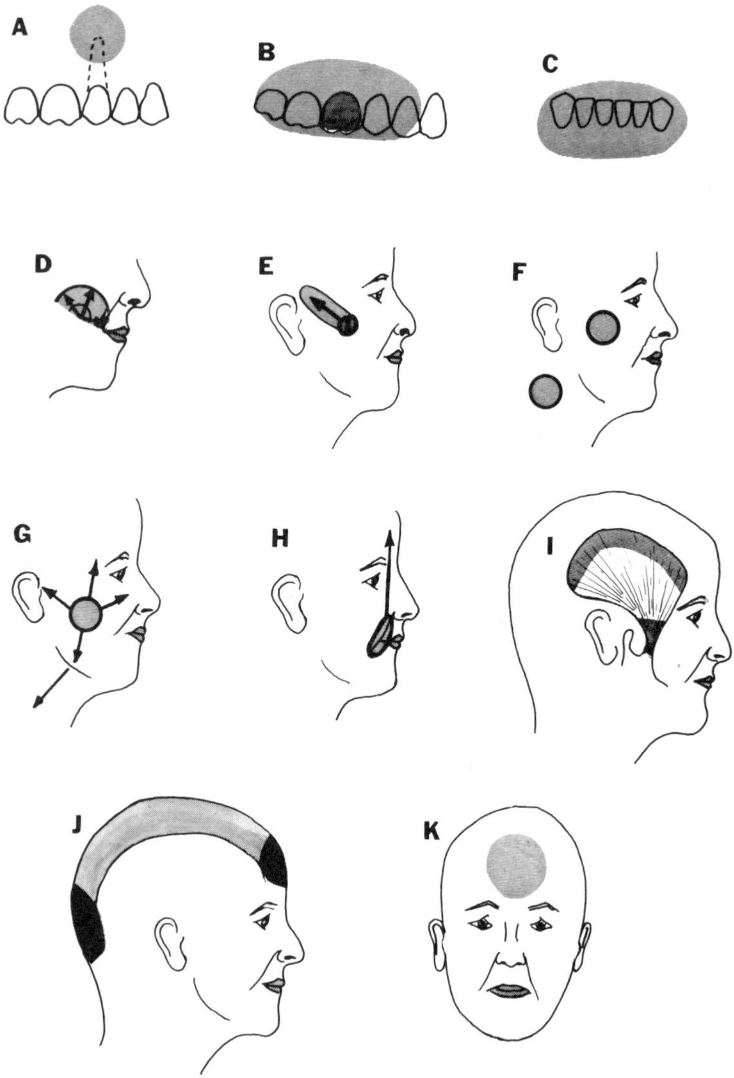


**Fig. 18.1**. Examples of pains that are not referred.

A. Localised pain at apex of a premolar.
B. Diffuse pain from a single diseased upper molar.
C. Diffuse pain from several teeth with sensitive cervical dentine.
D. Spreading pain which seems to glow.

**Fig. 18.1** (continued)

E. Pain which spreads slowly in one direction.
F. Pain at apex of an upper molar with pain in lymph gland due to spread of infection.
G. Radiating pain — different directions at different times.
H. Shooting pain (about a second) from trigger area.
I. Pain at origin of temporalis muscle as well as insertion.
J. With occipital pain it is said that pain is referred to the frontal area but it is simpler to think of the occipito-frontalis muscle acting as one.
K. Ice cream headache was supposed to be referred but it is simpler to think it is due to diminished blood supply.

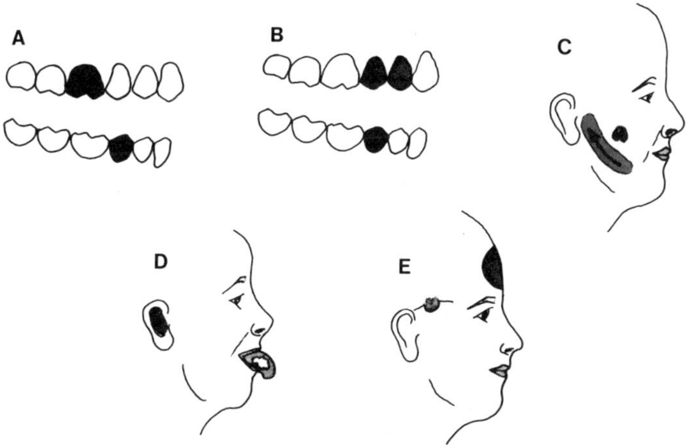


**Fig. 18.2**. Examples of referred pain.

A. Pain in lower premolar from diseased upper molar.
B. Pain in both upper premolars from diseased lower premolar.
C. Pain moving along lower jaw to TMJ due to acute pulpitis in the upper first molar.
D. Pain in ear from malignant ulcer of tongue.
E. Frontal headache from tumour in pituitary region.

defects being treated first. When patients are not told what is happening they lose confidence if the first steps in treatment fail to stop the pain.

Although the above examples were treated within one week, cases of referred pain do not occur with this frequency. In a way, this is surprising because dental disease is so prevalent that more cases of referred pain might be expected. On the other hand it could be argued that there is no obvious reason why such cases should ever occur, and the mechanism of referred pain is not completely understood (see later).

Sometimes pain occurs first in the diseased tooth and later passes to a tooth in the opposite jaw. Assuming that there is no disease in the latter tooth it might appear that this is spread of pain rather than referral, but in some cases the patient is aware of quite separate 'hemispheres' of pain.

Pain need not be referred from one tooth to another. Thus, a patient complained of pain extending along the lower jaw to the region of the temporomandibular joint (Fig. 18.2C). It was of such intensity and duration that she was crying, 'at the end of her tether'. Examination showed that there were no cheek teeth present in the lower jaw, and radiographs showed no abnormality. The upper first molar was found to have an exposed pulp and subsequent histological examination revealed an acute pulpitis. Although the referred pain ceased as a result of the extraction there was some delay, and the patient did not feel entirely free of pain until she awoke the next morning.

**Localisation of stimuli**

Friend and Glenwright (1968) investigated the ability of human subjects to localise pain in teeth caused by electrical stimulation, and found that it varied from one subject to another and from tooth to tooth. The site of stimulation was wrongly identified as being in the opposite jaw in 3·4 per cent of cases, approximately half being referrals from the maxilla to the mandible, and half referred in the opposite direction. Mumford and Newton (1971) made a similar investigation on maxillary teeth but obtained no referrals. The results of these two investigations appear to be contradictory, but Friend and Glenwright applied electrodes to both upper and lower teeth whereas Mumford and Newton applied electrodes only to upper teeth; it could therefore be that the subject's awareness of the electrode arrangements could have been a factor in localising the pain.

Kawamura *et al.* (1967) found that human subjects did not misjudge an upper tooth for a lower one when it was subjected to axial pressures.

**Character of pain referred between the jaws**

One of the chief features of referred pain is that it does not cross the midline (but see below). Its other characteristics depend upon the disease which give rise to it, the following being examples:

Pain experienced in a lower left premolar was found to be due to disease of the upper third molar on the same side. This was extracted, histological examination made, and it was found that there was a small pulp exposure with an underlying partial acute pulpitis. The referred pain occurred spontaneously, was a dull ache, lasted 20 minutes, and there was no sensitivity on percussion; this is what would be expected from a partial acute pulpitis.

Pain experienced in a lower molar was found to be referred from a carious upper molar. Pain occurred at intervals over a period of months, being caused by heat or cold, but not always. It was a dull ache lasting for some minutes to an hour, and ceased when the carious tooth was dressed.

**Pain referred across the midline**

It is generally accepted that pain is not referred across the midline but several factors suggest that this may not be strictly true.

Harris (1973) described an apparently authentic case in whom pain was experienced in the left lower first molar. Apart from a large amalgam filling with a cement lining, this tooth seemed normal. The right lower lateral incisor had a periapical rarefaction and infiltration anaesthesia by this incisor reduced pain in the left molar. An inferior dental injection on the right side stopped pain in the left molar (see below).

Mumford and Newton (1974a, b) stimulated each of the upper central incisors with a subthreshold electrical stimulus and this resulted in pain perception, suggesting spatial summation because of neuronal convergence from these two teeth. One explanation could be that nerve fibres from these teeth cross the midline. It was also shown that this effect extended to include the lateral incisor on the opposite side.

Starkie and Stewart (1931) found that in some cases the incisor nerves formed an incisor plexus within the mandible and some nerve fibres crossed the midline to the pulps of the contralateral incisors.

Returning to the case of Harris, a single case is interesting but it is essential to remember that coincidence could account for the condition. Also it would have been more interesting if pain had stopped following infiltration anaesthesia of the right incisor. This would have blocked neural impulses passing along overlapping nerve fibres of the left inferior dental nerve, thus preventing them from summating with neural impulses at subthreshold level from the left molar (with its large filling and unknown pulp condition). On this basis summation of neural impulses would have been in the spinal nucleus of the left trigeminal nerve. However, pain only stopped following an inferior dental injection on the right side. Excluding coincidence, this could only be explained by preventing neuronal convergence at higher levels than the trigeminal spinal nuclei, i.e. in the reticular system of the brain stem or higher.

## PAIN REFERRED FROM THE MOUTH TO OTHER SITES

### Earache

Pain in the ear can arise from dental disease, e.g. a patient suffering from an acute periapical periodontitis in the upper first premolar also had earache which ceased when the tooth was treated by pulp canal drainage, even though the tooth remained sensitive to biting for a further period. Another patient had pain only in the ear and this ceased when an upper first molar was extracted; histological examination revealed a subacute pulpitis.

When a carcinoma involves the tongue there may be pain referred to the ear — it used to be said that an old man with cotton wool in his ear would be found to have a lesion of the tongue (Fig. 18.2D).

The pharynx and nasopharynx must also be examined since a carcinoma here can cause earache, and not just old men but middle-aged patients (Ballentyne and Groves, 1972).

A sharp pain in the ear can also occur in association with herpes, and such a pain can precede the eruption by a day or even two days.

The innervation of the ear is rather complex, several nerves being involved. The auriculotemporal nerve conveys neural impulses from the tragus, the upper part of the auricle, principally the lateral surface, the external auditory meatus and the tympanic membrane. Since the auriculotemporal nerve is part of the mandibular division of the trigeminal system this anatomical arrangement presumably explains how earache can occur from disease of the lower teeth and tongue. It does not seem to provide such a good explanation for being referred to the ear from disease of the upper teeth as described above. However, the separation of the trigeminal nerve branches at the periphery does not preclude convergence of neural impulses from them more centrally.

The auditory tube (pharyngotympanic tube) is innervated by the pharyngeal branch derived from the pterygopalatine ganglion. The trigeminal system also supplies nerve fibres to the tympanic plexus via the otic ganglion.

The ear is also innervated by sensory fibres from the facial, glossopharyngeal, great auricular and lesser occipital nerves, and by the auricular branch of the vagus (Anson and Donaldson, 1973; Warwick and Williams, 1973). It is evident that an anatomical basis therefore exists for pain to be felt in the ear as a result of disease or dysfunction in various remote sites. It must also be supposed that pain could also be referred from the ear to these other sites.

**Eye pain**

When the upper anterior teeth are affected with acute periapical disease it is quite common for there to be tenderness in the infraorbital region and this is spread of inflammation; not referred pain, but occasionally patients complain of pain in the eye.

Pain in the eye can also occur from acute maxillary sinusitis or neoplasia of this sinus. This can be associated with a sense of numbness which extends from the infraorbital region into the orbit.

Supraorbital pain can occur from bruxism, as has been shown experimentally by Christensen (1967). Subjects performed intensive chewing movements for 20 minutes and this was followed, 2–3 hours later, by pain supraorbitally as well as in the area of the temporomandibular joints. This pain lasted for hours.

**Neck pain**

Pain may occur in the neck as a result of dental disease, e.g. a patient complained of pain in the right side of her face spreading down her neck, and was found to have deep caries exposing the pulp in her upper first molar. Histological examination revealed a localised acute pulpitis with abscess formation. Such pain is best described as spreading for it is not really referred pain. Since the neck pain was not present alone it afforded no problem.

**Headache**

The patient sometimes complains of pain in the temple. In some cases examination has revealed disease of teeth in either jaw, examples being a gangrenous pulp in a lower premolar, or an acute pulpitis in an upper third molar. Treatment of these stopped the pain in the temple. However, it is uncommon for headache to occur from dental disease without toothache being present at the same time. Nevertheless, a colleague always has an ache in his temple some hours to a day before the outbreak of herpes near his lips. Although this might be true referred pain it is probably due to dilatation of the anterior branch of the superficial temporal artery, or possibly tension in the anterior fibres of the temporalis muscle.

Temporal pain has been ascribed to the condyle of the mandible

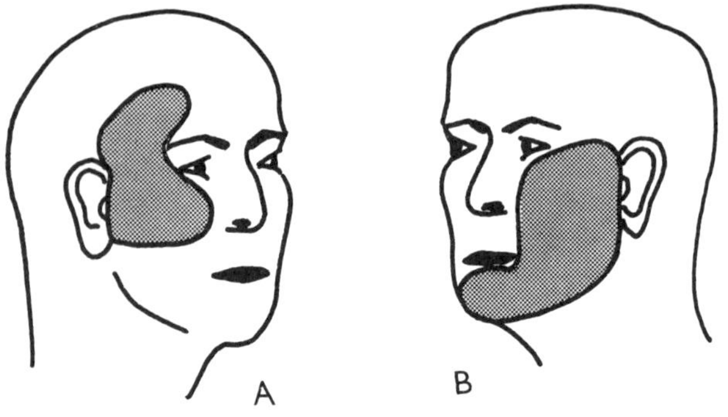


**Fig. 18.3.** A, Prolonged electrical stimulation of 5⌋ caused a sensation of numbness, fullness and stiffness in the area shaded. This occurred in 5 minutes. After 20 minutes there was a headache in the same area. B, After prolonged stimulation of ⌈4 the corresponding sensations were found in shaded area, also in 5, and 20 minutes. (After Wolff, 1963).

impinging on the auriculotemporal nerve, but the nerve is behind the neck of the mandible; not behind the condyle (Chapter 14).

Headache has been experimentally induced by prolonged electrical stimulation of human teeth (Robertson, Goodell and Wolff, 1947). Stimulation was maintained for 10 minutes causing pain which was sometimes the worst which the subject had experienced. After 5 minutes there was a sensation of pressure in the tooth, with fullness and numbness of the cheek, together with tightness and stiffness in the jaw, and fullness in the ear on the same side (Fig. 18.3). A headache developed after 20 minutes and lasted for several hours.

The author has stimulated many hundreds of teeth by electrical impulses in both patients and human experimental subjects. At the level of the pain perception threshold in no case was headache reported; nor was it expected. More recently, teeth in human subjects were stimulated to determine the pain perception threshold; the same teeth were then stimulated by currents of greater intensity until the subjects considered pain to be no longer tolerable, when stimulation was terminated (Newton and Mumford, 1972; Mumford, Newton and Ley, 1973). This pain tolerance level of current was approximately three times that at the pain perception threshold but in no case did the subject complain of a headache. However, it should be noted that in the investigation reported by Wolff the painful stimulation was maintained for as long as 10 minutes. The site of headache indicated by Wolff (Fig. 18.3, B) would probably not be called a headache.

The same semantic problem applies to the unilateral headaches of dental origin reported by Monica and Raymond (1957). They found that in 17 out of 18 cases unilateral headaches were relieved by oral rehabilitation. Although any ache in the head could be called a headache, the word should be reserved for the cranial portion of the head as it already is in common use, and it would be better to make greater use of the expression face ache.

In one case described by Wolff a headache occurred on the same side as an upper third molar which had just been extracted. Local anaesthesia applied to the third molar area caused the headache to stop 'at once' and it did not return until local anaesthesia ceased. Notice that this is the same result between the jaws. However, this is less clearly a case of referred pain, as indicated at the beginning of the chapter.

**Other sites**

Occasionally patients complain of pain going from the mouth to the 'stomach', the legs or elsewhere but these should not be thought of as referred pain. They are more likely to be cases of atypical facial pain (Chapter 19) and there is usually some feature of the case that is unusual. For example, one such patient complained of pain, of five years' duration, which started from a trigger point situated a centimetre above and distal to the gingival margin of an upper premolar. From here, he said, pain radiated to the temple and the stomach. When asked about his last extraction two years earlier, he produced the tooth from his pocket!

Nevertheless, one seemingly authentic case has been reported by Rood (1972). A 20-year-old patient complained of a 'gripping feeling across the lower part of the ribs — just above the stomach', which spread bilaterally to the lower jaw, being more severe on the right. Having first occurred 3 weeks earlier, pain lasted for a few minutes and was becoming more severe. There was no association with effort, no relief from antacids and no chest disease. The character of the pain was affected when he pressed his tongue on the lingual aspect of the right lower second premolar. The pulp was opened and pus drained away, followed by no further chest pain.

## OROFACIAL PAIN REFERRED FROM OTHER SITES

**Intracranial**

As mentioned in Chapter 1, all three divisions of the trigeminal nerve have branches to the dura mater and blood vessels of the anterior and middle cranial fossae, and also the superior surface of the tentorium cerebelli. When disease affects these sites it is therefore possible for pain to be experienced elsewhere in the cutaneous distribution of the nerves, often in the frontal, orbital and temporal areas (i.e. referred pain. Fig. 18.2E). This relationship has also been found following experimental stimulation of the dura mater and associated vessels (Dalessio, 1974, 1980).

Intracranial lesions can also cause pain by their direct involvement of the cranial nerves themselves, so pain in the face may be due to meningioma, tumours of the trigeminal nerve, acoustic neuroma, malignant tumours of the base of the skull, aneurysm or other vascular problems. It tends to be constant and is associated with paraesthesia together with various neurological signs which depend on the causative factor and its position. These include loss of sensation in the trigeminal area, the cornea being especially important because of the indirect threat of blindness due to corneal ulceration following loss of the corneal reflex. Muscle activity may be adversely affected following involvement of the motor nerves, so the eye movements may be modified, the masseters weakened, the muscles of facial expression affected. Smell, vision, taste and hearing may be changed.

Clinicians generally will note some or all of the above features but such a case is clearly for the neurologists and neurosurgeons. They will use various diagnostic methods including plain radiographs, angiography and computerised axial tomography. The latter method was used for a colleague's patient. She was a 77 year old

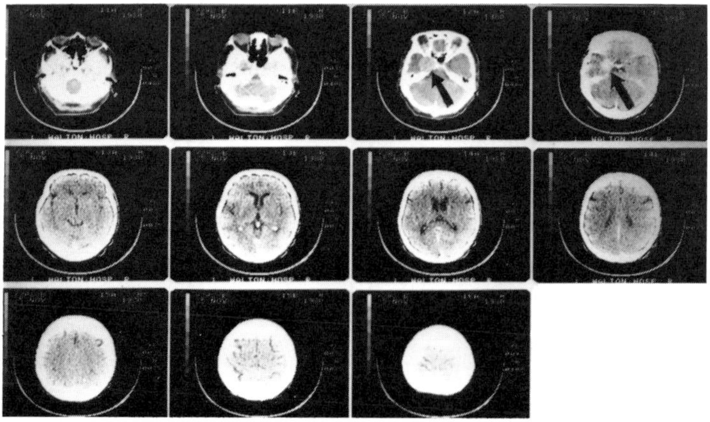

**Fig. 18.4**. Computerised axial tomographic scan showing a tumour in the middle cranial fossa (3rd and 4th on top row). The patient had pain in the face (Mr John Miles' case).

female with pain in the left side of her face for 3 years. It was constant but exacerbated by cold draughts, and worse at night. She complained of numbness in the face, and it was found that pinprick sensation was reduced in all of the trigeminal area on the left side. The corneal reflex was lost on this side, and there was a left sixth nerve palsy. Radiographs of the skull showed erosion of bone in the region of the left foramen ovale, the apex of the petrous ridge and the lesser wing of the sphenoid as well as widening of the left superior orbital fissure. Computerised tomographic scanning (Fig. 18.4) confirmed the bone erosion and demonstrated a round, solid, strongly enhancing mass responsible for this erosion. The mass, in the left para-sella region, was thought to be a meningioma but, at this age, operation was considered inappropriate even if it had been technically possible, so one ml of absolute alcohol was injected into the nerve to stop the pain.

**Diseases of the eye**

Glaucoma may be secondary to other eye disease, or it may be primary, one of the latter group being closed angle glaucoma. There is a history of coloured halos being seen around lights, associated with periodic obscuration of vision and it is immensely important to diagnose at this time for it can be treated. If not, the condition deteriorates in time until an acute congestive attack develops. There is severe pain which may spread beyond the eye to the entire distribution of the trigeminal nerve, associated with vomiting and irregular pulse. The eye is no longer white but congested because of the veins being dilated, and vision rapidly diminishes (Miller, 1978). The ophthalmologists have a problem. Strictly speaking, spread of pain in this way should not be described as referred.

The pain of iritis and iridocyclitis is deep and throbbing, and worse at night or early in the morning. It is sometimes referred to the teeth, sinuses or ear (Moses, 1970).

The trigeminal nerve ophthalmic division may be affected by granulomatous tissue within the orbit (Tolusa-Hunt syndrome) causing pain above and behind the eye, associated with ophthalmoplegia due to involvement of the oculomotor, trochlear and abducens nerves. This division might also be affected by a meningioma, pain being experienced in the forehead, possible with diminished sensation in this area. Sudden severe pain can occur if the division is affected by an enlarging aneurysm of the internal carotid or ophthalmic arteries.

**Diseases of ear, nose and throat**

The pain of otitis media is felt within the ear and ranges in character from a dull ache to sharp, lancinating spasms (Hall and Colman, 1971). Pain is worse if the middle ear becomes filled with inflammatory exudate and the tympanic membrane is stretched. Pain ceases if the membrane perforates spontaneously or is incised. There may be tenderness when pressure is applied over the tragus. According to Grossman (1965) there may be pain referred to the face or lower teeth.

In mastoiditis pain is similar to that of otitis media and there may also be tenderness on applying pressure over the mastoid process.

Disease of the external ear, including furunculosis, might be more confusing to the dentist because pain may be localised in front of or below the ear, or may spread into the jaws (Hall and Colman, 1971). There is also tenderness in front of and below the ear. In these conditions pain is made worse by moving the cartilage of the ear.

Pain referred from the nasal mucous membrane and the sinuses is localised along the zygomatic arch and around the eye (Rasmussen, 1965). Patients may volunteer information regarding previous attacks of sinusitis.

Acute sphenoidal sinusitis can produce pain in the jaws and teeth, and in the temporal and zygomatic areas (Ballentyne and Groves, 1971). In such a case there is likely to be pain between and behind the eyes, with rhinorrhoea and lacrimation. Disease of the ethmoidal sinuses may produce a similar result.

Pituitary ablation is one of the ways of treating patients suffering severe pain from hormone-dependent tumours. One method is to pass a rigid wide bore needle into the nostril and through the nasal cavity to the antero-inferior border of the sphenoid bone. The needle is then passed through the bone, using a surgical hammer, until it reaches the pituitary fossa. This sounds horrid but is not too bad and the patient could be conscious though sedated. In one case, as the needle was being tapped through the bone the patient complained of pain in the teeth. Being sedated she ignored efforts to have her localise the pain more clearly. This could be explained on the basis of the patient not normally being aware of the sphenoid area and interpreting the neural impulses as coming from the mouth and teeth which she is more aware of.

In acute tonsillitis the throat is raw, there is pain on swallowing, and a sensation of constriction in the throat. By the second day the tonsillar crypts become filled with debris, pus and desquamated epithelial cells. At this stage the condition is so obvious that there should be no confusion, but there can be an ache which stretches from the temple, down the side of the face and into the neck. As might be expected the regional lymph nodes are also swollen and tender

However, most difficult pain cases for whom otorhinolaryngological consultation is requested (by dentists) are found not to have ear, nose and throat conditions (Stell, 1967).

**Diseases of the neck**

Neoplasia affecting the upper cervical vertebrae may cause irritation of the corresponding cervical nerves resulting in pain or hyperaesthesia in the area of distribution. Since the trigeminal spinal nucleus extends through the medulla as far as the second cervical segment this nucleus may also be affected. The result may be pain all over one side of the head (Fig. 18.5). Such a case is difficult to diagnose and requires a multidisciplinary approach.

Pain around the eye has been ascribed to arthritis of the atlanto-occipital joint, possibly because of the proximity of the trigeminal spinal nucleus, but this explanation is not generally accepted.

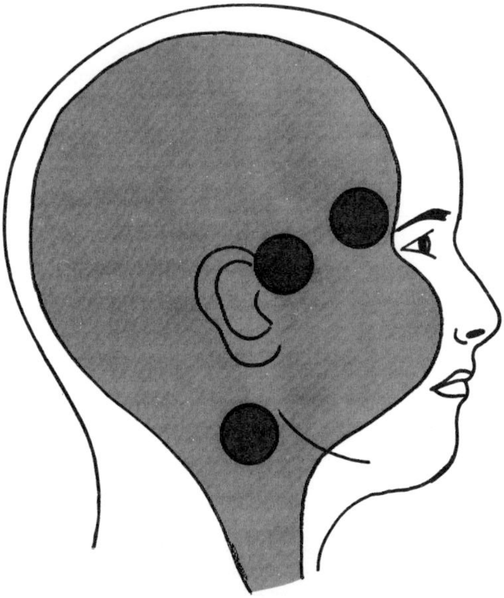

**Fig. 18.5.** Area of pain in a female patient with secondary tumours in the upper cervical vertebrae. The darker shaded areas are the site of most intense pain.

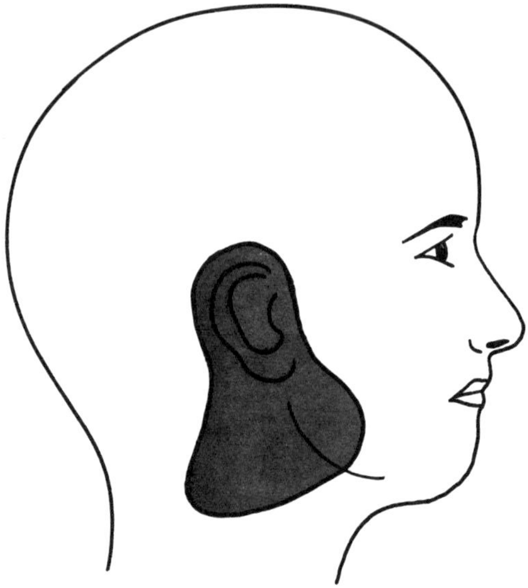

**Fig. 18.6**. Area of hyperalgesia occurring several years after a whiplash injury (after Frankel, 1972).

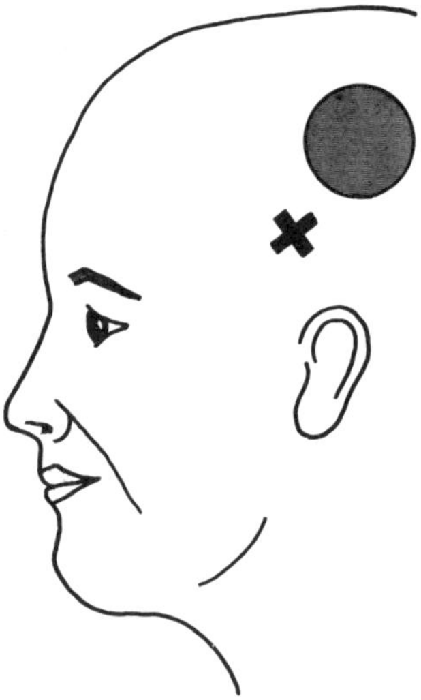

**Fig. 18.7**. Pain experienced in the parietal area could at first be stopped by pressing on the zone indicated with a cross, and this might have been a feature of the posterior branch of the superficial temporal artery. Then masticatory dysfunction syndrome was considered, but see Fig. 18.8 (Mr T. O. Tweedie's case).

The upper cervical vertebrae can also be affected in whiplash injury. This occurs when, one car being stationary at traffic lights, the following car crashes into it, usually at quite low speeds such as 15 m.p.h. As the first car is pushed forwards so are its seats and occupants, but the head tends to be left behind because of inertia. The result is that the neck is subjected to severe forces and the temporomandibular joint can also be stretched. There might be a lingering hyperaesthesia in part of the area supplied by the second and third cervical nerves (Fig. 18.6). Pain may not start until some years after the accident (Frankel, 1972) but then it might last for years. It may cover a larger area than shown in Fig. 18.6, can be more severe, and may be associated with myelopathy. All this can be confusing and made worse if there is also pain referred to the orbit (Crue, Kenton and Carregal, 1979).

A female patient had pain in the left parietal area which stopped, at first, when pressure was applied to the site indicated (Fig. 18.7).

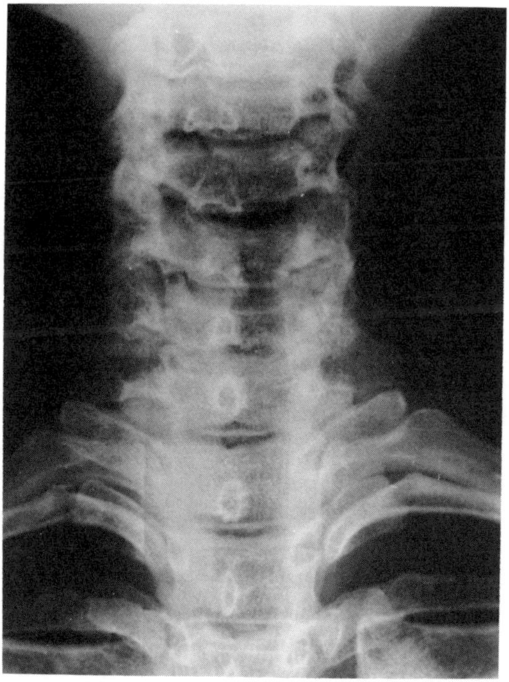

**Fig. 18.8**. A cervical spine radiograph revealed deviation of the cervical vertebrae and diffuse changes in the transverse processes. This accounted for the pain being in the lesser occipital nerve area (Fig. 18.7) (Mr T. O. Tweedie's case).

Since this occluded the posterior branch of the superficial temporal artery an arteritis was considered, but then the case was passed to a dentist who thought it was a case of masticatory dysfunction syndrome. He provided an occlusal splint (quite reasonably) and this seemed to work for a few days, the pain being considerably reduced, but the case deteriorated again. Since pain seemed to be in the sensory field of the lesser occipital nerve a spinal radiograph was taken and this showed distorted cervical vertebrae (Fig. 18.8).

Cervical muscle spasm can cause pain which may be associated with orofacial muscle pain, and referred to the mouth and face.

Bell and Ware (1971) describe a case where pain in the upper and lower molars and the infraorbital area became worse on palpating the middle of the sternocleidomastoid muscle on the same side. Injecting a local anaesthetic solution into the muscle site eliminated all pain.

Inflammation of the thyroid gland has been found to cause bilateral pain in the jaws and ears (Smith and Myall, 1977).

**Coronary artery disease**

In cases of myocardial ischaemia due to coronary artery disease exertion causes severe substernal pain which may radiate to the arms, throat, or jaws, and is relieved by rest or vasodilator drugs. Rarely the substernal element of this pain is missing and the patient may complain only of pain in the jaws (Taverner, 1959), which could be very confusing to the dentist, and this is a case for the patient's physician.

## MECHANISM OF REFERRED PAIN

Referred pain is pain experienced in a normal or apparently normal site as a result of disease somewhere else. This is a straightforward definition but the subject has been confused in various ways which may now be apparent.

The basic approach to referred pain postulates an 'irritable focus' in the spinal cord. This arises because of visceral disease which causes neural impulses to reach the dorsal horn setting up the irritable focus there. Neural impulses from normal skin in the same segment of the body arrive at the irritable focus and are more effective than usual in stimulating secondary neurones. This is because of spatial and temporal summation. The impulses, ascending via the secondary neurones and subsequent ones, reach the brain where they are interpreted as coming from the skin because the

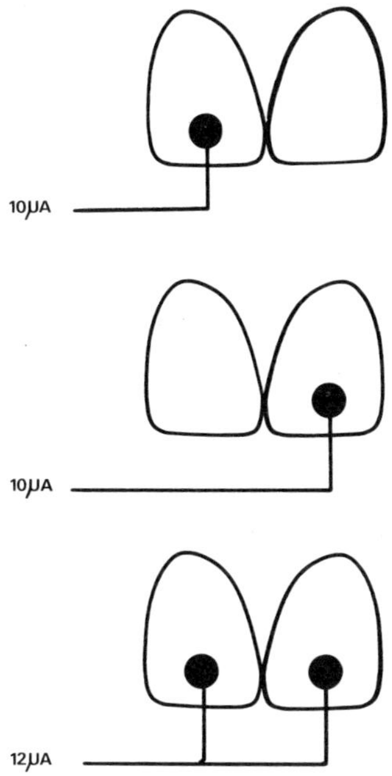


**Fig. 18.9.** Since the pain perception threshold was 10 μA for each central incisor the corresponding value for the two together should have been 20 μA, but was only 12 μA, or 60 per cent.

skin is well represented in the sensorium. For this reason disease of the skin does not cause pain referred in the opposite direction to the viscera. It seems to the author that this explanation might be sufficient without suggesting an 'irritable focus', but perhaps there is an irritable focus as well. There might also be a more diffuse influence of the central excitatory state. This depends upon neural impulses arriving in the central nervous system from all over the body — the normal continuous bodily activity. Because of spatial and temporal summation the central excitatory state allows fewer neural impulses from an area to be effective in producing onward transmission to higher centres. However, this background should be less influential than comparable activity within the same segment of the body than further afield.

The above influence of proximity has been demonstrated in the trigeminal system by using electrical stimulation of teeth (Mumford and Newton 1974a, b). The pain perception threshold of an incisor was determined and found to be, say, 10 microamps. It was also 10 microamps for the adjacent tooth. The factor that matters in electrical stimulation is not simply current intensity but the current density (current flowing through unit area). This means that doubling the electrode area should require double the current to reach the same current density. In other words stimulating two teeth simultaneously was expected to need 20 microamps. Instead, only 12 microamps were needed (Fig. 18.9).

This means that each tooth was receiving only 6 microamps which is well below the threshold level. Nevertheless, the current must still have been producing neural impulses, in themselves below the level of the perception threshold, but reaching the threshold once they are summated with comparable impulses from the adjacent tooth.

Looking at this another way there could be disease in one tooth producing subthreshold stimulation (and therefore not recognised). A small change in the adjacent tooth could then produce sufficient additional neural impulses to summate in the brain stem to a level required to reach consciousness, and the person might think that the second tooth was entirely responsible for the pain although the first tooth was really the one that mattered.

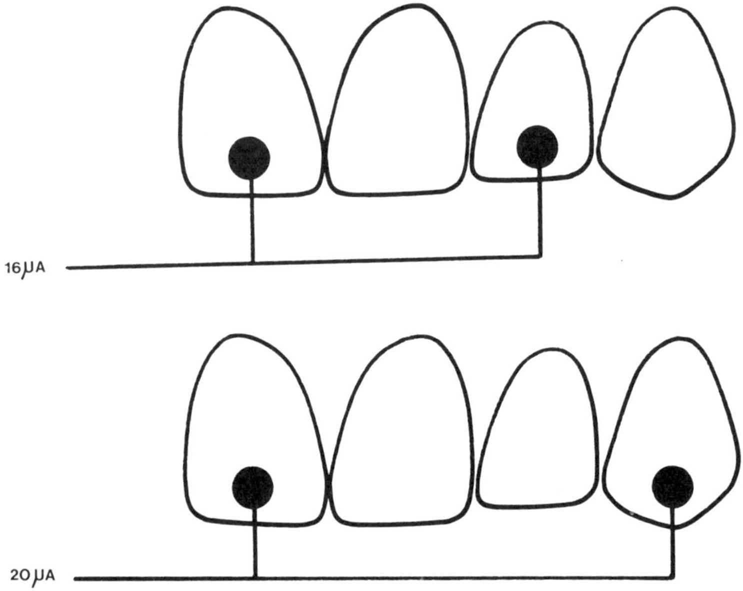


**Fig. 18.10.** *Upper*. For these two teeth the pain perception threshold was 80 per cent of what was expected.

*Lower*. For these two teeth it was 100 per cent, and this relationship seemed to correspond with the separation needed for 2-point discrimination.

Moving further away to the next tooth but one the influence of convergence is still present, but to a lesser extent. Stimulating these two teeth simultaneously required 16 microamps rather than what would have been 20 microamps (Fig. 18.10 upper).

Moving still further away (Fig. 18.10 lower) the full 20 microamps were needed, the influence of convergence being lost. At this stage the subject is also able to recognise that two separate teeth have been stimulated. Until then stimulation of adjacent teeth or nearby adjacent teeth produced only a sensation of one being stimulated.

This factor of convergence with spatial and temporal summation is clearly an important one, but it is certainly not the whole story since the essence of referred pain is that it is felt in an area separated from the one primarily responsible. Moreover, additional neural inputs do not always increase ongoing neural activity but may decrease it as suggested by the gate control theory. This effect goes beyond the single segment, as demonstrated (in some cases) by acupuncture; needling the foot has been shown to stop post-herpetic neuralgia in the trigeminal first division (Mann *et al.*, 1973) at least for a while in some cases. In such cases the possibility of coincidence or the placebo response must not be forgotten. Moreover, in the same group of experiments, acupuncture failed to stop a patient's toothache but brought on a renewed attack of her 'tennis elbow'.

Similar convergence effects have been found in clinical situations as in the following examples. A patient complained of an intermittent dull ache in the right upper quadrant of her mouth, and it was found to be referred pain from a lower right molar with an exposed pulp, but pain was also provoked by scaling the lower anterior teeth, presumably because this treatment provoked additional neural impulses. Another patient suffered pain which was eventually found to be due to an unlined amalgam filling in the left upper second molar. During the investigation, when a cold stimulus was applied to the first premolar pain was localised in the same tooth. When cold was applied to the second molar pain was localised in this tooth as expected, but it was also localised in this tooth when cold was applied to the first molar or even to the second premolar.

It sometimes seems to be thought that referred pair occurs because nerve fibres from the diseased site and from the site of referral join one another in a common trunk on their way to the central nervous system, as though neural impulses can somehow switch from one set of fibres to the other. This is not the case (except, perhaps, when adjacent fibres are damaged as mentioned in earlier chapters).

It has been suggested that axonal branching might account for it, stimulation of one terminal being erroneously interpreted as originating in the other terminal. If this view were correct referred pain should develop simultaneously but this is not always so.

Brodal (1969) seemed to hold the view that referred pain occurred only when the initial pain has lasted for some time, but dental cases have been seen where the diseased area was not painful, so perhaps referred pain might be classified as with or without primary pain.

In the mouth region it could be that the patient felt both primary and referred pains but that they were merged so could not be separated. In that case it would not be called referred pain because referred pain and primary pain are not continuous, by definition.

It has been suggested by Lewis (1942) that antidromic impulses (which travel along the nerve in the opposite direction from usual) might liberate a chemical at the site giving rise to referred pain, but if this were so pain should not cease on applying a local anesthetic to the area of the primary disease because the chemical would still be present at the referred pain site.

Another possible explanation is that the site where pain is experienced has been affected previously in some way so as to leave a 'memory trace', in the central nervous system. Noxious stimulation of a second site generates neural impulses which pass to the region of this 'memory trace', activating it so that pain is experienced in the referral site. Nathan (1977) cites interesting cases.

Hutchins and Reynolds (1947) and Reynolds and Hutchins (1948) noted that pain in the face occuring in high altitude flying was felt in many cases in the teeth and in the maxillary sinus, and was localised in teeth previously subjected to trauma (including cavity preparation). One of them therefore prepared and filled cavities. Later the other stimulated the mucosa near the ostium of the maxillary sinus by a needle prick and found that pain was felt at the site and also in the tooth treated 10–16 days earlier. They found that the same result could occur after preparing the cavities under general anaesthesia so it was not necessary for consciousness to be present; in other words it was not a psychological memory of pain. They considered that these results lent support to the concept of a 'memory trace' factor in referred pain, but it would appear from Wolff (1963) that stimulation of the ostium of the maxillary sinus can cause pain in the teeth anyway. Another explanation could be that the teeth were still generating impulses, but at sub-threshold level, which is enhanced by stimulation of the ostium. This could make the concept of a 'memory trace' unnecessary. However, it is believed that pre-existing pain can 'channel' referred pain to its own site (Hockaday and Whitty, 1967).

## REFERENCES


Anson, B. J. and Donaldson, J. A. (1973) *Surgical Anatomy of the Temporal Bone and Ear*, 2nd ed. Philadelphia: Saunders.

Ballentyne, J. and Groves, J. (1971) *Scott-Browns Diseases of the Ear, Nose and Throat*, Vol. 1. *Basic Sciences*, 3rd ed. London: Butterworths.

Ballentyne, J. and Groves, J. (1972) *Scott-Brown's Diseases of the Ear, Nose and Throat*, Vol. 2. *The Ear*, 3rd ed. London: Butterworths.

Bell, W. H. and Ware, W. H. (1971) Management of temporomandibular joint pain dysfunction syndrome. *Den. clin. N. Amer.*, **15**, 487–506.

Brodal, A. (1969) *Neurological Anatomy in Relation to Clinical Medicine*, 2nd edition. London: Oxford Univ. Press.

Christensen, L. V. (1967) Experimentelt provokerede ansigtssmerter fra kaebernes bevaegesystem ved bruksisme. *Saetryk af Tandlaegebladet*, **71**, 1171–1181. (English summary.)

Crue, B. L., Kenton, B. and Carregal, E. J. A. (1979) Neurophysiology of pain-peripheral aspects: speculation concerning the possibility of a unitary peripheral cutaneous input system for pressure, hot, cold, and tissue damage. In *Chronic Pain*, ed. Crue, B. L., pp. 59–96. New York: SP Medical and Scientific Books.

Dalessio, D. J. (1974) Mechanisms and biochemistry of headache. *Postgrad. Med.*, **56**, 55–62.

Dalessio, D. J. (1980) *Wolff's Headache and Other Head Pain*, 4th ed., ed. Dalessio, D. J. New York: Oxford.

Frankel, V. H. (1972) Whiplash injuries to the neck. In *Cervical Pain*, eds. Hirsch, C. and Zotterman, Y., pp. 97–112. Oxford: Pergamon.

Friend, L. A. and Glenwright, H. D. (1968) An experimental investigation into the localization of pain from the dental pulp. *Oral Surg.*, **25**, 765–774.

Grossman, L. I. (1965) *Endodontic Practice*, 6th edition. London: Kimpton.

Hall, I. S. and Colman, B. H. (1971) *Diseases of the Nose, Throat and Ear*. Edinburgh: Livingstone.

Harris, W. E. (1973) Endodontic pain referred across the mid-line. *J. Amer. dent. Ass.*, **87**, 1240–1243.

Hockaday, J. M. and Whitty, C. W. M. (1967) Patterns of referred pain in the normal subject. *Brain*, **90**, 481–496.

Hutchins, H. C. and Reynolds, O. E. (1947) Experimental investigation of referred pain of aerodontalgia. *J. dent. Res.*, **26**, 3–8.

Kawamura, Y., Nishiyama, T. and Funakoshi, M. (1967) A study of topognosis of human teeth. *J. Osaka Univ. dent. Sch.*, **7**, 1–5.

Lewis, T. (1942) *Pain*. New York: Macmillan.

Mann, F., Bowsher, D., Mumford, J., Lipton, S. and Miles, J. (1973) Treatment of intractable pain by acupuncture. *The Lancet*, July 14, 57–60.

Melzack, R. and Wall, P. D. (1965) Pain mechanisms; a new theory. *Science*, **150**, 971–979.

Miller, S. J. H. (1978) *Parson's Diseases of the Eye*, 16th ed. Edinburgh: Churchill Livingstone.

Monica, W. S. and Raymond, L. F. (1957) Unilateral headaches of dental origin; diagnosis and treatment. *J. New Jersey State dent. Soc.*, **29**, 14–16.

Moses, R. A. (1970) *Adler's physiology of the Eye: Clinical Application*, 5th ed. St Louis: Mosby.

Mumford, J. M. and Newton, A. V. (1971) Sensory convergence in the trigeminal system on stimulating human teeth. *Archs. oral Biol.*, 16, 1089–1097.

Mumford, J. M. and Newton, A. V. (1974a) Trigeminal convergence from human teeth: influence of contralateral stimulation and stimulus frequency on the pain perception threshold. *Archs. oral Biol.*, **19**, 145–149.

Mumford, J. M. and Newton, A. V. (1974b) Electrical stimulation of human teeth and convergence in the trigeminal system. In *International Symposium on Pain*, ed. Bonica, J. J., pp. 357–363. *Advances in Neurology*, Vol. 4. New York: Raven Press.

Mumford, J. M., Newton, A. V. and Ley, P. (1973) Personality, pain perception and pain tolerance. *Brit. J. Psychol.*, **64**, 105–107.

Nathan, P. W. (1977) Pain. *Brit. med. Bull.*, **33**, 149–156.

Newton, A. V. and Mumford, J. M. (1972) Lateral dominance, pain perception and pain tolerance. *J. dent. Res.*, **51**, 940–942.

Rasmussen, P. (1965) *Facial Pain*. Copenhagen: Munksgaard.

Reynolds, O. E. and Hutchins, H. C. (1948) Reduction of central hyper-irritability following block anaesthesia of peripheral nerve. *Amer. J. Physiol.*, **152**, 658–662.

Robertson, H. S., Goodell, H. and Wolff, H. G. (1947) Studies on headache: the teeth as a source of headache and other pain. *Arch. Neurol. Psychiat.*, **57**, 277. Quoted by Wolff, cited below.

Rood, J. P. (1972) Chest pain of dental origin. A case report. *Brit. dent. J.*, **133**, 110.

Smith, M. J. A. and Myall, R. W. T. (1977) Subacute thyroiditis as a cause of facial pain. *Oral Surg.*, **42**, 59–62.

Starkie, C. and Stewart, D. (1931) The intra-mandibular course of the inferior dental nerve. *J. Anat.*, **65**, 319–323.

Stell, P. M. (1967) Personal communication. 6 Feb. 1967.

Taverner, D. (1959) Facial pain. *Brit. dent. J.*, **106**, 65–71.

Warwick, R. and Williams, P. L. (eds) (1973) *Gray's Anatomy* 35th ed. London: Longman.

Wolff, H. G. (1963) *Headache and Other Head Pain*, 2nd edition. New York: Oxford Univ. Press.

# 19

# Atypical facial pain

The subject of atypical facial pain is one which worries many clinicians and this is not surprising because it is not a specific condition, but a collection of different conditions which have not been properly diagnosed. For this reason the expression undiagnosed facial pain would be better. An alternative expression, 'atypical facial neuralgia', is considered even less acceptable because in most cases pain is not neuralgic. The subject is obviously difficult and the following account is partly speculative.

Atypical facial pains can be divided into three categories.

## CATEGORY 1. INCOMPLETELY UNDERSTOOD CONDITIONS

In this group are cases which, if properly understood, would be diagnosed as one of the conditions described elsewhere in the book. This can only be achieved as a result of meticulous examination of the face, mouth and teeth, such an examination being time consuming and tedious. It is not like an ordinary examination in which, for example, a carious lesion missed on one occasion can be recognised next time. The trouble is that this missed lesion could be the cause of the pain. Moreover, the examination may demand the removal of existing fillings so that the floor and walls of each cavity can be examined afresh. All too often this reveals nothing definite but a dressing is placed, with hope diminishing as each new tooth is investigated. However, this procedure is sometimes successful in stopping the pain even though the reason is not known.

One explanation could be the existence of an area with unrecognised damage, and its subsequent protection. Another could be that each tooth had been the source of neural impulses insufficient in themselves to allow perception (i.e. below the pain perception threshold) but sufficient for neural impulses from several teeth to summate in the brain stem to produce ongoing impulses which were sufficient to allow perception threshold levels in subsequent neurones. Placing a dressing in one or more adjacent teeth could reduce the neural impulses sufficiently to keep even the summated impulses below threshold. This view is based on investigations of convergence in the trigeminal system by Mumford and Newton (1974a, b).

A fortunate example in this group of cases is that of a middle-aged female who complained of a flashing pain if the skin of her cheek was touched in the neigbourhood of the mental foramen. Since this is close to a main trigger point area of idiopathic trigeminal neuralgia this was considered as a possible diagnosis. However, a slightly defective silicate filling was found cervically in the lower canine. This was removed, a new filling was inserted, and the flashing pain ceased, much to the author's surprise.

Cases have been seen with flashing pain which lasted for only about a second at an intensity sufficiently strong to make the person stop all activity for a short time. Most of these have been found to be associated with a localised acute pulpitis (Chapter 11) but in other cases there has been no recognised disease, no treatment and no subsequent trouble. This is partly because teeth with large fillings tend to be left alone if possible. There could well be demonstration of disease to account for the pain if the teeth were extracted and subjected to histological examination, but this is not usually feasible.

In the early stages periodic migrainous neuralgia may be thought of as atypical facial pain, but its periodic nature, facial flushing and possible watering of the eye on the same side should help the correct diagnosis to be made (Chapter 17). Related to this, some people complain of a throbbing pain deep in the face, behind the eye, or at the back of the nose. It is thought that they have become aware of pulsation in the ophthalmic artery, the maxillary artery or one of its branches, and anxiety makes them focus more attention on it. Provided a careful examination has been made firm reassurance is given. It is easier to be brave in this way if the case has gone on for some time with no deterioration, and if other clinicians have examined the case with no abnormality detected.

Another condition which may be confusing, and wrongly described as atypical facial pain, is pain associated with the masticatory dysfunction syndrome. This can even cause a flashing pain which simulates idiopathic trigeminal neuralgia. Since it can be treated without resorting to surgery it is worth while constructing the necessary occlusal splint to see if this stops the pain (Chapter 14).

Pain in this group may also be due to a lesion further afield. An example is that of a middle-aged female with pain involving all one side of the head; pain did not cross the midline. The area involved was more than that which is normally caused in the masticatory dysfunction syndrome but, when muscles are painful, muscles farther afield may be recruited to 'help' ease the strain, so this patient was treated with an occlusal splint. The treatment failed because the diagnosis was wrong but she at least enjoyed the attention. Unfortunately she was found to have metastatic tumours in the cervical vertebrae. These caused irritation of both the upper cervical nerves and the trigeminal spinal nucleus, so the pain was widespread, involving the trigeminal area, the great auricular area and the areas covered by the lesser and greater occipital nerves (see Fig. 1.2).

Whenever there is pain in the side of the head and the back of the neck it is necessary to suspect a cervical spine condition, and local anaesthetic block of the second cervical nerve may stop the pain (Lipton, 1974).

Lesions of the oral mucosa can also be confusing, including some burning sensations, and pain that seems to be post-incisional (Chapter 15).

Intracranial conditions may be suspected and other sensory disturbances must be sought, including numbness, paraesthesia, muscular weakness, wasting or involuntary movements.

## CATEGORY 2. AUGMENTATION

In this category are people who are more aware of their face and mouth than is usual. Whilst they may seem peculiar and irritating to some clinicians they should be regarded as within the normal range. It is well known that some people are more than usually sensitive to certain clothing materials, e.g. wool irritates the skin of some people, and explanation could be that the individual is aware of neural impulses that others would not notice. This is at least partly a feature of attention and involves the reticular activating system. To some people who are trying to study, the tick of a clock can be distracting, at least until they become more involved in the subject being studied. People who seem to magnify external stimuli in this way have been called augmentors by Petrie (1967). At the other end of the spectrum are people who effectively diminish the input from external stimuli and Petrie called these reducers.

If a person is an augmentor and becomes aware of the face or mouth, perhaps as a result of a dental procedure or a Caldwell-Luc operation, then that area may loom larger in his thoughts and he becomes anxious, noticing small sensations that others would not notice. This might happen as a result of such a seemingly innocuous thing as washing the face too frequently, which produces an astringent effect with the result that the skin feels 'tight' and the person becomes unpleasantly aware of it, though he may be too embarrassed to say so.

It can even occur following a light touch when the touch sensation persists for some time, sometimes in an unpleasant way. By concentrating their attention on the area after the sensation has ceased some people can become aware once more of the sensation. As Melzack (1973) remarks, the presence of such a zone of awareness could mean that focusing attention on an area may facilitate transmission of neural impulses from that area. Mental activity can have a considerable influence upon the sympathetic outflow of the skin — there can be a tenfold increase in the total number of impulses per minute during periods of mental stress as compared with resting conditions (Hallin and Torebjörk, 1974). In some people the problem is partly one of uncertainty because any sensation may be only at the threshold level, and such uncertainty could increase anxiety.

When a person does complain, medical and dental examinations necessarily focus more attention on the 'affected part' and in some cases this is undesirable, but the difficulty is that the clinician may not know until too late. He may naturally wish to 'do something for the poor suffering patient' but is well advised to do nothing in the first place (and possibly nothing afterwards either). With such vague symptoms it is not surprising if the patient goes through the hands of specialists in several disciplines. This just makes matters worse for such attention serves to authenticate the 'fact' that there is something really wrong. Eventually the patient becomes afraid of what may be happening inside him, cancer being the thing most feared. If the person is being passed around in this way then, as soon as possible, some clinician has to be brave and tell himself that 'the buck stops here'. He could be wrong but, provided a thorough examination has been made, it is possible to reassure the person with an explanation along the lines suggested above. Where cancerphobia is present a firm reassurance must be given that no cancer exists.

It should not be forgotten that people in pain receive special attention, relief from duty, soothing medications, etc. which might motivate them to keep the pain (See Chapter 5).

It is not intended by the foregoing remarks to suggest that the pain or sensation is 'psychological'. Such an explanation is hurtful to many people, especially since it could imply that the pain does not really exist but is only 'in the mind', or that he is only malingering or cheating. It is essential to convince the patient that his sensations are only at one extreme of a normal range. It is also desirable to support the patient by getting this concept across to the nearest relatives. After several years of having a chronic pain case in the family the clinician must not leave them with the idea that it was all a spoof!

The difficulty for the clinician is how to decide whether a case is in this group or one of the other two groups. One feature that supports the decision is when the sensation is not too intense and when the patient can be distracted from it by his work or something else that interests him. Another feature of such a case (suggested by gate control theory) is that he should increase his facial and oral activity so that more neural impulses are transmitted in larger nerve fibres thus modulating activity in smaller nerve fibres and (hopefully) reducing pain sensation.

In such a case it is wise (if only for medico-legal reasons) to offer to see the patient again if he ever wishes to do so.

**Failure to habituate**

Two ways in which the body reduces the effect of stimulation are by adaptation and habituation. Adaptation is a peripheral mechanism and is a short-term reduction in response of nerve terminals to stimulation. Habituation is a central mechanism and is a reduced response to sensory input of longer duration. In effect, the body learns to stop responding to that sensory input. It seems possible that some forms of long-continued facial pain could be due to failure of habituation.

**Failure to forget**

Memory supposes an internal model which represents the world and, as circumstances change, this model requires modification. In other words, the model must be updated. Failure to do this might result in unnecessary remembering of the pain or sensation.

In general it is considered that pains are forgotten, but some cases of chronic pain could be due to a failure to forget. Short-term memory is thought to involve neural impulses circulating through some part of the nervous system and these have been called reverberatory chains. Eccles (1973) described the information as being carried by impulses traversing neurons weaving a pattern in space and time. Such electrochemical activity cannot account for long-term memory for this is retained even after suppression of neural activity by general anaesthesia or even coma. Long-term memory is therefore supposed to depend upon some permanent change in the nervous system and changes at the synapses are regarded as providing the most likely explanation. There is postulated a change in the way in which part of the nervous system is 'connected up'. This is brought about by an increase in the number of synapses, or an increase in size of synapses, or both, or a decrease in number or size, or both. (Although electrophysiological work seems to support this view there is, apparently, no firm support as yet from microscopic investigation.)

When activation of such a sub-system occurs neural impulses are generated in a spacio-temporal pattern like that which originally lead to the synaptic modification. In other words, there is memory of the original event which might have been a pain. What triggers the memory? One possibility is thinking about it or being afraid of it (and therefore thinking about it). This means that one part of treatment needs to be directed towards producing a break in such undesirable activity (breaking the vicious circle) and this may require drugs. Another part of treatment is reassurance to diminish the fear and therefore the incidence of recall.

## CATEGORY 3. PAIN OF PSYCHOLOGICAL ORIGIN

In this group are cases of pain which are more easily explained by the concepts of psychology and psychiatry than by those of neurophysiology. Pain in these cases does not follow a distribution that would usually be expected for it is neither along nerves nor distributed along blood vessels. On the contrary, it is usually ill-defined and may spread to involve the other side of the face. It can also spread into the neck and mastoid region and even other areas of the body (Cohen, 1959). Kay (1974) described it as a peripatetic pain, crossing the midline with blatant impunity. The patient describes it as a continuous dull pain lasting days, months or even years. It is felt deep in the soft tissues or in the bone rather than superficially (Lascelles, 1966). It is not affected by facial movement or contact but is aggravated by fatigue, worry, tension and emotional upset (McArdie, 1970).

In some of these cases the patient over-dramatises, describing the symptoms in a bizarre way (Moulton, 1968). He may also be anxious about other things; for example, he is worried because opening his mouth pulls down the skin around his eyes, and he gives a demonstration. He may complain of difficulty in swallowing, a sense of nausea, fullness in the stomach or that there is a sensation in his legs of insects crawling on the skin.

All of the above does not necessarily come out at the first visit, and only a limited area of pain may at first be complained of. The dentist therefore treats the case in a standard manner and this is likely to involve some surgery. The patient is happy enough to have this treatment and only in time does the nature of the case become apparent, possibly after the unnecessary loss of several teeth.

Much waste of time can sometimes be avoided by good cooperation between the patients' physician and dentist. The physician might, for instance, give timely advice that 'the patient will gladly keep you listening to him all day if you let him'. Since there is a strong psychological component in these cases, a careful assessment must be made as soon as possible, and may include help from a psychiatrist.

According to Merskey (1974a) the psychiatrist's first task is to diagnose and treat patients with psychological illness who have pain as a result of their emotional state. The second task is to treat patients whose pains would not be troublesome if the patients were not anxious or emotionally disturbed. Such treatment may be by means of psychotherapy, psychotropic drugs or even electro-convulsive therapy.

It is not really possible to understand atypical facial pain in this group without having some idea of abnormal behaviour states, and the following brief account may be helpful. It is necessarily incomplete.

## NEUROSES

The neuroses are a group of conditions in which the person, though abnormal, remains in touch with reality. He is aware of his sickness and would like to overcome it though he may be unable to do so. More than one kind of neurosis can occur at the same time; thus, anxiety and depression may coincide (Bond, 1979).

### Depression

Cases of depression form the most important group, in terms of numbers (Lascelles, 1966). The facial pain is frequently associated with disturbance of sleep, and also with fatigue and irritability. The pain in such cases is interpreted as developing as an appeal for help (Walters, 1966); i.e. help over and above that which is normally being requested by any patient complaining of pain.

In such a case of reactive depression questioning the patient will reveal some incident to account for it, e.g. a bereavement or loss of his job. Unsatisfactory housing is another depressing problem and one young mother used to appear with a vague facial pain which seemed to arise whenever her mother-in-law made too frequent appearances. Endogenous depression is classified with the functional psychoses which are mentioned later.

Reactive depression can continue for an unduly long time so cases need early co-operation with the patient's physician. On this basis the dentist is able to help, and it should not be forgotten that any orofacial pain may be primary rather than secondary to the depression. If such pain has continued for a long time the patient is 'entitled' to feel depressed by it, especially if many different medical specialists have failed to find an organic cause. Occasionally, the dentist has been partly to blame, e.g. by failing to record incomplete extractions. When subsequent clinicians see an edentulous mouth they may suppose there is no dental cause of pain, yet there may be retained roots sufficient to account for it (Fig. 19.1). If these are on both sides of the midline they would account for pain on both sides although bilateral pain is often re-

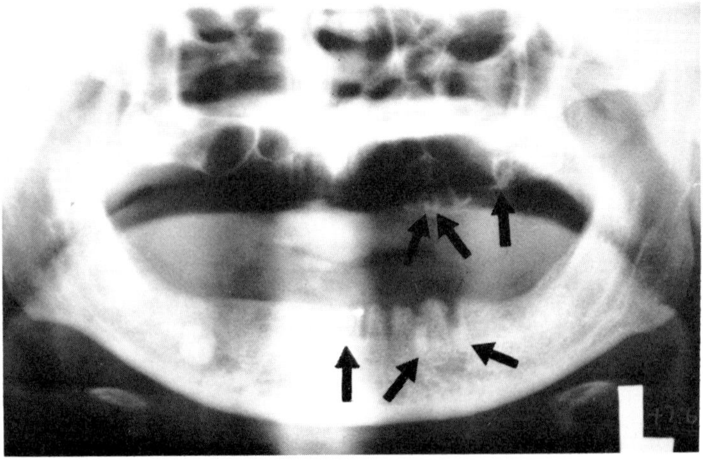

**Fig. 19.1.** Patient described as having atypical facial pain but there were various buried roots sufficient to account for her pain.

garded as being a feature of pain of psychological origin. The patient whose jaws are illustrated (Fig. 19.1) complained of bilateral toothaches, bilateral face aches and bilateral headaches before the radiographically visible roots were removed, and it was expected that these pains would cease. Unfortunately, they did not and she remained depressed. Her case history notes described her as having a 'functional overlay or even a psychotic delusion' but a further radiograph taken four years after the first one showed additional roots (Fig. 19.2). These had been missed, partly because of

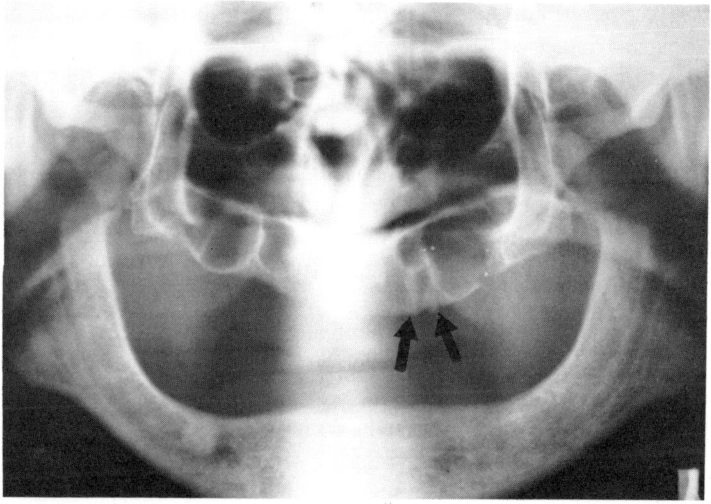

**Fig. 19.2** Same patient as in Fig. 19.1. Taken some years later, there are still two buried roots so it was hardly fair to suggest that pain was neurotic or even a psychotic delusion!

technical features of the original radiograph, and partly because they may have become more visible as a result of surrounding rarefying osteitis. These roots were extracted, and it would be nice to report that the depression ceased but a further appointment was not made in the hope that she might feel cured, and also to avoid any unnecessary further attention to the area.

*Treatment*

Time is the great healer and the process is helped by sympathetic listening. This is all that the patient's physician may need to do, and the dentist can help. Unfortunately, bad housing and other problems are often ongoing, and tricyclic antidepressants may be needed; these are said to relieve the pain due to depression (Lascelles, 1966; Rees and Harris, 1979). If these drugs do not work a drug free interval of one week is allowed and then monoamine oxidase inhibitors are used (Watts, 1976). It is suggested by Pilowsky and Spence (1976) that the clinician needs to adjust his attitude according to whether the repeated expressions of pain represent a masochistic dependence or an expression of hostility for the loss suffered.

**Hysteria**

The state usually described in lay terms as being hysterical is when a person makes a great fuss about very little. Behaviour becomes histrionic with crying, moaning and even screaming, and behaviour like this can be disruptive but this is not, strictly speaking, the kind of case that the term hysteria applies to.

Hysteria is really the state in which a person suffers functional abnormalities of apparently neurological origin even though no neurological abnormality can be found. These functional abnormalites are called conversion symptoms, examples being hysterical paralysis, blindness, deafness, painful or anaesthetic states. An essential feature is that the area involved does not correlate with the known anatomical arrangement of nerves.

Conversion pains are said to occur most frequently in the face (Spear, 1964) and this is probably because the face ranks highly in its significance to the individual. To have a pain in the face is important, and deserving of sympathy which may be more readily obtained in this way than by expression of other anxiety. As aptly stated by Harris (1974), hysteria is a state in which psychological benefit is derived from physiological loss. There then arises the paradox that successful treatment of the pain is not necessarily desirable because the pain actually stands between the patient and some intolerable life situation which he prefers not to know about. This may be guilt, and it has been suggested that pain may protect the patient by attenuating his sense of guilt and shame (Serafetinides, 1968); in other words he wants to suffer to expiate the guilt. Alternatively, the symptoms might have developed as an appeal for help (Walter, 1966).

A female patient had the two lower premolars extracted without difficulty but developed numbness in the face in that area. Years before, she was pregnant but when she saw another woman's lipstick on her husband's collar she obtained an abortion in a fit of pique. Unfortunately, she saw the foetus and thought it beautiful. A Roman Catholic, she then felt guilty and when the next child died of cardiovascular disease at the tender age of three she thought this was God's punishment. Her husband rejected her sexually and described her as an 'ugly moron' (incorrectly on both counts). The facial numbness in this case could have been either an expression of guilt or a plea for a little kindness — or both.

Lascelles (1966) did not find hysteria to be important in his group of 93 cases with prolonged facial pain, but Merskey (1974b) did in his group of 100 cases.

**Obsessive compulsive states**

Many people are careful and particular about how things about them should be arranged, and such an attitude is normal for them. Behaviour must be uncontrollable before it is called obsessional, the person being unable to stop; if he does stop he becomes assailed with anxiety. In dentistry cases are seen when the patient is obsessional about dentures, continually worrying about them and making the dentist alter them in one way or another. Part of the anxiety may be because of pain caused by the dentures, either directly or by altered muscular activity. In other cases there may simply be vague pain.

In Lascelle's (1966) group of 93 patients suffering from atypical facial pain most appeared to have good previous personalities and tended to be 'obsessive' in that they were meticulous and over-conscientious in their approach to life. Lascelles found that patients in this category responded well to treatment.

Some patients in this category have pain which they are able to treat themselves in a way which is ritualistic. For example, Gayford (1969) reported a case where the patient was able to relieve pain by stroking the mucosa of the buccal sulcus. Two strokes produced considerable relief but it was always the third stroke that gave complete relief. (We call it ritualistic but perhaps the patient was only making use of gate control theory!)

**Anxiety state**

There is a long-lasting diffuse state of anxiety which spoils the person's sleep, reduces his ability to concentrate and impairs his performance, all of which makes him feel worse. There may be intermittent dull facial pains in such a case and these cause a further deterioration since they give rise to additional anxiety. Provided the orofacial condition justifies it firm reassurance is indicated.

Anxiety may express itself more narrowly as a phobia and this is quite likely to relate to orofacial pain. The needle and the drill figure largely and occasionally a patient writes long letters preparing the ground for a coming dental appointment, possibly requesting both a local and a general anaesthetic to make sure there is no pain, the letter having parts heavily underlined. However, the first letter may seem reasonably normal and not until further letters arrive does the dentist recognise abnormality.

Some patients complain of burning or metallic sensations in the mouth. For example, a recently married woman complained of a burning pain associated with a bridge replacing the lower incisors. The pain was thought to be of psychological origin, since the teeth and mucosa looked normal, and she expressed some anxiety about her husband practising oral sex, this anxiety being made worse by her fear that the bridge would have to be removed. Fortunately, radiographic examination revealed a retained root under the bridge and also some periodontal inflammation (Fig. 19.3). The root was surgically removed and the diseased periodontal area curetted during the same operation, after which pain ceased.

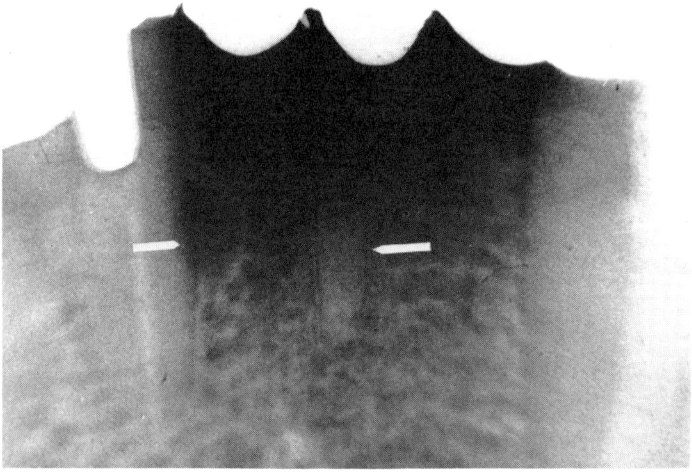

**Fig. 19.3.** A burning pain under a bridge was associated with a buried root and a chronic lateral periodontal inflammation. When these were treated pain ceased.

*Treatment*

Anxiety may be only a little more than normal and can sometimes be assuaged by sympathetic understanding, explanation and reassurance. It is reasonable in some cases to use general anaesthesia if the patient wishes and this initial success helps raise their morale so that local anaesthesia suffices in future. Minor tranquillisers such as diazepam help but, nowadays, are prescribed for only a short period of time. It is worth checking on the quantity of tea and coffee being drunk because the patient may be taking too much caffeine.

**Hypochondriasis**

This is a state of anxiety about health. The patient worries about things such as the heart-beat that is probably normal, and small pains may be magnified. In the mouth, the vallate papillae, on being seen for the first time, may be a source of great anxiety. The medical practitioner is more likely to suffer from such people than is the dentist. The latter is shielded from wasting time with too many hypochrondriacs because dentists are much more likely to operate than is the medical practitioner. Nevertheless, the dentist should make a proper examination, unlike one who dismissed a medical student's orofacial pain as being of psychological origin provoked by an approaching anatomy examination, although the teeth turned out to be grossly carious (Fig. 19.4).

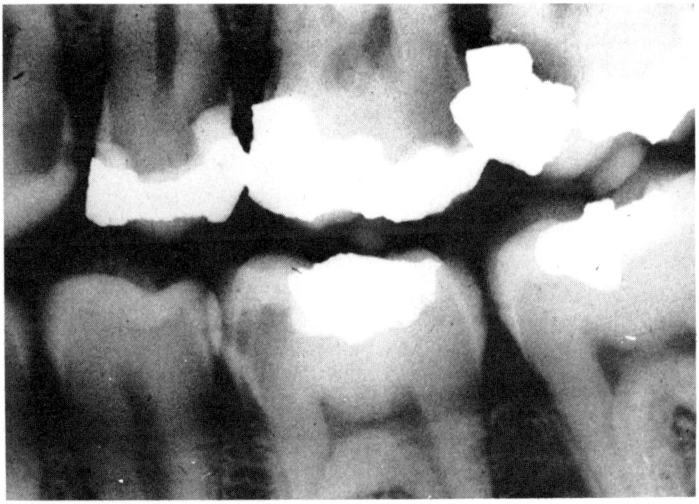

**Fig. 19.4**. Pain in this medical student was dismissed as psychological, being attributed by the dentist to the approaching anatomy examination. There are five extensive carious lesions any one of which would be sufficient to account for pain.

## PSYCHOSES

Whereas the neurotic person retains touch with reality the psychotic is divorced from reality. He is 'not in this world' and his speech and description of symptoms, including pain, may be bizarre. The prognosis for psychotics is less favourable.

**Schizophrenia**

This is a functional psychosis, possibly due to overactivity in the brain dopamine systems (Iversen, 1979), and it is of great importance for it has been estimated to affect about 1 per cent of the population over many different countries. In the simple form the person loses interest and gradually withdraws, preferring to be left alone. In the catatonic form the patient sits quietly and motionless. The paranoid form is when the patient suffers delusions of persecution (see case below).

In schizophrenia there is disorganisation of personality and incongruity of ideas. There is loss of contact with reality so that the person's speech loses meaning or may be repetitious, with the result that it is difficult to terminate a diagnosing session, the schizophrenic wishing to keep the interview going. It is misleading to think of the personality as undergoing a two-way split as in the split personality of popular fiction e.g. Dr Jekyll and Mr Hyde. Such a rare condition is regarded as being a manifestation of hysteria rather than schizophrenia.

In schizophrenia, patients are said to be very tolerant of pain (Petrie, 1967) but they may also have some peculiar ideas about it. One used to write letters asking for appointments and describing his pain at great length in a way which was disconcerting until his mental condition was recognised. He wrote that he 'suffered a severe attack of pain at three o'clock in the morning; it was sharp, hot and lasted about three minutes, probably due to a dislocated stapes'. In another letter he described it as 'a short duration diathermy radio transferred heat pain, the old jew having had one of my teeth wired up with a diathermy brace tacked up to his hypercussion radar sections for operating in or against the Port of Liverpool's aerial defence systems in order to trigger electrical dynamite in the gambling quantum scheme of America and Canada, etc., etc.'.

In cases such as this psychiatric assistance is clearly needed, although the above paranoid schizophrenic was already well known in the department of psychiatric medicine. Merskey and Spear (1967) point out that such painful hallucinations only occur in a minority of schizophrenics and depressives. Moreover, it should not be forgotton that bizarre descriptions of pain can occur in cases of organic disease as well as psychological ones.

*Treatment*

These patients need support, especially within the family. Tranquillisers also help.

**Manic-depression**

This is another important functional psychosis, the patient being sometimes manic and sometimes depressed. In the manic state he is elated, carefree, optimistic, full of energy and friendly. However, the mood can swing to depression, annoyance, irritability or even violence.

Depression may be associated with low levels of amine transmitters at brain synapses, whereas mania may be associated with excessively high levels of these transmitters (Iversen, 1979).

**Endogenous depression**

The person feels sad, helpless and hopeless, loses self esteem, and feels guilty. He is apathetic about food and sex and may feel suicidal. This state overlaps that of reactive depression, the difference being the appropriateness of the mood and its duration. The facial sensations tend to vary from one appointment to the next, and Fig. 19.5 illustrates a case. This man was divorced but said

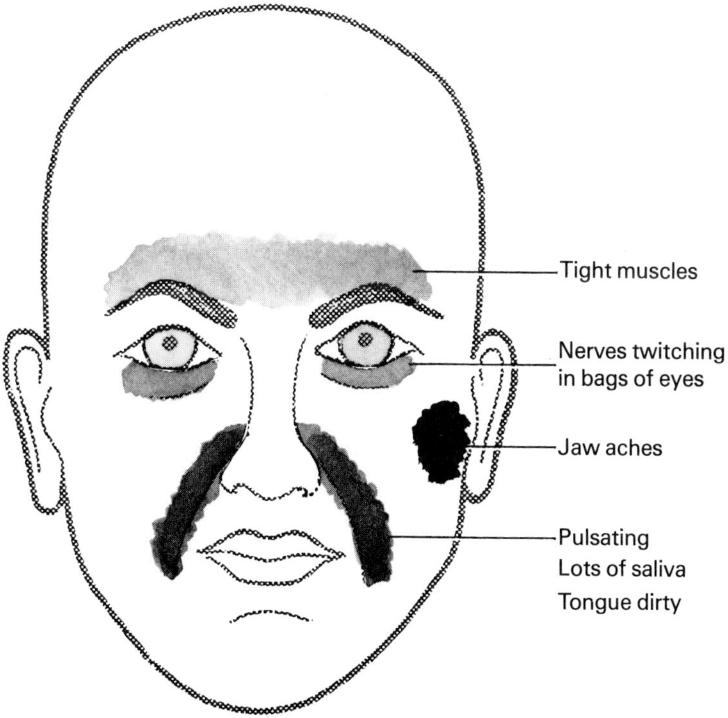


**Fig. 19.5**. This male patient was seen by a psychiatrist and wept throughout the interview. It was not known if his depression preceded his alcoholism or vice versa.

that he did not miss his wife or even his small daughter, though such a separation might well justify a state of depression. He also consumed 8 pints of beer a night, and the psychiatrist did not know if the alcohol was a primary cause or secondary to the depression. The patient cried during the psychiatric interview.

In such cases pain in the face may be suffered in an attempt to expiate the persons guilt; extra care is needed in dealing with the patient.

**Even psychopaths get toothache!**

One of the main objectives of this chapter has been to draw attention to the fact that people complaining of pain in the face and mouth may be suffering primarily from a psychological complaint. It should not be forgotten that people with psychological complaints, even severe ones, may have pain due to ordinary orofacial conditions.

**One last word**

Because pain of psychological origin has been placed at the end of this book it should not be supposed that the diagnosis of such a condition is a last resort. Naturally, great care must be taken to exclude organic disease, but if psychological illness is suspected it is obviously desirable to find out definitely as soon as possible. Apart from the need to know, this can avoid unnecessary surgery, and the shorter the duration of the illness the easier it is to treat (Lascelles, 1966). Finally, there should be a willingness to review the situation from time to time in case fresh evidence emerges, especially if treatment does not progress as well as was expected (Merskey, 1974b).

REFERENCES

Bond, M. R. (1979) *Pain. Its nature, analysis and treatment.* Edinburgh: Churchill Livingstone.

Cohen, H. (1959) Facial neuralgias. *Brit. dent. J.*, **107**, 9–18.

Eccles, J. C. (1973) *The Understanding of the Brain.* New York: McGraw-Hill.

Gayford, J. J. (1969) The aetiology of atypical facial pain and its relation to prognosis and treatment. *Brit. J. oral Surg.*, 7, 202–207.

Hallin, R. G. and Torebjörk, H. E. (1974) Single unit sympathetic activity in human skin nerves during rest and various manoeuvres. *Acta Physiol. Scand.*, **92**, 303–317.

Harris, M. (1974) Psychological aspects of facial pain. *Brit. dent. J.*, **136**, 199–202.

Iversen, L. L. (1979) The chemistry of the brain. *Scient. Amer.*, **241**, 118–129.

Kay, L. W. (1974) The location, control and treatment of pain. In *Restorative Procedures for the Practising Dentist,* ed. Harty, F. J. and Roberts, D. H., pp. 21–45. Bristol: Wright.

Lascelles, R. G. (1966) Atypical facial pain and depression. *Brit. J. Psychiat.*, **112**, 651–659.
Lipton, S. (1974) Personal communication. 1 Nov. 1974.
McArdie, M. J. (1970) Atypical facial neuralgia. In *Trigeminal Neuralgia Pathogenesis and Pathophysiology*, ed. Hassler, R. and Walker, A. E., pp. 35–42. Stuttgart: Thieme.
Melzack, R. (1973) *The Puzzle of Pain*. Harmondsworth, England: Penguin Books.
Merskey, H. (1974a) The contribution of the psychiatrist to the treatment of pain. In *International Symposium on Pain*, ed. Bonica, J. J., pp. 605–609. *Advances in Neurology*, Vol. 4. New York: Raven Press..
Merskey, H. (1974b) Psychological aspects of pain relief; hypnotherapy; psychotropic drugs. In *Relief of Intractable Pain*, ed. Swerdlow, M., pp. 90–115. Amsterdam: Excerpta Medica.
Merskey, H. and Spear, F. G. (1967) Pain, Psychological and Psychiatric Aspects. London: Baillière, Tindall and Cassell.
Moulton, R. (1968) Emotional factors in non-organic temporomandibular joint pain. In *Facial Pain and Mandibular Dysfunction*, ed. Schwarts, L. and Chayes, C. M., pp. 318–334. Philadelphia: Saunders.
Mumford, J. M. and Newton, A. V. (1974a) Trigeminal convergence from human teeth: influence of contralateral stimulation and stimulus frequency on the pain perception threshold. *Archs. oral Biol.*, **19**, 145–149.
Mumford, J. M. and Newton, A. V. (1974b) Electrical stimulation of human teeth and convergence in the trigeminal system. In *International Symposium on Pain*, ed. Bonica, J. J., pp. 357–363. *Advances in Neurology*, Vol. 4. New York: Raven Press.
Petrie, A. (1967) *Individuality in Pain and Suffering*. Chicago: Univ. Chicago Press.
Pilowsky, I. and Spence, N. D. (1976) Illness behaviour syndromes associated with intractable pain. *Pain*, 2, 61–71.
Rees, R. T. and Harris, M. (1979) Atypical odontalgia. *Brit. J. oral Surg.*, **16**, 212–218.
Serafetinides, E. A. (1968) Neuropsychiatric aspects of pain. In *Pain*, ed. Soulairac, A., Cahn, J. and Charpentier, J., pp. 61–92. London: Academic Press.
Spear, F. G. (1964) *A Study of pain as a Symptom in Psychiatric Illness*. M. D. Thesis, Bristol University. Quoted by Merskey, H. and Spear, F. G. cited above.
Walters, A. (1966) The psychogenic regional pain syndrome and its diagnosis. In *Pain*, ed. Knighton, R. S. and Dumke, P. R., pp. 439–456. London: Churchill.
Watts, C. A.H. (1976) Treatment of depression in general practice. *Prescriber's J.*, **16**, 145–149.

# Index